Willard Maxley
66. Walter Road.
Drawy Ca.
28.10.17.

PROGRESS IN
CLINICAL SURGERY

PROGRESS IN
CLINICAL SURGERY

BY VARIOUS AUTHORS

Edited by

RODNEY SMITH

M.S., F.R.C.S.

Surgeon, St. George's Hospital, London

With 112 Illustrations

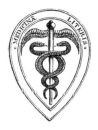

LONDON

J. & A. CHURCHILL LTD.

104 GLOUCESTER PLACE, W.1

1954

PREFACE

In writing a book on clinical surgery it is today manifestly impossible to cover the subject completely, omitting nothing, unless it is intended to devote to it several volumes and upwards of a million words. There is, of course, nothing basically wrong in an ambitious approach of this kind, but the result inevitably becomes a reference work, apt to spend the evening upon a shelf rather than the knee of the student. If, on the other hand, a book of readable length is the aim, much must be left out and it becomes of basic importance to decide at the outset for whom the book is to be written and what standard of knowledge is to be reached.

In the preparation of this book it has been my object to produce a volume of help, particularly, to the postgraduate student working for his final F.R.C.S. examination and the younger surgeon with a recent hospital appointment. It is thus intended to supplement, and not to replace, the standard surgical textbooks in general use in preparation for qualifying examinations. It is assumed that the reader already possesses sufficient knowledge to aim at a Fellowship and a surgical career. My object has been to build upon this and to raise his knowledge to the desired level by selecting for discussion those subjects in which it seemed that a big gap existed between the rather compressed information generally available outside specialized articles in surgical journals and the standard expected in the Fellowship, and in particular to spotlight surgical progress of the last ten or fifteen years.

Thus, in this book many common subjects will not even be mentioned if it is felt that they are adequately covered in standard works, or that no important progress calls for description. The student will, for instance, search in vain for accounts of appendicitis, biliary and renal calculi and the differential diagnosis of cystic swellings of the neck. He will, however, find considerable space devoted to the expanding subjects of cardiac and vascular surgery, and he will find certain organs, such as the œsophagus and the pancreas, which have only recently become possible let alone profitable fields for major surgery, discussed in detail.

Several subjects obviously pick themselves. Surgery since the war has so clearly advanced in consequence of improvements in anæsthetic technique and measures for the control of fluid and electrolytic balance that a relatively detailed account is obligatory. Various subjects, such as acute intestinal obstruction, ulcerative colitis, general peritonitis and, in particular, malignant disease of diverse organs, are not new ones and figure prominently in all previous standard books, but have been included on account of recent new work or because some change in general opinion upon some important aspect has become manifest. Other subjects, apart from those mentioned, such as hypertension, portal hypertension and the adrenal glands are comparatively new, but undoubtedly the province of the general surgeon and therefore not to be omitted. It may be argued that respiratory and cranial surgery is the province of the specialist and might have been left out, but I do not hold this view. Very great advances have been made in both of these branches of surgery which should be appreciated by all general surgeons, for the route to specialization in either of these off-shoots of general surgery should *invariably* lie through a proper general surgical training.

Finally, one or two subjects have been selected for discussion because it has been thought that their importance has not hitherto received adequate recognition. Thus, views on amputations, particularly for vascular disease, have changed and the new principles which seem to emerge are worth stating. The infected hand clearly merits discussion, whilst the somewhat detailed account of the injured hand seems to me an important inclusion, for this subject has hitherto been properly dealt with only in highly specialized journals and the average general surgeon has, frankly, little idea of how much can be done with injuries of the hand, particularly gross mutilating injuries occurring in, for instance, workers in heavy industry, even though it is, rightly, to the general surgeon that these patients first come.

Inevitably each individual reader will find some subject omitted which he would like to have seen included, and attempts to make this impossible would at least have doubled the length of this book. In apologizing now for such omissions as may appear significant, I hope that the deeds of my contributors will compensate for the misdeeds of their editor, and take this opportunity of thanking them for all the care and trouble they have taken to cover so fully and concisely these selected subjects.

RODNEY SMITH

CONTRIBUTORS

IAN AIRD, Ch.M., F.R.C.S.
>Professor of Surgery, University of London.
>Director of the Surgical Unit, Postgraduate Medical School, London.

H. F. ANDERSON, M.A., F.R.C.S.
>Surgeon and Surgeon-in-Charge Infected Hand Clinic, St. George's Hospital.

J. R. BELCHER, M.S., F.R.C.S.
>Surgeon, The London Chest Hospital.
>Consultant Thoracic Surgeon, North West Metropolitan Regional Hospital Board.

SOL. M. COHEN, M.A., F.R.C.S.
>Surgeon, Gravesend and North Kent Hospital.
>Surgeon-in-Charge of Peripheral Vascular Centre, Joyce Green Hospital, Dartford.
>Late Hunterian Professor R.C.S.

E. MERVYN EVANS, M.A., F.R.C.S.
>Orthopædic Surgeon, Glentawe and West Wales Hospital Management Committee.
>Late Surgeon, Birmingham Accident Hospital.
>Late Hunterian Professor R.C.S.

R. H. FRANKLIN, F.R.C.S.
>Consultant Surgeon, Kingston Hospital.
>Senior Lecturer and Surgeon, Postgraduate Medical School, London.
>Late Hunterian Professor R.C.S.

ALAN H. HUNT, M.A., D.M., M.Ch., F.R.C.S.
>Surgeon, St. Bartholomew's Hospital.
>Surgeon, Royal Cancer Hospital.

MARTIN HYNES, M.D., M.R.C.P.
>Pathologist, Royal Northern Group of Hospitals.

ROLAND N. JONES, M.A., M.Ch., F.R.C.S.
>Consultant Surgeon, Colchester Group of Hospitals.

ERNEST LANDAU, D.A., F.F.A., R.C.S.
>Anæsthetist, St. George's Hospital.
>Anæsthetist, Victoria Hospital for Children, Tite Street.

VALENTINE LOGUE, F.R.C.S., M.R.C.P.
Neurological Surgeon, St. George's Hospital.
Neurological Surgeon, The Maida Vale Hospital for Nervous Diseases.
Neurological Surgeon, The Royal National Orthopædic Hospital.

E. G. MUIR, M.S., F.R.C.S.
Surgeon, King's College Hospital.
Surgeon, Bolingbroke Hospital.

M. F. NICHOLLS, *C.B.E.*, M.A., M.Chir., F.R.C.S.
Surgeon and Surgeon-in-Charge of the Genito-Urinary Department, St. George's Hospital.
Surgeon, Royal National Orthopædic Hospital.

RONALD W. RAVEN, *O.B.E.*, M.D., F.R.C.S.
Surgeon, Westminster (Gordon) Hospital.
Surgeon, Royal Cancer Hospital.

VICTOR RIDDELL, M.A., M.D., F.R.C.S.
Surgeon, St. George's Hospital.
Late Hunterian Professor R.C.S.

C. G. ROB, *M.C.*, M.A., M.Chir., F.R.C.S.
Professor of Surgery, London University.
Director of the Surgical Unit, St. Mary's Hospital.
Late Hunterian Professor R.C.S.

A. H. M. SIDDONS, M.Chir., F.R.C.S., M.R.C.P.
Thoracic Surgeon, St. George's Hospital.
Surgeon, Royal Chest Hospital.

RODNEY SMITH, M.S., F.R.C.S.
Surgeon, St. George's Hospital.
Surgeon, Victoria Hospital for Children, Tite Street.
Consultant Surgeon, Wimbledon Hospital.
Late Hunterian Professor R.C.S.

A. S. TILL, M.A., M.Chir., F.R.C.S.
Surgeon, Radcliffe Infirmary, Oxford.

E. G. TUCKWELL, M.Ch., F.R.C.S.
Surgeon, St. Bartholomew's Hospital.

CONTENTS

CONTENTS

CHAPTER I

FLUID REPLACEMENT IN THE SURGICAL PATIENT

It is possible that nearly as many patients are killed by fluid replacement as are cured by it. The reason for this sad state of affairs is not that fluid replacement is of itself a bad thing but that surgeons do not understand this subject and the patients die as a result of this ignorance. The obvious route for introducing anything into the body is through the mouth. In this chapter the treatment of patients who are unable to take their nourishment in this way will be discussed, but it is stressed that the aim of all good pre- and post-operative care is to restore mouth feeding as quickly as possible.

Throughout this chapter the concentrations of electrolytes will be expressed in milli-equivalents per litre and not in grams per litre. The normal levels in the blood plasma are sodium 140 mEq., potassium 5 mEq., chloride 100 mEq. and bicarbonate 27 mEq. per litre. The milli-equivalent of a substance is obtained by dividing the number of milligrams per litre of the substance by its atomic weight for monovalent elements and by its atomic weight divided by 2 for divalent elements. What is the advantage of this? A good illustration is given by physiological or isotonic saline; in the body sodium acts as a base and chloride as an acid—this is the important thing. A litre of physiological saline contains 3·54 gm. of sodium and 5·45 gm. of chloride; this means something to a chemist but little to a clinician, in fact most of us would think that there was more of the acid chloride ion than of the base ion sodium. Converting to milli-equivalents produces the following result:

3·54 gm. Na ÷ 23 (atomic weight)=154 mEq. per litre.

5·45 gm. Cl : 35·5 (atomic weight)=154 mEq. per litre.

It now becomes clear that such a solution contains equal quantities of the acid chloride ion and the base ion sodium. If one is not a chemist it is easier to understand changes in the body's electrolytes when the figures are expressed in this manner.

After a moderately severe surgical operation such as a partial gastrectomy the following changes occur in the patient's metabolism: The patient produces little or no urine for the first 12 hours, in some patients there may be oliguria for as long as 48 hours. The urinary excretion of sodium is decreased for 2 to 5 days and the excretion of potassium is increased; after this there is potassium retention and increased sodium loss. The body loses nitrogen for 5 to 7 days and weight is lost, probably due to the oxidation of fat. Recovery is rapid and in the absence of complications no special treatment is needed. The great thing is to avoid doing harm by unnecessary fluid or electrolyte replacement.

Water. It is of importance to remember that the output of urine is diminished after an operation. The following case history illustrates the dangers of water intoxication. A vagotomy was performed for an anastomotic ulcer; after the operation the patient was given a continuous infusion of tap water per rectum. He absorbed this and so he was given more, in all he received 9 litres in 24 hours. He passed no urine for 48 hours. Allowing for 1 litre per day of insensible loss he had a positive water balance of 8 litres at the end of 24 hours and 7 litres after 48 hours. What happened? He had a series of epileptic fits and passed into coma. The plasma electrolyte readings before operation were: hæmatocrit 46, sodium 145 mEq., chloride 102 mEq.; after the 9 litres of rectal tap water they were: hæmatocrit 33, sodium 110 mEq., chloride 78 mEq. We treated him by stopping his intake of water and giving him 450 mEq. of sodium chloride in 450 ml. of water; he recovered from his coma, had a diuresis but remained disorientated for days.

The lesson from this case is that it is possible to poison a patient with rectal tap water. It has been stated that you cannot give too much fluid per rectum because the body will reject the excess. This is not true; fluids per rectum in the immediate post-operative period can be as dangerous as fluids into a vein. A simple fluid intake and output chart indicates the water balance and attention to this will prevent water intoxication.

Sodium and Chloride. A fairly common complication of a partial gastrectomy is for the stoma to remain obstructed for several days after the operation. This presents special problems. These patients lose by gastric aspiration about 100 mEq. of chloride and 40 mEq. of sodium per day (less if the gastrectomy has been subtotal). As a result they develop a subtraction alkalosis because of the aspiration of more chloride than sodium. At the same time they develop sodium depletion due to the absence of any intake by mouth, the loss in the aspirate from the stomach and the fact that after 4 or 5 days the kidneys excrete sodium in the urine even when the patient is depleted. Potassium is also lost in the aspirate and the urine. The treatment of these patients may be grouped under the following headings:

Correct the alkalosis.
Correct the sodium and potassium depletion.
Give adequate calories.
Do not give excess water.

On the Surgical Unit at St. Mary's Hospital we give these patients

2 litres of fluid per day by intravenous infusion (more if the insensible fluid loss is increased). This 2 litres consists of 1 litre of physiological saline which contains 154 mEq. of sodium chloride, and 1 litre of a solution containing 50 mEq. of potassium chloride, 50 mEq. of sodium chloride and 50 mEq. of ammonium chloride. This provides every 24 hours 2 litres of water, 204 mEq. of sodium, 304 mEq. chloride, 50 mEq. potassium and 50 mEq. ammonia. To provide calories we add to each litre enough glucose to make a 5 per cent. solution (200 calories), enough fructose to make a 5 per cent. solution (200 calories), and enough alcohol to make a 6 per cent. solution (240 calories). This gives a daily intake of 1,280 calories. It is stressed that this is not our routine post-operative management after a partial gastrectomy, but the regime we adopt if the stoma remains closed for three or more days.

Alcohol is a very valuable addition to an intravenous infusion. It provides calories, produces euphoria, causes a diuresis and assists sleep. It is not irritant to the veins. If ever I have to have an intravenous infusion I shall ask for it.

Sodium. An excessive sodium intake causes œdema. This is particularly likely to occur in the immediate post-operative period when the kidney is not excreting sodium. In the words of Moore and Ball (1952), "The provision of sodium is too easy". On the other hand, sodium depletion must be corrected. Loss by gastric aspiration has been discussed, in addition bile contains about 150 mEq. per litre, an ileostomy discharge 50 to 140 mEq. per litre and the fæces in diarrhœa between 200 and 300 mEq. per day.

A low plasma sodium may be due to dilution of the blood (over-hydration) or true sodium depletion. It is important to distinguish between these two conditions. The main points of clinical difference are listed below.

	Low Sodium due to Dilution	Low Sodium due to Depletion
General State	Drowsy. Mental Changes. Fits.	Alert. Apprehensive. Weak.
Tongue.	Moist.	Usually dry.
Eyeball Tension	Normal.	Low.
Pulse Rate	Normal	Raised
Temperature	Normal.	Low.
Blood Pressure	Normal.	Low.
Urine Volume	Normal.	Usually low.
Urine S.G.	Low.	High.
Urine Electrolytes	Low.	Low.
Hæmatocrit	Low.	High.

The treatment of a patient suffering from over-hydration is to limit the intake of water and in severe cases too give a concentrated solution of sodium chloride. The treatment of a patient suffering from sodium depletion is complicated by the fact that these patients are usually dehydrated and deficient in other electrolytes as well. The plasma potassium should be estimated and if low the patient given potassium chloride about 50 mEq. per day, but only after the sodium depletion has been corrected and the renal function re-established. The sodium should be replaced as both sodium chloride and sodium lactate and these patients nearly always benefit from a blood transfusion. To quote again from the writings of Moore (1952), "whole blood comes high on the list of treatment for sodium depletion. The moral is, treat the patient not the sodium concentration".

Potassium. This is chiefly an intracellular ion. In addition to that excreted in the urine potassium may be lost in gastric or intestinal aspiration, the fæces, etc. A low serum potassium is particularly liable to develop in any patient who cannot take food by mouth, because the kidney is unable to conserve this substance and the urinary output of about 50 mEq. per day continues in the face of depletion. Clinically a patient suffering from potassium depletion is weak, apathetic and even comatosed, the pulse is rapid and paralytic ileus is common. Replacement must be controlled with care, particularly in patients with oliguria or an impaired renal function.

Protein and Blood. After a surgical operation the patient loses protein and in an uncomplicated case the nitrogen balance will be negative for about seven days, this is followed by a period of positive balance and recovery. It is of value to realize that protein either by mouth or intravenously is poorly utilized in the immediate post-operative period. It is largely a waste of time and energy to try to correct the negative nitrogen balance at this stage. Conversely after this period protein given either by mouth or intravenously is a valuable aid to recovery but it is unnecessary to give it in excess of requirements.

Acute protein loss results from hæmorrhage, tissue damage as in burns or severe infections such as general peritonitis. If the loss is severe enough the patient passes into the clinical state known as surgical shock. Replacement is an urgent necessity. Of the factors responsible for the degree of shock hæmorrhage is by far the most important, so that early and adequate whole blood transfusion is the most valuable remedy. There is a tendency to underestimate the amount of blood lost during a surgical operation, it is for example nearly 1 litre in the average radical mastectomy and may reach 2 litres in a difficult case. Grant and Reeve (1951) when commenting on the treatment of those war wounds classed as very large state that their high mortality was due to the failure to recognize the grossness of the hæmorrhage and to give sufficient blood early and quickly.

Plasma transfusions are often life saving in acute protein loss associated with burns or severe peritonitis. The best guide to the quantity of plasma required is the blood pressure, and it is desirable to give sufficient plasma or whole blood to restore the blood pressure and hæmatocrit readings to normal and keep them there. The disadvantage of human plasma is the risk of homologous serum jaundice; this has been reduced because the plasma is now made in small batches and not from large pools as before. Plasma substitutes such as dextran or plasmosan are of value in the treatment of surgical shock in that they restore the blood pressure and lower the hæmatocrit reading.

Protein hydrolysates are of little value in patients suffering from acute protein loss or during the first few days after a surgical operation, but they have a valuable place in the treatment of patients suffering from chronic protein deficiency and in patients who some days after a surgical operation are still unable to absorb protein from the alimentary tract. In these latter patients the intravenous administration of a protein hydrolysate is of use.

Fats. These are the most prolific source of calories. The production of a fat emulsion suitable for intravenous use will be a great advantage. Such an emulsion exists and has been used with success in the form of a 15 per cent. fat emulsion containing 1,350 calories per litre, but it is not yet available for general use either in America or Britain.

Technique

When food cannot be taken by mouth one of the following routes should be used as an alternative.

A Nasal, Gastrostomy or Jejunostomy Tube. Here a tube is introduced into the upper alimentary tract and the patient fed through it. In the past complicated diets were worked out so that these patients could be given an adequate food intake; the domestic food liquefier has made them less necessary. All that is needed now is for the ward sister to place in the food liquefier the daily diet as supplied by the hospital kitchen plus such obvious additions as water, salt, etc. After liquefaction it is fed down the tube in the usual manner. If the patient is in need of more food he can be given a second helping.

Rectal Infusions. There is a tendency in some parts of the world to abandon this route, perhaps because it is old fashioned, having been used since Roman times. It is, however, an excellent route for the administration of water, and after many operations a rectal infusion of 2 litres of tap water per day is all the patient needs until mouth feeding can begin again. The dangers of overdosage have been mentioned.

Subcutaneous and Intramuscular Infusions. These are of value in infants and young children, particularly if hyaluronidase is added to promote absorption. Isotonic sodium chloride may be given by this route but glucose should be avoided.

Intravenous Infusions. These are superior to rectal or subcutaneous infusions because of the great variety of substances which can be introduced with safety into a vein. This route should be used whenever an adult patient has to be fed parenterally for more than 48 hours. The use of a fine polythene tube in place of a metal cannula or needle has been an advance. A fairly large needle is introduced into a vein and the polythene tube passed through the needle into the vein for a distance of about 12 inches. The needle is then withdrawn from the vein, the polythene tube temporarily disconnected from the infusion apparatus and the needle removed. The advantage of a polythene tube over a metal cannula or needle is that such an infusion will run for days or even weeks without thrombosing the vein, a complication which can be reduced still further by adding 25 mg. of heparin to each litre of fluid; this amount does not influence the coaguability in the general blood stream.

Intra-Arterial Blood Transfusion. This is of value in the treatment of severe oligæmic shock and the resuscitation of the apparently moribund. The aim is to force blood into the ascending aorta so that the circulation in the coronary vessels is re-established. In some cases the need for this method of transfusion arises during an operation on the thorax or abdomen; under these circumstances a needle can be introduced into the aorta under direct vision. In most other patients it is easier to insert a large needle into the aorta via the lumbar route, as used in aortography, than to try to enter the lumen of a peripheral artery which is likely to be contracted.

Biochemical Estimations. The patient's water requirements can be calculated from a fluid balance chart and a study of this chart is an essential part of all fluid and electrolyte replacement. In the past the estimation of the sodium and potassium content of blood plasma was difficult and time consuming. The result was that clinicians used the easily estimated urinary chloride to predict the more important sodium value. This method of predicting the sodium level from the chloride has proved unsatisfactory and it should be abandoned in all hospitals large enough to possess a flame photometer. The sodium and potassium content of any body fluid can be obtained rapidly and easily with this apparatus. Our photometer on the Surgical Unit at St. Mary's Hospital cost £70 to make and we are all able to use it.

C. G. ROB

References

1. GRANT, R. T., and REEVE, E. B. (1951) "Observations on the General Effects of Injury in Man." Spec. Rep. Ser. med. Res. Coun., Lond. No. 277. H.M.S.O.
2. MOORE, F. D., and BALL, M. R. (1952) "The Metabolic Response to Surgery." Springfield, Ill. Charles C. Thomas.

CHAPTER II

RECENT DEVELOPMENTS IN ANÆSTHESIA

THE past decade has been an important period in the development of anæsthesia, and has been remarkable for the introduction of new drugs and techniques and the advancement of the science and art of anæsthesia to a specialty with a status equal to that of other branches of medicine. With this improvement in status, the responsibilities of the anæsthetist have expanded to include the management of the surgical patient before operation, and during the often critical hours following operation. Whilst this aspect of his duties has become more important as the scope of surgery has increased, it is proposed in this chapter to discuss only those developments in anæsthesia which have a practical application in modern anæsthetic methods.

General Anæsthesia

There can be no question but that of the new drugs introduced into anæsthesia in recent years, intravenous relaxants have been the most important.

Whilst modern inhalation methods of anæsthesia may be used for maintaining moderate degrees of relaxation for prolonged periods, or extreme muscular relaxation for short periods without harmful effects, the maintenance of prolonged relaxation solely by inhalation methods may produce a degree of generalized depression of cellular function of vital organs which many anæsthetists consider undesirable and in some cases even prejudicial to the patient's recovery. They have therefore sought alternative methods of producing relaxation in these circumstances. The intravenous short-acting barbiturates, though not analgesics, when given in combination with Nitrous Oxide : Oxygen will provide adequate relaxation for short abdominal operations and will give excellent results when administered by those familiar with the limitations of these drugs. They are not degraded as quickly as was previously thought, and can be recovered from body fat 2 to 3 hours after administration (Brodie *et al.*, 1950); their slow redistribution from this reservoir may delay recovery and produce a prolonged period of post-operative depression. They are therefore unsuitable for major abdominal surgery.

In the past some anæsthetists and surgeons have preferred spinal analgesia (subarachnoid block) or local analgesia, combined with splanchnic block when indicated, for the more extensive and "shock" producing operations, for surgery for relief of intestinal obstruction, or when inhalation methods for other reasons have been considered undesirable. It is probable that but for the introduction of the "Curare" drugs the newer methods of regional analgesia, to which reference is made below, would be more extensively used than they are at present.

The introduction of the relaxants has provided a new solution of this problem, in that muscular relaxation can now be maintained by means of a drug administered intravenously. Rees and Gray (1952) describe this new concept of anæsthesia as a triad, the components of which are Narcosis, Analgesia and Relaxation; thus it is now a common practice to induce sleep with a small dose of an intravenous barbiturate, to maintain narcosis and analgesia at a light level of anæsthesia and provide relaxation with a "curarizing" agent.

The first of these agents to be employed successfully in anæsthesia, the alkaloid d-tubocurarine chloride, was crystallized from crude "tube" curare by H. King of the Institute of Medical Research in London in 1935. In 1939, working in New York with McIntyre and Gill, he prepared a purified extract of curare named Intocostrin, the active principle of which is d-tubocurarine. Following the successful use of this substance in surgery by Griffith and Johnson of Montreal (1942), Gray and Halton of Liverpool (1946) published their report of "Tubarine", an aqueous solution of d-tubocurarine chloride, and "Curare" was firmly established in anæsthesia.

In clinical dosage d-tubocurarine produces muscular paresis or paralysis by its inhibitory effect on the acetylcholine mechanism of nerve impulse transmission at the neuromuscular junction. It is suggested that a similar inhibitory action on the preganglionic synapses of the sympathetic and parasympathetic nervous systems accounts for the absence of "shock" following surgery on curarized patients under light anæsthesia. D-tubocurarine has a slight histaminic action, manifested by a small and transient hypotension and occasionally by bronchospasm. It has a negligible lipoid solubility and therefore does not easily penetrate the cells of the body (Keele, 1952). The exact method of elimination is not yet known: it is partly excreted unchanged in the urine, and partly according to Collier (1948) broken down in the liver and intestines.

Following the introduction of d-tubocurarine a number of synthetic relaxants have been produced. Myanesin, the first of these to be used in anæsthesia, has not a curariform action in that it depresses the interneurons of the central nervous system. It differs from the "curares" by producing muscular relaxation whilst sparing the muscles of respiration. It sometimes causes hæmoglobinuria, and as a result of reports of fatal cases of anuria following its use, its employment in anæsthesia has been abandoned, and its use limited to the treatment of spastic diseases of the central nervous system.

Gallamine triodide (Flaxedil, Syncurarine), first investigated by Bovet et al. (1947) is the most important of the synthetic long-acting "curares" in use at the present time. Its action is shorter and it has less histaminic action than the natural drug. It has a vagolytic action, but its tendency to produce tachycardia is considered a disadvantage. Apart from economic considerations it would seem to have no advantage over curare in clinical usage.

Decamethonium iodide (C.10) has a clinical action very similar to that of curare. Paton and Zaimis (1950) showed that it produces a neuromuscular block by an excess of depolarization at the neuromuscular junction end. It may occasionally produce prolonged apnœa, and as there is no known antidote its use, too, has been largely abandoned.

More recently Succinylcholine iodide (Suxamethonium iodide, Celocurin) which has an action similar to, but shorter than that of C.10, has been purified in Sweden and used clinically by Thesleff (1951). Succinycholine chloride (Suxamethonium chloride, Scoline) is being used extensively in this country. A single dose will produce complete relaxation from one to ten minutes, and is useful for intubation, the setting of fractures and other procedures requiring a short period of intense relaxation. It may be used for producing relaxation towards the end of an operation in preference to gallamine triodide or d-tubo-curarine, the lissive action of which persists for from 20 to 30 minutes, to ensure the return of muscular tone before the patient leaves the theatre. To prolong relaxation the dose may be repeated or the drug given in a continuous intravenous "drip" infusion, and it is now being used in this way for major abdominal surgery with excellent results.

Succinylcholine is rapidly hydrolysed in the body by cholinesterase and acetylcholinesterase into succinylic acid and choline, which are natural metabolites, and a marked feature of the drug is the complete and rapid return of full respiratory movements and muscular tone even after its prolonged use. There have, however, recently been reported cases of prolonged apnœa following injection of this drug, and it is suggested that patients sensitive to the action of succinylcholine have a low pseudocholinesterase blood content. It is, however, possible that some of these cases have been due to overdosage, to hyperventilation, or to the use of anticholinesterase drugs, which will prolong its action.

A number of other synthetic curarizing substances with long and short actions are being investigated, but so far none has been produced which has advantages over those mentioned.

Controlled Respiration

The management of hypopnœa and apnœa associated with curarization is based on experience gained in the use of techniques described by Guedel (1934) and Nosworthy (1941) involving planned apnœa with closed circuit anæsthesia. Nosworthy's method of "Controlled Respiration", was designed primarily to prevent mediastinal "flap" and paradoxical respiratory movements, and to provide a quiet field, during surgery of the open chest. By a combination of moderate depression of the respiratory centre and a period of hyperventilation with carbon dioxide absorption, apnœa is produced at a light level of cyclopropane anæsthesia with an excess of oxygen, and thereafter the patient is ventilated by manipulation of the breathing bag. The apnœa produced by curarization is managed in the same way, when paralysis of respiratory muscles is complete respiration is controlled, when only partial, assisted. Furthermore, curarization by paralyzing the respiratory muscles and ablating intrathoracic reflexes will not only permit controlled respiration to be initiated at a lighter level and with greater ease, but makes it possible to substitute a less toxic and non-explosive nitrous oxide and oxygen mixture for cyclopropane previously used in this technique.

For surgery in the open chest the advantages of complete control of respiration are now generally conceded. For major thoracic surgery three methods designed to protect the sound lung or lobes from infection or drowning by blood, pus or fluid content of cysts are in common use (Nosworthy, 1951). The affected lobes or lung may be isolated by ballooned suction blockers of the Magill or Thompson type positioned under bronchoscopic vision or by a solid plastic blocker passed blind (Pinson). The sound bronchus may be protected by a ballooned endotrachcal tube passed blind (Waters and Gale, 1932) or under vision by means of a special bronchoscope designed by Magill (1936). The third method, useful for children or for upper lobectomies in adults, depends on postural drainage to provide the gravitational free drainage of secretions (Beecher, 1940; Parry Brown, 1948).

The rapid increase in the scope of cardiac surgery which now includes operations on the heart itself, has presented new problems to anæsthetist and surgeon. Many of the patients undergoing surgery on the heart are very poor risks, and do not tolerate well disturbances of respiratory or cardiac rhythm during induction of anæsthesia. Premedication is directed towards lowering the metabolic rate by comparatively large doses of opiate and barbiturate, and children especially should be kept cool during operation on a chilled water bed (Millar, 1951). A tranquil induction is assured by means of thiopentone intravenously, and intubation performed, after topical analgesia of the upper respiratory tract, with the assistance of a relaxant.

Anæsthesia is maintained under complete respiratory control, with a high percentage of oxygen and minimal supplements of volatile anæsthetic or intravenous analgesic; many anæsthetists consider ether with maximum oxygen preferable to other anæsthetic combinations for the "bad" risk patient. Cardiac arrhythmias are controlled by the prophylactic administration of quinidine before operation, and procaine intravenously during operation (Burstein, 1940, 1946; Hutton, 1951). Should dangerous hypotension develop, the procaine drip is temporarily stopped, and a vasopressor injected if necessary. Blood is usually given throughout operation, massive transfusions into two veins simultaneously are sometimes required to replace the rapid and profuse hæmorrhage which, though at present an unavoidable hazard in operations on the heart, may soon become controllable (see Chapter XXVI).

It is the opinion of some anæsthetists that for surgery below the diaphragm controlled respiration, more particularly if excessive pressure is applied to the rebreathing bag, may impede the venous return, and so prevent adequate cardiac filling and lead to a diminution of cardiac output, and that alveolar gaseous exchange is more efficient when spontaneous respiratory movements are permitted to persist. They therefore prefer either to maintain anæsthesia and secure relaxation with well-established agents and methods, and to complete relaxation with a curarizing drug only in difficult or resistant subjects, or to induce and maintain anæsthesia at a light level, and by injection of the curarizing agent in fractional doses to provide relaxation without complete apnœa. Others consider that complete control of respiration is preferable because of the technical difficulty of synchronizing pressure on the breathing bag with the patient's inspiratory efforts, and of the potential dangers of injudicious attempts to inflate the lungs during the expiratory phase. Gray and Rees (1952) recommend controlled respiration for all abdominal surgery, and find that smaller doses of relaxant and anæsthetic agent are required when this technique is used.

Curarization will permit anæsthesia to be maintained with nitrous oxide-oxygen mixtures containing at least 20 per cent. oxygen, supplemented when required by minimal concentrations of a volatile agent or fractional doses of thiopentone The substitution of pethidine hydrochloride for thiopentone, the analgesic action of which reinforces the weak analgesic action of nitrous oxide, allows narcosis to be maintained with a minimum of respiratory depression and without hypoxia. This method first described by Neff, Mayer and Perales (1947) and by Neff, Mayer and Thompson (1950), was introduced into this country by Mushin and Rendell-Baker (1949) and has gained rapidly in popularity. It is now being used extensively in the maintenance of anæsthesia for all types of operations.

The need to maintain artificial respiration, often for prolonged periods, and the difficulty of regulating the phases of respiration efficiently by manipulation of the rebreathing bag, has led to the development of machines designed to ventilate the patient automatically. Following the researches of Giertz in Stockholm, the Swedish surgeons Freckner and Crafoord, in collaboration with the Anderson of the Swedish firm AGA, designed a combined anæsthetic and ventilating apparatus, which was successfully used by Gordh and Mørch for major thoracic surgery; Mørch later designed a simpler machine in which the phases of respiration were controlled by means of a pump. In this country Pinson (1944) described a "pulmonary pump" of his own design and in 1949 reported its successful use over a period of four years. Musgrove (1952), after reviewing the results of research on mechanical and automatic control of respiration, describes the essential mechanism of a British machine which is now in commercial production, the Blease pulmoflator. This machine will measure and reproduce the tidal volume of the patient, can be regulated to synchronize with the patient's own respiratory efforts when these are present, and will reproduce them when controlled respiration is instituted; all phases of respiration can be varied at will, and at such pressure as is required. Esplen (1952) and Williams (1952) have designed machines with similar features which will soon be in production on a commercial scale.

Though at present many anæsthetists express a preference for manual methods of control, the advantages of rhythmic ventilation at a fixed and adequate level and the quiet surgical field produced by mechanical regulation are such that it is probably but a matter of time before automatic control will be regarded as essential for all major intrathoracic and upper abdominal operations.

Controlled Hypotension

There are three methods at present being investigated to secure a comparatively bloodless field for operations in which otherwise uncontrollable blood loss may endanger the life of the patient, the vitality of delicate structures, or obscure the surgical field.

Griffiths and Gillies (1948) describe their method of inducing hypotension for splanchnicectomy and sympathectomy, based on experimental work of Vehrs (1931). A low intradural concentration of procaine is used to produce differential spinal block; total sympathetic block is produced with loss of arteriolar tone and a minimum of sensory and motor paralysis. The patient is put in a steep Trendelenburg position, and the operation completed under light narcosis in the lateral jack-knife position, pooling of blood occurs in the dependent parts, gravitational drainage ensures adequate filling of the heart, and artificial ventilation a high concentration of oxygen in the blood. Bromage (1951) achieves a similar result using extradural block according to the method of Dogliotti.

Enderby (Enderby, 1950; Enderby and Pelmore, 1951) has introduced a method of producing sympathetic block and consequent loss of arteriolar tone by the intravenous injection of hexamethonium Bromide (C.6) or Pentamethonium Iodide (C.5). The patient is positioned, after induction of anæsthesia, so that the site of operation is elevated and an appreciable volume of blood drained into the atonic arterioles, the method of inducing hypotension is essentially the same as that described above.

The third method involves bleeding of the patient from an artery, generally the radial, until the blood pressure has dropped to the desired level, the blood suitably stored is returned to the circulation under pressure towards the end of the operation or sooner should the need arise. Bilsland (1951) using an apparatus based on that described by Hale (1948), has used this method for cranial surgery. Mortimer (1951) has devised an improved apparatus which permits the return of the blood with less risk of contamination, and which he claims lessens the risk of emboli occurring in the region of the arterial cannula by providing a slow intra-arterial continuous heparin drip.

Controlled hypotension is now being widely employed in many branches of surgery, and surgeons who have experience of this technique speak enthusiastically of it. Thus Mercer and Scott (1952) state that they have been using methonium hypotension for all major procedures, particularly on hip and spine, and McIndoe (1952) considers this technique "makes certain lengthy procedures (for plastic repairs of face and neck) both expeditious and safe". The dangers of induced hypotension are, however, recognized; Hayward (1952) referring to the risk of cardiac insufficiency developing in patients with coronary disease, states that this condition may be present in apparently healthy patients with normal electrocardiograms. Shackman *et al.* (1952) have shown that, during methonium hypotension (with cyclopropane anæsthesia), cardiac output may be diminished and indicate the danger of anoxia of the cerebral, coronary and hepatic circulations, should a reduced cardiac output be associated with an absence of vaso-constriction in the renal vessels or vessels of the body and skin. There is no doubt that fatal and non-fatal accidents have occurred following the use of controlled hypotension, and until more is known of the risk involved, it would seem clear that this technique should be reserved for those cases in which hæmorrhage cannot be controlled by safer methods, and for which such control is considered to be essential for the safety of the patient or the success of the operation planned.

Regional Analgesia

An interesting development in recent years has been the more extensive use made by anæsthetists of regional analgesic methods, often combined with light covering narcosis. Local infiltration combined with subcostal, paravertebral and brachial plexus block is preferred by some anæsthetists and surgeons for the modern operations for thoracoplasty, though others now consider that light general anæsthesia with control of cough reflexes by curarization afford greater protection against spread of infection. Rowbotham's method (Rowbotham, 1945) of combined local infiltration and general anæsthesia for surgery of the thyroid is well established and similar techniques have been developed for surgery in other regions (Dodds, 1949). As a result of experience gained in methods of local analgesia, anæsthetists are to an increasing extent being called upon to carry out therapeutic and diagnostic blocks; Minnitt and Gillies (1948) survey some of the conditions for which blocks are now being used.

Spinal analgesia (subarachnoid block) has never been as extensively used in this country as on the Continent and in America, though some anæsthetists and surgeons employ it in preference to other techniques for abdominal and pelvic surgery; in general it has been reserved for selected cases for which it is considered to be specially indicated. Following a wave of enthusiasm in the period between the two wars, during which Howard-Jones (1930) and Etherington-Wilson (1934) made important contributions to the technique, reports of meningitis and other serious neurological sequelæ discouraged many anæsthetists from using this method and the recently introduced methods of fractional spinal anæsthesia (Lemmon and Paschal, 1942; Tuohy, 1945) which necessitate injection of the repeated doses of anæsthetic drug into the subarachnoid space either by way of a malleable needle or catheter left *in situ* have only been used to a limited extent in this country. Extradural block (epidural block) of the spinal nerves marks an important advance in technique; as the analgesic solution is injected into the epidural space, the risk of damage to the cord or of meningitis is avoided, and the incidence of headaches much less frequent. First suggested by Pages (1921), the method has been developed in Italy by Dogliotti (1933), by Gutierrez of Argentina (1933) and Odom of the U.S.A. (1936), and introduced into this country by Dawkins (1945, 1949). Durrans (1947) has used a high block for thoracic surgery, and Bromage (1951), basing his conclusions on the results of 355 cases of major surgery over a period of three years, considers the operating conditions obtaining with this method and the immediate post-operative conditions of the patients "the best available at the present time". Ablett, Dawkins and Steel (1951), using xylocain, a recently introduced substitute for procaine (Gordh, 1949; Wilson and Gordon, 1952), have lowered the failure rate from 6 to 3 per cent. and claim a greater degree of analgesia compared with other analgesic drugs, and state that in their opinion this method of achieving relief from pain in major surgery is better than any yet devised for the bad risk patient. The disadvantages of this method are the occasional failures even in the hands of those experienced in the technique, the danger of accidental injection into the subarachnoid space with a possibly fatal outcome, or into the ligamentum flavum when sloughing of the skin may result (Dawkins, 1951).

Caudal analgesia produced by depositing the analgesic in the epidural space by way of the sacral hiatus has gained some popularity in this country. Whilst it is most useful for obstetric procedures (Hingson, 1949), Thorne (1950) has used it with success for prostatectomy and hæmorrhoidectomy, two surgical operations for which it is particularly suitable.

At the present time epidural analgesia is being used to an increasing extent, and is displacing subarachnoid block as a method of choice when regional analgesia is indicated.

The place of the newer techniques in modern anæsthetic practice has not yet been determined; methods involving extreme physiological disturbances are subject to criticism, and the use of simpler methods often urged for occasions on which these newer techniques are not specifically indicated. If, as now seems probable, control of cardiac rhythm is to be added to the other "controls" which are such a marked feature of present-day anæsthesia, more accurate means of assessing the patient's condition during operation would seem to be essential. Control of the depth of anæsthesia by electro-encephalographic recordings (Courtin *et al.*, 1950; Kiersey *et al.*, 1951; Bickford, 1951) and serial estimations of oxygen tension in the circulating blood and carbon dioxide in the expired gases (Brinkman, 1952; R. van Eck, 1952) are methods now being developed to provide accurate data from which the state of the patient may be deduced during induction, maintenance and recovery from anæsthesia. It is to be hoped that further developments on these lines will ensure the reversibility of suspended physiological functions and the safe emergence of the patient from anæsthesia.

ERNEST LANDAU

References

ABLETT, J. J. L., DAWKINS, C. J. MASSEY and STEEL, G. C. (1951) *Anæsthesia* **6**, 159.
BEECHER, H. K. (1940) *J. thorac. Surg.* **10**, 202.
BICKFORD, R. B. (1951) *Collected papers of Mayo Clinic* **42**, 613.
BILSLAND, W. L. (1951) *Anæsthesia* **6**, 20.
BOVET, D. *et al.* (1947) *C.R. Acad. Sci. Paris* **225**, 74.
BRINKMAN, R. (1952) *Anesthésie et Analgésie* **9**, 23.
BRODIE, B. B., MARK, LESTER C., PAPPER, E. M., LIEF, PHILIP A., BERNSTEIN, ELENORE, and ROVENSTINE, E. A. (1950) *J. Pharmacol.* **98**, 85.
BROMAGE, P. R. (1951) *Anæsthesia* **6**, 26.
BROWN, A. I. PARRY (1948) *Thorax* **3**, 161.
BURSTEIN, C. L. (1940) *Anæsthesiology* **7**, 133.
COLLIER, H. O. (1948) *Nature*, **161**, 817.
COURTIN, R. F., BICKFORD, R. G., and FAULCONER, J. (1950) *Proc. Mayo Clin.* **25**, 197.
DAWKINS, C. J. MASSEY (1945) *Proc. R. Soc. Med.* **38**, 299.
DAWKINS, C. J. MASSEY (1949) "Modern Practice in Anæsthesia." London, Butterworth & Co. Ltd.
DODDS, H. (1949) *Ibid.*
DOGLIOTTI, A. M. (1933) *Amer. J. Surg.* **20**, 107.
DURRANS, S. F. (1947) *Anæsthesia* **2**, 106.
ECK, RITSEMA VAN (1952) *Anesthésie et Analgésie* **8**, 691.
ENDERBY, G. HALE, and PELMORE, J. F. (1950) *Lancet* **ii**, 45.
ENDERBY, G. HALE, and PELMORE, J. F. (1951) *Lancet* **i**, 663.
ESPLEN, J. R. (1952) *Brit. med. J.* **ii**, 896.
ETHERINGTON-WILSON, W. (1934) *Brit. J. Anæsth.* **11**, 43.
GALE, J. W., and WATERS, R. M. (1932) *J. thorac. Surg.* **1**, 432.
GORDH, T. (1949) *Anæsthesia* **4**, 4.
GRAY, T. C., and HALTON, J. (1946) *Proc. R. Soc. Med.* **41**, 559.
GRAY, T. C., and REES, G. J. (1952) *Brit. med. J.* **ii**, 891.
GRIFFITH, H. R., and JOHNSON, G. E. (1942) *Anæsthesiology* **3**, 418.
GRIFFITHS, H. W. C., and GILLIES, J. (1948) *Anæsthesia* **3**, 134.
GUEDEL, A. E. (1934) *Curr. Research, Anesthesia and Analgesia* **13**, 263.
GUTIERREZ, A. (1933) *Anæsthesia Extradural, Buenos Aires.*
HALE, D. E. (1948) *Anæsthesiology* **9**, 498.
HAYWARD, G. W. (1952) *Anæsthesia* **7**, 67.
HINGSON, R. A. (1949) *Brit. med. J.* **ii**, 777.
HOWARD-JONES, W. (1930) *Proc. R. Soc. Med.* **23**, 919.
HUTTON, A. M. (1951) *Anæsthesia* **6**, 4.
KEELE, C. A. (1952) *Proc. R. Soc. Med.* **45**, 245.
KIERSEY, D. K., BICKFORD, R. G., and Faulconer, A. (1951) *Brit. J. Anæsth.* **23**, 3.
KING, H. (1935) *Nature* **135**, 469.
KING, H. (1935) *J. Chem. Soc.* 1381.
LEMMON, W. T., and PASCHAL, C. W. (1942) *Surg. Gynec. Obstet.* **74**, 948.

McINDOE, A. H. (1952) *Practitioner* **169,** 427.
MAGILL, I. W. (1936) *Proc. R. Soc. Med.* **29,** 643.
MERCER, W., and SCOTT, J. H. S. (1952) *Practitioner* **169,**
MILLAR, E. J. (1951) *Proc. R. Soc. Med.* **45,** 51.
MINNITT, R. J., and GILLIES, J. (1948) "Textbook of Anæsthetics." p. 522.
    Edinburgh, E. & S. Livingstone Ltd.
MORTIMER, P. L. (1951) *Anæsthesia* **6,** 128.
MUSGROVE, A. H. (1952) *Anæsthesia* **7,** 77.
MUSHIN, W. W., and RENDELL-BAKER, L. (1949) *Brit. med. J.* **ii,** 472.
NEFF, W., MAYER, E. C., and PERALES, M. (1947) *Calif. Med.* **66,** 67.
NEFF, W., MAYER, E. C., and THOMPSON, R. (1950) *Brit. med. J.* **i,** 1400.
NOSWORTHY M. D. (1941) *Proc. R. Soc. Med.* **34,** 479.
NOSWORTHY, M. D. (1951) *Anæsthesia* **6,** 211.
ODOM, C. B. (1936) *Amer. J. Surg.* **34,** 547.
PAGES, F. (1921) *Rev. Sanid Milit. Lima* **11,** 351.
PATON, W. D. M., and ZAIMIS, E. J. (1950) *Lancet* **ii,** 568.
PINSON, K. B., and BRYCE, A. G. (1944) *Brit. J. Anæsth.* **19,** 53.
PINSON, K. B. (1949) *Anæsthesia* **7,** 232.
ROWBOTHAM, S. (1945) "Anæsthesia in Operations for Goitre."
SHACKMAN, R., GRABER, I. G., MELRISE, D. G., and SMITH, J. (1952) *Anæsthesia* **7,** 217.
THESLEFF, S. (1951) *Nord. Med.* **27,** 1045.
THORNE (1950) *Brit. med. J.* **i,** 414.
TUOHY, E. B. (1945) *J. Amer. med. Ass.* **128,** 262.
VEHRS, G. R. (1931) *Northwest Med.* **30,** 256, 322.
WILLIAMS, S. (1952) *Brit. J. Anæsth.* **24,** 3.
WILSON, H. B., and GORDON, H. E. (1952) *Anæsthesia* **7,** 157.

CHAPTER III

CANCER OF THE MOUTH AND PHARYNX

PATIENTS with cancer of the mouth and pharynx comprise slightly less than 3 per cent. of the total number of those dying from cancer in England and Wales at the present time. In recent years as a result of advances in the methods of treatment the outlook for patients with the disease is more favourable, especially when they are treated during an early stage.

Cancer of the Mouth

Carcinoma is the commonest form of malignant tumour encountered in the mouth and is therefore chiefly considered. It affects males three times more often than females and they are usually over 60. The frequency with which the various parts of the mouth are affected is shown by the figures set out in Table 1.

TABLE 1

CANCER OF THE MOUTH. SITE INCIDENCE. (Raven, 1933.)

Site	No. of Cases	Per cent.
Tongue	219	65·0
Floor	75	22·2
Lip ..	20	5·9
Roof	10	3·0
Cheek	7	2·1
Alveolus	6	1·8
Total ..	337	100·0

The disease manifests many comparable features in all these sites, but the treatment differs in certain respects, and the end-results achieved vary according to the situation and extent of the growth.

Etiological Factors and Pre-cancerous Lesions. During the seventeenth century there was a great increase in the number of patients with carcinoma of the tongue in this country, and D'Arcy Power (1919) thought this reflected the increased incidence of syphilis, and the habits of smoking tobacco and consuming alcoholic spirits which had grown during the sixteenth century. He put forward the view that the predisposing cause of this form of carcinoma is degeneration caused by spirochætal infection which is accentuated by increasing age and

19

alcohol, the exciting cause being local irritation of the tissues by tobacco and infection.

Precancerous lesions include traumatic ulcers caused by irritation from sharp teeth or badly fitting dentures, leucoplakia, and benign tumours, especially papillomas. The cause of a traumatic ulcer should be removed and a biopsy performed. The treatment of leucoplakia includes the elimination of any obvious irritating cause and keeping the patient under observation so that a biopsy of any suspicious hypertrophic area can be done. Patients with leucoplakia of short duration appear more likely to develop carcinoma in it. The onset of malignancy in benign lesions is usually shown by ulceration, induration and rapid extension; they are removed before these changes supervene.

Symptoms and Signs. A full description of these is unnecessary as they are well known, but attention is called to the appearances of the early lesion. A small ulcer usually appears in the buccal mucous membrane with an indurated edge and it soon develops the features of a destructive neoplasm. In others there is a papilliferous tumour with an indurated base which is covered by intact mucous membrane. Rarely a flat plaque is found covered by smooth mucous membrane. Sometimes there is a diffuse carcinoma which causes contraction and fixity of the tongue, or multiple neoplasms appear in the tongue or in other parts of the mouth.

Spread of the Disease. This occurs by direct extension to adjacent tissues in the mouth and oro-pharynx, by the lymphatics to the regional lymph nodes in the neck, less commonly by the blood stream, and rarely by direct implantation lower down the alimentary canal in the pharynx or œsophagus. There is a rich lymphatic drainage from the tongue and floor of the mouth and the lymph nodes in the neck are closely connected so that the more malignant neoplasms in this region may metastasize widely in both sides of the neck. The lymphatic drainage of the lip is less rich and the regional lymph nodes are less numerous. The frequency with which carcinoma of different parts of the mouth gives rise to lymph node metastases is variable, and a number of factors may account for it. These include local tissue resistance; the richness of the lymphatic drainage; the microscopic type of the neoplasm and its biological properties. The relative frequency is in this order—carcinoma of the tongue and floor of the mouth, the buccal mucosa, the lower gingiva, and the lip.

Treatment. In these patients there is often a severe degree of oral sepsis and caries of the teeth which must be treated. When the Wassermann reaction is positive a course of anti-syphilitic treatment is given and the patient's general health is built up as much as possible by the usual means. The treatment of the individual lesions in the mouth is considered separately, and finally the treatment of the regional cervical lymph nodes is described.

Carcinoma of the Tongue

The treatment of specific varieties according to site is described as follows.

An early carcinoma, especially of the papilliferous type, which is situated at, or near, the tip. A wide local wedge excision is recommended with reconstruction of the tongue. The incisions are placed at least 2·5 cm. away from the macroscopic edge of the growth.

A carcinoma situated in the lateral border of the middle part. This is treated by radiotherapy using interstitial radium needles which are inserted vertically into the tongue 1 cm. apart around the circumference of the growth.

A carcinoma in the body. This is treated in a similar way with interstitial radium needles.

A carcinoma in the posterior third. A course of teleradium, or high voltage X-ray therapy is advised as this region is relatively inaccessible through the mouth and tumours in this situation are usually radiosensitive.

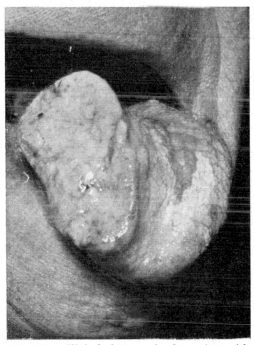

A diffuse carcinoma. A total glossectomy is advised when the patient's general condition is satisfactory and the cervical lymph nodes are operable.

Multiple carcinomas. A pre-operative course of teleradium, or high voltage X-ray therapy is given followed by a total glossectomy when the patient's general condition is satisfactory and the cervical lymph nodes are operable (Figs. 1 and 2).

A carcinoma in the under

FIG. 3.1.   Clinical photograph of a patient with two carcinomas of the tongue. There is a large carcinoma involving the anterior two-thirds of the right side; the smaller growth in the left border is not shown. The whole tongue is unhealthy with multiple fissures and leucoplakia.

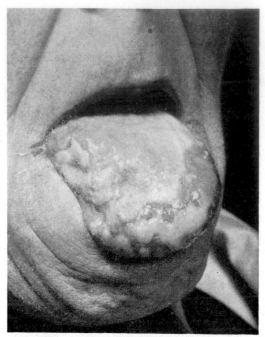

FIG. 3.2. Clinical photograph of the same patient (Fig. 1) after a course of high-voltage X-irradiation to the tongue, total dose 2250 R in 21 days.
Regression of the carcinomas has occurred and the irradiation reaction is shown, the tongue being smooth and a membrane has formed. Subtotal glossectomy and bilateral block dissection of the neck were performed subsequently in stages.

aspect. A course of teleradium therapy is recommended.

A carcinoma infiltrating contiguous tissues. These infiltrated tissues include the floor of the mouth, the mucous membrane of the alveolus and mandible, the fauces and tonsil and the hypopharynx. If the bone is not involved a course of teleradium therapy is advised. When the mandible is infiltrated it may be possible to combine a resection of the involved portion of the jaw with a partial glossectomy if the cervical lymph nodes are operable.

A recurrent carcinoma or one uncontrolled by irradiation treatment. When the patient's general condition is satisfactory and the local disease can be eradicated with the regional lymph nodes, a partial or total glossectomy should be done.

Floor of Mouth

The treatment given depends upon the extent of the disease, and the following clinical types are described.

A small carcinoma confined to the Floor of Mouth. This is treated by interstitial irradiation with radium needles.

An extensive carcinoma confined to the Floor of Mouth. A course of irradiation with teleradium is given (Fig. 3).

A carcinoma which has spread to the Mandible. When the adjacent bone is invaded irradiation is unsuitable because of the risk of bone necrosis. Therefore if the patient's general condition is satisfactory and the regional lymph nodes are operable, a radical excision of the floor of the mouth and the involved part of the mandible is done. The mandible can be reconstructed using a polythene graft; but the disability is not great when this is not done, for example in an elderly patient.

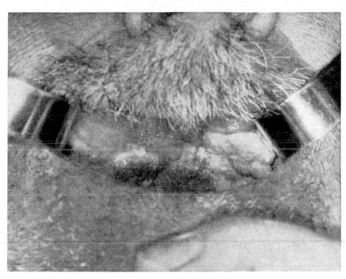

FIG. 3.3.   Clinical photograph of a patient with an extensive carcinoma in the floor of mouth. This was treated with teleradium; maximum dose of 6504 R was given to the primary growth and 4780 R to the regional lymph nodes in 58 days.

Recurrent carcinoma or carcinoma which is uncontrolled by irradiation treatment. If the patient's general condition is suitable for a major operation and the regional lymph nodes are operable, a radical excision of the floor of the mouth should be performed.

Buccal Aspect of the Cheek

There are two main types of carcinoma to consider.

Carcinoma involving the angle of the Mouth. The best method of treatment is irradiation of the growth by interstitial radium needles inserted as follows. One-half of the upper and lower lips on the affected side of the mouth are sutured together with interrupted sutures of nylon to form a solid block of tissue in which the neoplasm is situated. Radium needles are then inserted horizontally at a distance of 1 cm. apart uniformly in the tumour and surrounding tissues (Figs. 4 and 5).

Carcinoma in the centre of the Cheek. This is usually treated by a course of teleradium. If the disease is not controlled by this means, or it recurs later, the area is destroyed by the diathermy cautery.

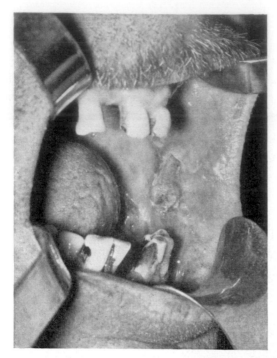

FIG. 3.4. Clinical photograph of a patient with a carcinoma in the buccal aspect of the left cheek.

FIG. 3.5. Clinical photograph of the same patient (Fig. 4) after treatment with interstitial radium needles, the dose given was 6400 R.

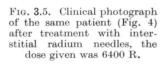
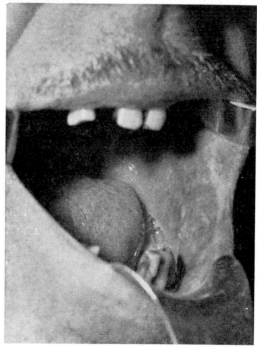

Roof of Mouth

A carcinoma may occur in the hard or soft palate, and it is usually treated by a course of teleradium. If this treatment fails, radical surgical excision should be carried out provided the regional lymph nodes are operable.

The Alveolus

A distinction is made between a carcinoma confined to the mucous membrane and one which infiltrates the subjacent bone. The former is treated by a course of irradiation with teleradium. When the bone is involved wide surgical excision should be performed if the regional lymph nodes are operable. Reconstruction of the mandible with a polythene graft may be done at the same operation.

The Lip

Carcinoma of the lip varies in its extent and different forms of treatment are required.

A carcinoma less than 1·5 *cm. diameter.* A wedge-shaped excision of the affected part of the lip is performed with reconstruction.

A carcinoma greater than 1·5 *cm. diameter.* This lesion also penetrates deeper into the substance of the lip and a course of irradiation with teleradium is given. Surgical excision would produce too much deformity.

Recurrent, or a carcinoma uncontrolled by irradiation. A wide surgical resection of the involved part of the lip is necessary followed by a plastic reconstruction.

The Treatment of the Regional Lymph Nodes in the Neck in Carcinoma of the Mouth

General Considerations. The cervical lymph vessels and nodes which drain the buccal cavity especially the tongue and floor of mouth are numerous and form a large intercommunicating network in the neck. The lymphatics of the lip are more localized. When the carcinoma crosses the midline of the mouth, the lymph nodes in both sides of the neck may contain metastases; this sometimes occurs with unilateral disease. If a cervical block dissection is required, it must be a complete operation. This is done when the lymph nodes are found to be enlarged on clinical examination except when one of the following contra-indications is present. The primary carcinoma cannot be controlled; distant metastases are present; the lymph nodes are fixed to deeper structures which cannot be removed; the patient's general condition precludes the operation.

When the lymph nodes are not palpable the patient is kept under observation and examined every month for the first year and at increasing intervals afterwards. If any enlargement of the lymph nodes occurs a block dissection of the neck is done at once.

Special Considerations. The complete block dissection operation includes the removal of the submental nodes (when the anterior structures in the mouth are affected), the submaxillary nodes with the superficial part of the submaxillary salivary gland, and the upper and lower deep cervical lymph nodes. Care is taken to remove any of the submaxillary lymph nodes which lie on the outer side of the mandible close to the facial artery. In addition to these structures the following are also excised: the platysma, sternomastoid, omohyoid, posterior belly of the digastric and stylohyoid muscles, and the internal jugular vein. The connective tissues are excised over an area which extends from the mastoid process and horizontal ramus of the mandible above to the clavicle below and from the midline of the neck to the anterior border of the trapezius muscle. A group of lymph nodes are arranged in relation to the spinal accessory nerve, which is removed with them, and all the tissues are removed in one piece.

When a bilateral block dissection is necessary it is advisable to do this in two stages and both internal jugular veins may be removed if this is required. An interval of two weeks separates the two operations.

The Combined Cervico-Buccal Operation. When a carcinoma of the floor of the mouth is invading the mandible, or a carcinoma of the alveolus infiltrates the adjacent bone of the mandible, and the cervical lymph nodes are enlarged, a combined operation can be done to excise the primary growth and lymph node metastases in continuity in one piece.

Palliative Treatment. Some degree of regression of the primary carcinoma is often achieved with radiotherapy, and fungation of lymph node metastases in the neck may be minimized or prevented. The sepsis in the mouth should be controlled by the usual means. Pain may be very severe, especially when it shoots up to the ear, and analgesics are necessary. Various types of neurectomy may be required for its relief, including section of the sensory root of the Gasserian ganglion, or alternatively alcoholic injection. When eating is difficult tube feeding must be instituted to maintain the patient's nutrition.

End-results of Treatment. The prognosis in carcinoma of the mouth varies with the situation and the stage at which treatment is given. The most important factor influencing it is the presence of metastases in the regional lymph nodes.

TABLE 2

CARCINOMA OF THE MOUTH. END-RESULTS IN 800 CASES TREATED AT THE ROYAL
CANCER HOSPITAL. (Ledlie and Harmer, 1950)

Site	5 Year net survival rate with all methods of treatment	
	Without lymph node metastases	With lymph node metastases
Lip	81%	28·0%
Posterior third tongue .. .. Whole tongue Anterior Pillar Fauces .. .. Soft Palate Tonsil	35%	7·5%
Anterior two-thirds tongue	32%	9·0%
Upper alveolus and hard palate, lower alveolus, buccal mucosa, floor of mouth and inferior surface of tongue	38%	13·5%

Cancer of the Pharynx

This is one of the most serious forms of malignant disease, as it is associated with a high mortality and a severe degree of suffering for the patient. The disease will be considered in each part of the pharynx.

The Nasopharynx

A number of malignant tumours occur in this situation and include teratoma, endothelioma, lymphoepithelioma, lymphosarcoma, myxosarcoma, chondrosarcoma, fibrosarcoma and carcinoma. Those which are more commonly seen are described.

Lymphoepithelioma. This tumour probably arises from structures called lymphoepithelial organs which are collections of lymphoid tissue in the mouth and pharynx. It develops at a relatively slow rate and is frequently small when first seen, with a nodular and superficially ulcerated surface which bleeds easily. A prominent feature is the early enlargement of the cervical lymph nodes which are usually discrete and mobile and may become large later.

The larger tumours cause symptoms which include difficulty in breathing, speaking and swallowing. Direct invasion of neighbouring tissues also occurs and widespread metastases may develop later, especially in the spine.

Treatment. The tumour is very radiosensitive and treatment by irradiation of the primary growth and regional lymph nodes is carried out. The best results are achieved when there are no lymph node metastases, but recurrence is frequent at the primary site.

Endothelioma. This tumour occurs in young adults as well as in those of more advanced age. It has marked infiltrating properties and invasion of the base of the skull usually occurs. Initially a small sessile tumour forms in the lateral wall of the nasopharynx which spreads widely in the submucous tissues without causing any ulceration, and other structures, including various cranial nerves, are involved. The patient may present with enlarged cervical lymph nodes which are often tender and discrete, but later become hard and fixed.

The early symptoms include pain in the face and head over the area supplied by the trigeminal nerve, deafness, and hæmorrhage from the nose or mouth.

Treatment. The primary neoplasm is treated by irradiation, and when this is controlled a block dissection of the cervical lymph nodes is performed if they are enlarged. For the relief of the trigeminal neuralgia an injection of the Gasserian ganglion with alcohol may be required.

The prognosis is poor unless treatment is given when the disease is small in extent and localized.

Carcinoma. This usually occurs in elderly patients although those in the younger age groups may be affected. There are two varieties, namely, a malignant ulcer and a tumour mass. The former has the features of an ulcerating squamous-cell carcinoma; the latter proliferates and forms a large swelling which ulcerates later on the surface (Fig. 6).

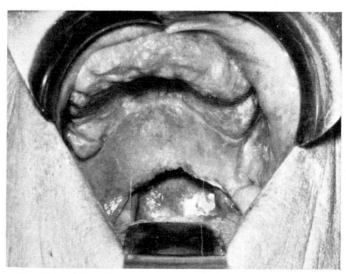

Fɪɢ. **3.6.**   Clinical photograph of a patient with an ulcerating
squamous carcinoma of the nasopharynx.

Symptoms and Signs. These patients suffer from a number of symptoms several of which are not pharyngeal in nature. The most common is pain in the ear, face, or side of the head. Others have generalized headaches, tinnitus and paræsthesia of the face. In some transient ocular palsies occur. The usual nasopharyngeal symptoms include nasal obstruction, bleeding and discharge.

Later other symptoms and signs appear which are grouped together as follows.

Associated with the eye. Diplopia, ptosis of the upper eyelid, ophthalmoplegia, choked disc and optic atrophy.

Associated with the ear. Deafness, tinnitus and a discharge.

Associated with cranial nerves. Paralysis of the sixth, ninth, tenth, eleventh and twelfth cranial nerves. In some patients the tumour infiltrates the Gasserian ganglion and there is pain and paræsthesia in the distribution of the fifth cranial nerve (Fig. 7).

Associated with the neck. The patient may present for treatment with a swelling in the neck due to lymph node metastases.

Other symptoms include dysphagia, aphonia, mental disturbances, syncopal and epileptiform attacks.

Investigations. In all patients with a neoplasm in the nasopharynx an anterior and posterior rhinoscopy are performed and a biopsy is carried out to determine its histology. In some a digital exploration of the nasopharynx is necessary under general anæsthesia to determine the extent of

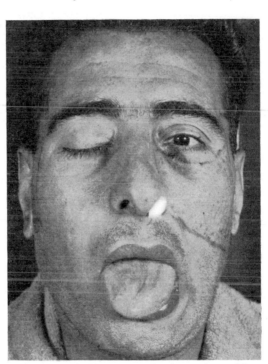

FIG. 3.7. Clinical photograph of a patient with a squamous carcinoma of the nasopharynx causing extensive cranial nerve palsies as follows: right 3rd, 4th, 6th, 7th, 9th, 12th; sensory changes of the left 5th and weakness of the 6th. There was a deep malignant ulcer occupying the right lateral wall, the post-nasal space and extending to the left lateral wall. Enlarged cervical lymph nodes. Treatment by high-voltage X-irradiation, total dose to the primary growth was 6020 R, and to the regional lymph nodes 5040 R in 65 days.

the malignant process. A radiological examination of the nasopharynx, base of the skull and the accessory air sinuses may show evidence of further infiltration.

Treatment. 1. *The primary carcinoma.* This is treated by irradiation with either high voltage X-irradiation or teleradium. At the same time the retro-pharyngeal lymph nodes also receive irradiation.

2. *The cervical lymph nodes.* When the primary tumour is controlled and the cervical lymph nodes are enlarged, a block dissection is carried out.

End-results. The prognosis is grave with present methods of treatment.

The Oropharynx

Various types of malignant disease occur in this situation and include carcinoma, both of the squamous- and transitional-cell varieties; lymphoepithelioma; lymphosarcoma; and malignant melanoma. These lesions usually commence in the tonsil or faucial pillars.

Carcinoma. This is the most common type, occurs in elderly patients and affects males more than females. A small ulcer appears in the tonsil or faucial pillars causing excavation as it increases in size.

Symptoms and Signs. The patient often notices referred pain to the ear on the side of the lesion. There may be a sensation of a lump in the throat with a constant desire to clear it. Later thickness of the voice, increased salivation, and dysphagia develop. Some patients present for treatment with a swelling in the neck at the angle of the mandible due to a lymph node metastasis. A typical ulcerating carcinoma is seen involving the tonsil or a faucial pillar and enlarged lymph nodes may be present in the neck.

Spread of the Disease. The disease spreads to contiguous tissues including the posterior aspect of the tongue, soft palate, posterior pharyngeal wall, upper and lower alveolus. Metastases occur in the upper deep cervical lymph nodes, and later the other groups are affected. Hæmatogenous metastases are uncommon, but have been described in the lungs and liver.

Treatment. Until recently there were two methods of treatment, but the results were far from satisfactory. Diathermy coagulation of the growth was used, but total ablation of the disease by this means was very uncertain with a risk of penetrating through the pharyngeal wall causing injury to the internal carotid artery which is in close proximity. Irradiation by teleradium or high voltage X-irradiation has also been used in many patients with unsatisfactory end-results. These considerations led to the development of a radical surgical operation—a combined cervico-buccal partial pharyngectomy with a radical block dissection of the regional lymph nodes—whereby the affected tissues are removed as a monoblock procedure (Raven, 1952). The excisional and reconstructional parts of the operation are performed in one stage so that the pharynx is closed and normal deglutition is re-established after a few days. This procedure is also recommended when irradiation treatment has failed to control the primary growth, providing the regional lymph nodes are operable.

End-results. These are poor with diathermy coagulation and radio-therapy. It is hoped that they will improve with radical surgery. I have one patient well and at work nearly four years later after operation (Fig. 8). He had an advanced squamous carcinoma of the oropharynx with spread to the soft palate and base of the tongue and metastases in the cervical lymph nodes. The disease was considered unsuitable for radiotherapy.

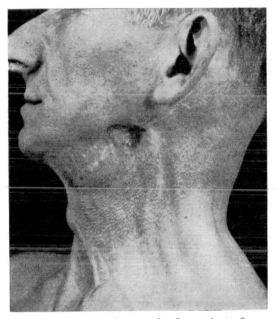

Fig. **3.8.** Clinical photograph of a patient after a cervico-buccal partial pharyngectomy for an extensive carcinoma in the left side of the oropharynx and metastases in the left deep cervical lymph nodes. The patient is well and at work nearly 4 years after the operation.
(Reproduced from the *Brit. J. Surg.* by kind permission.)

Lymphoepithelioma. This has the same general features here as in the nasopharynx, and treatment by irradiation is given.

Lymphosarcoma. This is not uncommon in the tonsil and is usually bilateral. It causes a uniform, fleshy, red swelling of the tonsils, which are firm in consistency. Metastases occur in the regional lymph nodes and are also blood-borne to distant organs. Irradiation treatment is given to the primary growth and regional lymph nodes. The disease usually regresses as a result, but it soon recurs.

The Hypopharynx

Malignant disease in this part of the pharynx is nearly always a squamous-cell carcinoma.

Pre-cancerous Lesion. The Plummer-Vinson syndrome occurs in women and is considered to be a deficiency state. It is associated with anæmia characterized by iron deficiency, often accompanied by achlorhydria, dysphagia, splenomegaly and spoon-shaped finger nails. The mucous membrane of the mouth and pharynx becomes red, smooth and atrophic and carcinoma may supervene in these structures. A post-cricoid neoplasm is especially liable to develop.

Symptoms and Signs. The early symptoms are usually vague and the patient may find difficulty in describing them. A sensation of a foreign body is present in the throat causing a constant desire to clear it. There is discomfort with deglutition and thickness of the voice develops. The symptoms gradually become more serious and later include dysphagia, dyspnœa, stridor, hoarseness of the voice and a persistent cough. A swelling may be present in the neck due to metastases in the deep cervical lymph nodes. The signs of advanced disease include fixity of the hypopharynx, lateral infiltration of the neck, engorged jugular veins and fixed cervical lymph nodes.

Investigations. The usual general investigations are made. Patients with dyspnœa should not undergo pre-operative direct pharyngoscopy and laryngoscopy; spraying the pharynx and larynx with a solution of cocaine may cause urgent dyspnœa requiring an immediate tracheotomy and this should be avoided. In other patients pharyngoscopy will give information regarding the site and upward extent of the growth. It may be localized in any of the following situations, the epiglottis, glosso-epiglottic fold, ary-epiglottic fold, pyriform fossa, posterior pharyngeal wall and the post-cricoid region. Laryngoscopy shows œdema and any anterior extension. Radiological examination with plain X-rays, a barium swallow and tomograms, gives additional information of its extent, and posterior infiltration through the pharyngeal wall and into the œsophagus may be discovered. The extent of involvement of the œsophagus must be known to decide if it can be divided at a safe level below the growth. This is usually determined on exploring the neck when the final decision regarding performing a radical operation is made.

Special Problems. *Dyspnœa and Stridor*. These symptoms are present with the more extensive neoplasms and nothing is done which may cause an exacerbation necessitating a tracheotomy before the radical operation is done. The latter causes several technical difficulties including infection around it. No instrumentation is carried out until the patient is in the operating theatre for the major operation when biopsy and histological examination by the frozen section technique is done. In the presence of severe respiratory obstruction a tracheotomy under local anæsthesia is instituted as the first step in the radical operation; after this a general anæsthetic is given by the endotracheal method and the procedure is continued.

Dysphagia. When the growth involves the pharyngo-œsophageal junction severe dysphagia is present. When the patient's nutrition is satisfactory special intravenous feeding is given for a few days before the operation, but if it is poor a temporary gastrostomy is advisable to build up the patient's general condition.

Spread of the Disease. Carcinoma of the hypopharynx possesses a high degree of malignancy and spreads rapidly as shown in Table 3.

TABLE 3

CARCINOMA OF HYPOPHARYNX—SPREAD OF THE DISEASE

Direct Extension.	Vertically in the wall to oro-pharynx and cervical œsophagus. Anteriorly into larynx and trachea. Laterally into thyroid gland and internal jugular veins. Posteriorly into prevertebral muscles and cervical vertebrae.
Lymphatic Metastases.	Deep cervical, recurrent laryngeal and superior mediastinal groups of nodes.
Hæmatogenous Metastases.	Lungs, Liver.

A rich lymphatic network is present and metastases occur in the nodes during an early stage of the disease. In my series these were present in 50 per cent. of the patients at operation. Even with a carcinoma localized in one-half of the hypopharynx lymph nodes may be affected in the opposite side of the neck. Lymph nodes in both sides have intercommunicating vessels so that widespread metastases can easily occur.

Treatment. As a result of my experience of patients with this disease I have no doubt that surgery has an important place in the treatment as it provides the best palliation and the possibility of a cure, especially when operation is done before lymphatic metastases are present. The end-results of all forms of radiotherapy are poor and patients with dyspnœa and stridor are unfit to undergo it.

The Radical 2-Stage Operation. Laryngo-pharyngectomy and Laryngo-œsophago-pharyngectomy

Excision Stage. A quadrilateral flap of skin is raised from the neck and the tissues excised include the hypopharynx and larynx, with the hyoid in high growths and the cervical œsophagus in low growths. A total thyroidectomy is performed if the thyroid is infiltrated. Bilateral excision of the cervical lymph nodes is essential when they are enlarged.

The Cervical Lymph Nodes. Multiple affected lymph nodes may be found at operation which were not palpable clinically and they are dealt with first. With a unilateral primary growth the lymph nodes may only be affected on that side, but the other side must always be explored and any enlarged nodes removed. With bilateral involvement I have found the nodes are usually bigger and more numerous on one side and a complete block dissection is required. On the other side when the nodes are small I leave the internal jugular vein and sterno-mastoid muscle but a complete removal of the nodes is essential. They extend from beneath the posterior belly of the digastric muscle, along the internal jugular vein downwards to the recurrent laryngeal group. In some patients the internal jugular vein is directly invaded, pulled over to the pharynx and must be excised.

The Hypopharynx. It is advisable to remove the regional lymph nodes, hypopharynx and larynx as a monoblock operation. With the higher growths the hyoid is removed and the lower section passes through the pharyngo-œsophageal junction. With the lower growths the hyoid remains and the cervical œsophagus is divided at the thoracic inlet. If there is doubt regarding clearance of the growth, immediate histological examination by the frozen section technique of the divided pharynx and œsophagus is useful. The trachea is divided between the second and third rings for the higher growths and between the third and fourth for the lower ones. When total thyroidectomy is required, the parathyroids may be included; one of my patients developed mild tetany which was easily controlled.

Reconstructional Stage. The quadrilateral skin flap is anastomosed to the divided oro- or hypo-pharynx above and the cervical œsophagus below to form a new skin tube which is temporarily left open laterally. The raw areas in the neck are covered with split-thickness skin grafts from the thigh. A polythene tube is inserted through the œsophageal opening into the stomach for feeding purposes (Fig. 9). An interval of six weeks elapses before the final stage is performed.

At the second operation the lateral cervical fistula is closed and the new skin hypopharynx is covered by whole thickness skin using rotated or hinged flaps from the neck, or acromio-pectoral tubed pedicle grafts. A period of three weeks is allowed for healing and the patient can then swallow (Figs. 10, 11 and 12).

1-Stage Operations with Primary Closure of the Pharynx

It is sometimes possible to perform this type of operation. For example, I have excised the hypopharynx and larynx and performed an end-to-end anastomosis between the upper segment of the divided

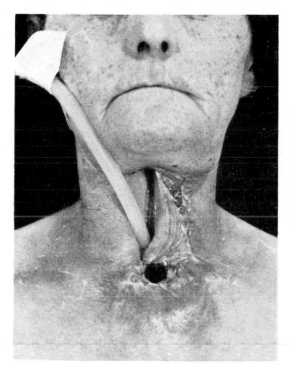

Fig. 3.9. Clinical photograph of a patient who had a carcinoma in the hypopharynx treated by laryngo-oesophago-pharyngectomy in two stages. This photograph shows the neck after the first stage; there is a lateral cervical fistula and the patient is fed through the polythene tube inserted through the œsophagus into the stomach.

Fig. 3.10. Clinical photograph of the same patient (Fig. 9) after the second stage operation. The patient has a permanent tracheostomy; she can swallow everything normally and is well 2 years later.

(Reproduced from the *Brit. med. J.* by kind permission.)

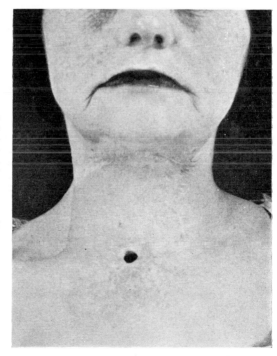

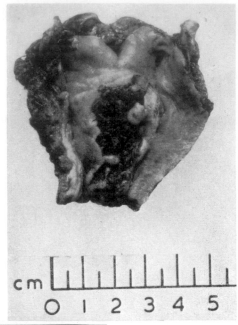

Fig. 3.11. Photograph of the specimen removed by laryngo-œsophago-pharyngectomy from the same patient (Fig. 9) showing an extensive post-cricoid carcinoma involving the cervical œsophagus and the anterior wall of the hypopharynx to the arytenoid region.

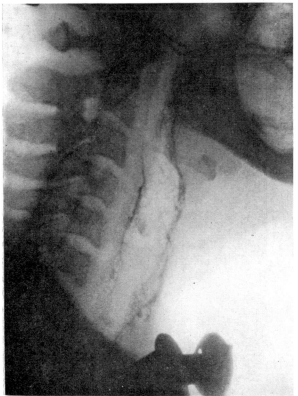

Fig. 3.12. X-ray photograph of the same patient (Fig. 9) after a barium swallow outlining the new skin hypopharynx.

hypopharynx and the pharyngo-œsophageal junction. This patient had a fixed cervical kyphosis which made the operation possible, and he swallowed perfectly after five weeks. For another patient with an early carcinoma in the left pyriform fossa I performed a partial pharyngectomy with conservation of the larynx and reconstructed the pharynx. Bilateral excision of the cervical lymph nodes is always necessary when they are enlarged.

Staged Operations after Radiotherapy

When radical surgery is required after radiotherapy there is a number of difficult technical problems to overcome. The main one is to obtain sufficient viable skin to cover the cervical prevertebral muscles and form a posterior wall for the new pharynx. Great care is taken to conserve the blood supply to the quadrilateral skin flap and its width is restricted so that sufficient will survive to form the posterior wall. When this has been secured the anterior wall is constructed with acromio-pectoral skin grafts. If the vitality of the skin of the neck is markedly impaired these skin grafts must be prepared beforehand and be ready for use when the excision of the hypopharynx is done. Sometimes the position and extent of the carcinoma allows the surgeon to leave a strip of the posterior wall and suture its edges to the skin forming a median cervical fistula. This is closed later by hinged skin flaps or acromio-pectoral tubed pedicle skin grafts.

These procedures take a long period of time and I have inserted a portex tube in the new pharynx to enable a number of patients to swallow until it was finally constructed.

End-results with Radical Operation

The periods of survival in 23 patients after these operations are shown in Table 4. One additional patient was found to be inoperable on exploration of the neck. There was no operation mortality.

TABLE 4

CARCINOMA OF THE HYPOPHARYNX. END-RESULTS WITH ALL TYPES OF OPERATION

	Period in Months after Operation									
Ten patients alive	3	5	6	7	9	23	23	26	26	45
Ten patients died of cancer	4	4	8	12	12	12	20	23	23	33
Three patients died of other cause ..	2	11	30							

The patient who has survived 45 months at present, had an advanced carcinoma for which a palliative gastrostomy was performed elsewhere;

she is well and swallows perfectly. For the majority of them no other treatment but surgery was possible and they were given complete relief from the distress of dyspnœa, stridor or dysphagia. After operation they are in good general condition, can swallow everything perfectly, live reasonably normal lives, and some return to work. Their ability to speak varies but is not so good as following laryngectomy. No patients developed a fibrous stricture at the junction of the skin pharynx and œsophagus.

RONALD W. RAVEN

References

LEDLIE, E. M., and HARMER, M. H. (1950) *Brit. J. Cancer* **4**, 6.
POWER, D'ARCY (1919) *Brit. J. Surg.* **6**, 336.
RAVEN, R. W. (1933) *St. Bart. Hosp. Reps.* **66**, 65.
RAVEN, R. W. (1952) *Brit. J. Surg.* **39**, 503.
RAVEN, R. W. (1952) *Brit. med. J.* **1**, 951.

CHAPTER IV

THE SURGERY OF THE ŒSOPHAGUS

Congenital Anomalies

THE œsophagus is developed from the primitive foregut in common with the larynx and trachea. The division of the œsophagus from the larynx and trachea is produced by two lateral grooves, which run in a longitudinal direction and which join internally between the fifth and sixth weeks of intra-uterine life. The errors of fusion produce various congenital anomalies, the most common and important of which is atresia with tracheo-œsophageal fistula (Fig. 1). This type of anomaly accounts for 80 per cent. of all cases of atresia of the œsophagus. Other types of anomaly associated with the œsophagus are shown in Fig. 2.

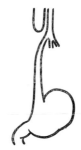

Fig. 4.1. Congenital atresia of the œsophagus showing the lower segment of the œsophagus arising from the trachea. This is the most common type of congenital anomaly of the gullet.

Congenital atresia of the œsophagus was described in 1697 by Gibson, who was army physician and grandson of Oliver Cromwell, but the subject never attracted great interest although it was referred to sporadically subsequently. Of recent years there has been a wider recognition of the anomaly and it has been realized also that the condition probably occurs about once in every 2,600 births.

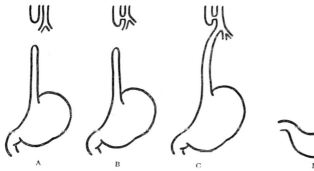

A   B   C   D

FIG. 4.2. (A) Congenital atresia without fistula. Twenty per cent of patients suffering from congenital atresia are of this variety.

(B)
(C) } Other rare forms of congenital anomaly.
(D)

Successful operations to relieve the condition were carried out by Ladd and Leven in 1939 and 1940 by using staged operations, and in 1941 Haight and Townsley reported the first successful direct anastomosis. Since then there have been a number of successes.

Diagnosis

The characteristic feature of infants suffering from this anomaly is cyanosis, which occurs whenever feeding is attempted, but it should usually be possible to suspect and confirm the diagnosis before the infant has had repeated attacks of this kind, each of which results in material entering into the respiratory system and has a deleterious effect on the lungs. Many children require aspiration of mucus from the nasopharynx soon after they are born, and it is suggested that the opportunity should be taken of introducing a well-lubricated rubber catheter and, when the pharynx has been emptied of mucus, to slide the catheter down into the stomach. If the catheter is arrested at a distance of 10 to 12 cm. from the anterior alveolar margin, it is almost certain that congenital atresia of the œsophagus is present.

Once the tentative diagnosis has been made there should be no further attempts at feeding, but arrangements should be made to transfer the child to a centre where both the confirmation of the diagnosis and surgical treatment can be carried out. A delay of some hours at this stage is of little consequence, provided that the nasopharynx is kept clear of mucus and the child's position is changed constantly in order to maintain aeration of both lungs. It is wise to administer an antibiotic by injection. The diagnosis is confirmed by radiological examination. The infant is screened and the condition of

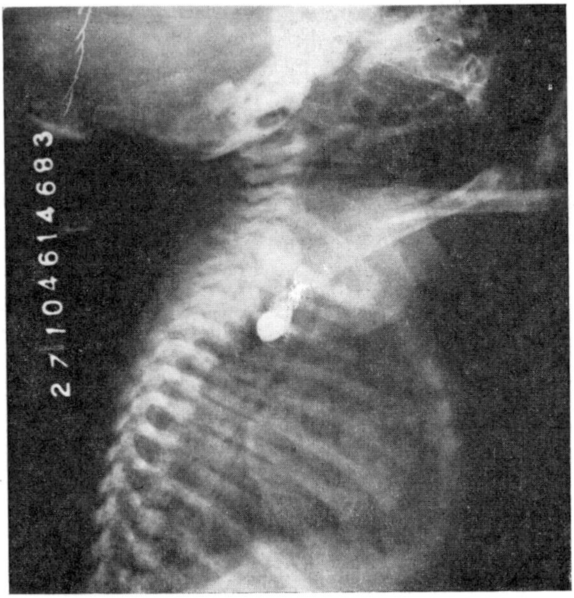

FIG. 4.3. X-ray appearance of congenital atresia of the œsophagus showing the blind upper segment filled with lipiodol.

the lungs noted, and the presence of air in the stomach and intestines looked for. This is of great importance, because in the presence of an atresia it implies that a tracheal fistula must exist. A catheter is introduced into the upper segment and $\frac{1}{2}$ ml. of iodized oil injected slowly. The appearance of an atresia is typical (Fig. 3) and when it has been confirmed that no upper fistula is present the iodized oil is withdrawn.

Operative Management

The anomaly is incompatible with life and for this reason an attempt should always be made to correct the deformity surgically.

The operation is best carried out under a general anæsthetic administered through an endo-tracheal tube. The child is placed in the left lateral position and a curved incision made just below the right scapula, which is then drawn forward to allow the thorax to be entered through the fourth intercostal space. The intercostal space is opened up by means of a special retractor, or, if this is not available, a mastoid retractor may be used for the purpose. The anæsthetist is asked to deflate the lung and it is then usually quite easy to find the vena azygos arch, which marks the approximate site of the anomaly. It is usually advisable to divide the azygos arch between thread ligatures, but occasionally the operation may be completed without doing this. If it seems clear that the arch will get in the way of the subsequent procedures, division should be carried out at this stage. It is most important that the ligatures should be applied sufficiently far apart so that when the arch is divided there is no risk of one of them slipping off, as this is an accident which may easily cause the death of the infant. The blind upper segment can usually be found without difficulty, but if it is not obvious a catheter introduced from the mouth will usually reveal its position. As soon as the blind upper segment is seen two stay sutures should be introduced so as to be able to manipulate it without producing any unnecessary damage. The sutures used for this purpose and for the anastomosis itself, are 5/0 silk carried on very small eyeless needles and they should be lubricated with liquid paraffin before use. Finding the lower segment is not always easy, and when the lower segment has been identified a search must be made for the exact point at which it arises from the trachea, the object being to separate it from the trachea, avoiding on the one hand the production of a tracheal stricture and on the other, the wasting of too much œsophagus. When the fistula has been clearly demonstrated it is divided and the opening into the trachea closed with a stitch of the same fine silk as is used throughout the operation. The lower segment of the œsophagus is controlled with stay sutures in exactly the same way as in the case of the upper segment. An opening is now made in the upper segment and three or four through and through interrupted sutures introduced and tied so as to complete the posterior part of the anastomosis. A sterile rubber catheter is now introduced into the anastomosis and one end passed into the stomach and the other up into the mouth where it is recovered. The presence of this catheter makes the completion of the anastomosis very much easier. As soon as a further three or four sutures have been introduced and tied, the stomach is emptied of air by aspirating the catheter, which is then withdrawn completely while the chest is still open. The lungs are expanded with care and the chest closed with a waterseal drain. It is wise to have an intravenous drip going during the operation and the infant usually benefits from a small blood transfusion (40 ml. to 60 ml.). If the intravenous therapy can be maintained, nothing need be given by mouth for 48 hours and the first feeds should consist of one drachm of penicillin solution. The child should be kept well under antibiotic control.

Investigation of Dysphagia in the Adult

The history of the patient's illness is of great importance and should be taken with accuracy.

Nature of Onset. Spastic conditions often first give trouble with fluids and later with solids. The converse is usually true in the case of cancer.

Duration. A long history is suggestive that the condition has been simple in the first instance, but it must be remembered that malignancy sometimes supervenes on a longstanding cardiospasm.

Remission of Symptoms. If there are repeated remissions and in each remission there is complete return to normal swallowing, the underlying cause is probably simple, but a single remission may occur in malignant disease when the growth originates in a neighbouring portion of the stomach, producing a temporary dysphagia by spasm which may disappear for some weeks, only to recur as the growth extends upwards to the œsophagus.

Site of Obstruction. The subjective feeling of the patient cannot be depended upon to determine the level of the lesion, although if pain is also present the position in which the pain is felt may give some indication of the site of obstruction.

Other Symptoms. Gurgling in the neck is highly suggestive of the presence of a pharyngeal pouch.

General Examination. Wasting may be the only abnormal physical sign, but a careful search should be made at the root of the neck where a malignant node may sometimes be found, in the abdomen where evidence of hepatic enlargement may be obvious or a cancer of the stomach may be felt and, rectally, where secondary malignant nodules may be palpable. The examination should be completed by watching the patient attempt to eat and drink.

Special Investigations. The first special examination should always be an X-ray examination with a barium swallow, and it will usually be necessary to follow this up by œsophagoscopy. Œsophagoscopy is particularly important if dysphagia is present and no cause can be found on X-ray examination. Œsophagoscopy should not be attempted in the presence of an aneurysm or if gross spinal curvature is present, and it must be remembered that it is potentially dangerous at all times and should be carried out with extreme gentleness.

Injuries of the Œsophagus

Swallowing of Corrosives

Empty beer or lemonade bottles are often used to store corrosive liquids and this is a practice which frequently leads to accidents and cannot be too strongly deprecated. Corrosives are also taken for suicidal purposes and in rare cases they may be administered homicidally.

The injury produced by a corrosive is usually most marked in the post-cricoid region or at the level of the arch of the aorta and at the cardiac end, because at these points there is often a delay in the passage of the fluid. The important feature of corrosive injuries is that the resultant burn seldom destroys the epithelium completely at any one level, because small islets of cells are protected by the longitudinal folds of oesophageal epithelium.

First-aid Treatment. The appropriate antidote should be given when possible and in the case of most corrosives it is safe to administer milk or olive oil as a demulcent. Following an injury of this nature the patient should be kept on a liquid or semi-solid diet for ten days and after each feed sterile water should be given followed by sips of penicillin solution. After ten days a normal diet may be resumed if no pain is produced on swallowing. If it seems likely that a severe injury has occurred, and this is suggested if persistent pain is produced when swallowing is attempted, or if dysphagia is considerable, a temporary gastrostomy should be made. No attempt at dilatation should be made until eight weeks after the accident.

Treatment of a Stricture following a Corrosive Injury. It has been advocated that the early passage of instruments is desirable after a corrosive injury, because after the lapse of several weeks the treatment of a stricture of this nature becomes one of great difficulty. This has not been the author's experience and most strictures resulting from corrosives can be cured by the method of auto-dilatation. This treatment consists in teaching the patient to swallow a gum elastic œsophageal bougie and it is essential that no force be used. The advantage of this method over endoscopic dilatation is that it can be carried out two or three times a day and the help given by the peristaltic movements of the œsophagus is not abolished by the presence of the œsophagoscope.

In very difficult cases it is a help if a gastrostomy is carried out in the first instance and the patient is then encouraged to swallow a ureteric catheter. This is seldom impossible, although the process may take a considerable number of hours and the patient may need a great deal of encouragement in order to achieve it. Once the ureteric catheter has negotiated the œsophagus it may be recovered from the gastro-stomy and replaced by a soft rubber tube, one end of which emerges from the patient's mouth and the other from the gastrostomy opening. By attaching a gum elastic bougie to one or other end of this tube "guided dilatation" may be carried out. When this can be done with ease the gastrostomy is allowed to close. Auto-dilatation with bougies should normally be done two or three times a day for the first few weeks, and it is important not to attempt to reach too big a size of bougie too quickly. As the treatment progresses the interval between dilatations can be increased. After a few weeks it may not be necessary to pass the bougie more often than once or twice a week. It is important not to stop dilatation prematurely and most strictures of this nature will require treatment for about a year at least. However tedious dilatation with bougies may appear, it is fair to say that if the œsophagus is dilated in this manner the final outcome is a restoration to normal swallowing and this cannot be said of any operation which replaces the normal œsophagus with some other viscus.

Foreign Bodies

Foreign bodies may injure the œsophagus during their passage and this type of injury has been referred to by Grey Turner as "transit" injuries. Even if the foreign body has been successfully removed through the œsophagoscope an injury may result, either because of the shape of the object, or sometimes because removal has been carried out roughly, and in either case a stricture may result. This type of stricture can be treated in the same way as one which has arisen as the result of corrosives.

Instrumental Injuries

If the œsophagoscope is used unskilfully it is possible to produce an injury at the pharyngo-œsophageal junction, and Goligher has reported such an injury which was recognized without delay and which was repaired by immediate exploration. In this particular case the occurrence of cervical emphysema led to a rapid diagnosis, but in other cases the indications for an immediate operation may be less clear because the onset of symptoms is gradual, and in such cases it is justifiable to administer antibiotics and to treat the patient expectantly. If this course is decided upon, it is wise to make a gastrostomy and to nurse the patient in the Trendelenburg position to lessen the risk of a spreading mediastinitis.

The œsophagoscope may also injure the œsophagus at or near the site of a carcinoma and the risk of producing such an injury must sometimes be taken when the object of the procedure is to introduce a Souttar's tube.

Injuries with the gastroscope also occur but with the early models the injury was more likely to be in the stomach, but post-cricoid damage may be produced even with the flexible gastroscope.

Whichever instrument is being employed, care should be taken to avoid over extension of the neck in the early stages of the examination and to exercise particular care in patients in whom the X-ray has shown the presence of cervical spurs.

Wounds of the Neck and Thorax

The œsophagus may be injured in wounds of this nature but very often the concomitant injuries cause the damage to the gullet to be overlooked.

Crush Injuries and Injuries by Compressed Air

These are similar in their effect with spontaneous rupture of the œsophagus.

Spontaneous Rupture of the Œsophagus

This condition implies the rupture of a previously healthy œsophagus. The accident occurs in men more frequently than in women and usually follows violent vomiting often associated with alcoholism. The effect of the alcohol is first to give rise to efforts of vomiting and, secondly, it may interfere with the co-ordinated muscular action of the œsophagus so that a greatly increased pressure is produced in the lumen. Clinically the condition causes violent pain which may simulate a perforation of a duodenal or gastric ulcer. It differs from the perforated ulcer, however, in that cyanosis, grunting respiration and excessive thirst are features of spontaneous rupture of the œsophagus. Emphysema at the root of the neck under these circumstances is diagnostic, but an attempt should be made to make an earlier diagnosis if possible before emphysema can be seen externally and, if the condition is suspected, X-ray examination may show emphysema in the posterior mediastinum and evidence of fluid or air in the thorax. The only satisfactory treatment is to carry out an immediate thoracotomy and to repair the œsophagus and provide waterseal drainage. Antibiotics must be given.

Hiatal Hernia and Reflux Œsophagitis

Inflammation of the œsophagus may accompany the specific fevers and other infections, but all these varieties of inflammation are unimportant compared with the condition of reflux œsophagitis, which was not clearly recognized in the past. The work of Allison, Barrett and others has clarified the position in recent years.

Reflux œsophagitis is an inflammatory condition of the œsophagus which starts at the lower end and is presumably caused by some irritating factor in the gastric juices. It is better to avoid the term "peptic ulceration" for this condition, because the use of the term implies that the ulceration occurs in ectopic islets of gastric mucosa. This probably does occur on very rare occasions, but it is of little clinical importance and the ectopic islets may occur at any level, whereas reflux œsophagitis always starts at the lower end. The regurgitation of gastric contents occurs occasionally in normal people and it is only when regurgitation is excessive, and when the gastric juices are irritating, that harm results. The causes of reflux œsophagitis may be excessive vomiting, as may happen in pregnancy, or after surgical operations and from other causes, but the most important cause is failure of the "cardiac sphincter" which normally prevents regurgitation from the stomach. The exact nature of this sphincter is open to doubt, but it seems that the fibres of the right crus of the diaphragm which embrace the lower end of the œsophagus in a manner comparable with the way in which the pubo-rectalis fibres of the levator ani embrace the ano-rectal junction, and the angle of insertion of the œsophagus into the stomach, are the two most important features. The causes of failure of the cardiac sphincter are the presence of a hiatal hernia, illnesses which weaken the muscular tone, and certain operations which destroy the sphincter. Of these causes one of the most interesting is the presence of a hiatal hernia, which impairs or destroys the sphincter by increasing the acute angle of insertion of the œsophagus and making the action of the right crus of the diaphragm ineffective. As a result of the herniation, the œsophago-gastric junction comes to lie above the opening in the diaphragm and the patient then presents a "short œsophagus" which used to be regarded as the primary abnormality. True examples of congenital short œsophagus may occur but it must be remembered that the condition is commonly seen in middle-aged and elderly patients, less frequently in infants and very rarely in young adult life. For this reason it seems probable that most examples of so-called congenital short œsophagus are really instances of secondary shortening, resulting from the changes associated with reflux œsophagitis which itself has been caused by the presence of the hernia.

Pathological Changes in Reflux Œsophagitis

The ulceration which is characteristic, is usually superficial and starts in the lowest part of the œsophagus, and when seen through the œsophagoscope the epithelium appears reddened in patches and may show superficial abrasions. Hæmorrhage occurs readily. The abrasions may coalesce and extend up the œsophagus so that a considerable part becomes involved. The condition has a natural tendency to heal and break down again so that the appearances vary with subsequent examinations. The œsophageal muscle is affected first by spasm and later by fibrosis. These processes result in shortening of the longitudinal fibres, drawing the œsophago-gastric junction still further into the chest, and spasm and fibrosis of the circular muscles may lead to stricture formation.

Symptoms

The characteristic symptoms are pain, dysphagia and anæmia. These symptoms may occur together or they may occur separately, and there is great variation in the severity of any of them. Pain is the most common symptom and is usually described by the patient as "heart burn". This heart burn may be severe and may radiate through to the back or up into the neck and down the arms. Heart burn is often attributed to the presence of a duodenal ulcer, but it seems more probable that it usually represents the presence of œsophagitis although the two conditions may occur together. When radiation up into the neck or down into the arms occurs, the suggestion of coronary disease may be made and it is quite understandable how, in the past, œsophagitis has been confused with other conditions and has not been recognized as a separate entity. Often the symptoms have been passed off as being "neurotic" in origin. The dysphagia is due to spasm in the first instance and later fibrosis may occur. Bleeding is often slight but continuous, and may produce a considerable anæmia without obvious evidence of hæmorrhage. Severe hæmorrhage is unusual with œsophagitis and is more often due to hæmorrhage from a chronic ulcer situated in the thoracic stomach.

Diagnosis

A careful assessment of the symptoms may suggest the presence of œsophagitis but whenever possible it should be confirmed by œsophago-scopic examination. The findings are characteristic. There is ulceration which is always most marked at the lower end of the œsophagus, and fluid constantly regurgitates from the stomach during examination. It is important to make sure that there is not a carcinoma lying just below the ulcerated area.

Treatment

The treatment of the condition is very similar to that which is successful for a duodenal ulcer, and for this reason many patients have been undiagnosed in the past, but have been cured by the medical regime instituted for what was supposed to be a peptic ulcer. In addition to a medical regime of regularity of meals, avoiding too long an interval, and eliminating sources of anxiety, it is important to advise the patient to avoid stooping or lying down or carrying out any movements which favour the regurgitation of material from the stomach into the œsophagus. Alkali powder should be prescribed and it is useful to suck an alkaline tablet which may be prescribed combined with dried milk. Olive oil before going to bed is a help. If this treatment is carried out thoroughly, many patients will become free from symptoms and will not require any operative intervention. If medical treatment has been tried and failed, or if serious stricture formation occurs, or if there have been episodes of severe bleeding, it is likely that surgery will be required.

Operations for the Relief of Reflux Œsophagitis

The ideal surgical treatment is to attack the underlying cause and repair the diaphragm in such a way that the stomach lies completely in the abdominal cavity and the anatomical arrangements of the cardiac sphincter are returned to normal. This ideal method, however, cannot always be followed, because the extent of the stricture and the degree of shortening may make any restoration of the normal anatomical arrangements impracticable. Under these circumstances it may be

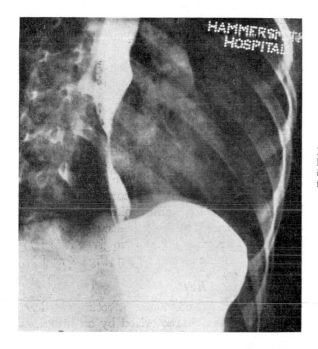

Fig. 4.4. Hiatal hernia leading to reflux œsophagitis and extensive stricture formation which ultimately required resection.

Fig. 4.5. The same patient as shown in Fig. 4. Resection has been carried out and the stomach anastomosed to the œsophagus above the arch of the aorta.

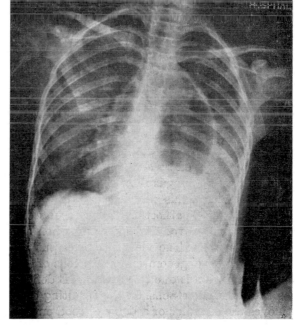

necessary to resect a considerable part of the œsophagus and restore continuity, either by use of the small bowel or stomach. Utilizing the stomach has the disadvantage that the stage is set for the further development of œsophagitis at a higher level, but it is a risk which may have to be taken and, if the patient is elderly and is controlled by a suitable medical regime after operation, no further ill-effects may occur. Where a high resection is to be carried out in children, there is always a fear that reflux œsophagitis may develop subsequently. Sufficient time has not yet elapsed to know how serious this risk is. Another method which is suitable in some cases, is to treat the condition by an abdominal partial gastrectomy which lowers the acidity of the regurgitating fluid. If the gastrectomy is carried out by the Billroth I method, it may also exert a mechanical effect in preventing herniation. The presence of a stricture does not necessarily mean that resection must be carried out and provided alkalis are given it is sometimes satisfactory to treat these patients by dilatation (Figs. 4 and 5).

Cardiospasm or Achalasia

This term should be restricted to a condition affecting the lower two-thirds of the œsophagus, which is characterized by an imbalance between the sympathetic and vagal innervation, with the result that resistance at the cardiac sphincter is increased and the œsophagus above it tends to undergo dilatation. Local causes of cardiospasm, such as an ulcer or carcinoma in the vicinity, should be excluded.

The ætiology of the condition is not simple, but it seems clear that for a bolus of food to pass smoothly down the œsophagus into the stomach a complex series of processes must be properly co-ordinated. The swallowing of the bolus is a voluntary act but once the food reaches the pharynx the condition becomes an involuntary reflex, and it seems to be essential in the first instance that the crico-pharyngeus muscle should relax and allow the bolus to enter the upper œsophagus. At this point the passage down the gullet is brought about by a wave of peristalsis, preceded by a wave of relaxation.

Section of the vagus in cats produces a condition comparable with cardiospasm and this ill-effect can be prevented experimentally by simultaneous sympathectomy. The results of the animal experiments, however, have proved disappointing when applied to the relief of the condition in man. The view has been put forward that one cause of the condition is degeneration of the cells of Auerbach's plexus and that this degeneration is due to a vitamin B deficiency. Once the condition has become well established the resulting dilatation of the œsophagus removes the stimulus of a bolus of food entering the gullet.

Clinical Course

Occasionally well-developed cardiospasm may be present without the patient complaining of any symptoms concerned with swallowing, but usually the first symptoms are subjective dysphagia, later, attacks of regurgitation may occur and, at a still later stage when there is considerable dilatation of the œsophagus, regurgitation may be less frequent but larger in amount. Another symptom which causes great distress is the regurgitation of food into the mouth when the patient is half asleep, and by this means aspiration of food into the trachea may occur and pulmonary complications result. In a longstanding case toxic absorption may take place and the patient may develop osteoarthropathy. Occasionally malignant disease supervenes.

X-ray Examination

The œsophagus is usually dilated and tapers to a point at the level of the diaphragm (Fig. 6). When a certain hydrostatic pressure has been reached in the œsophagus fluid passes into the stomach, and it is important to note that the lower end of the œsophagus is quite smooth in outline and contrasts with the appearance seen in cancer, when the lumen is displaced and irregular. The gastric air bubble is usually absent in cases of cardiospasm.

Confirmation of the diagnosis should be made with the œsophagoscope unless this is contra-indicated by the presence of an aneurysm, advanced age of the patient, or gross spinal deformity. Œsophagoscopy shows a normal epithelium in most cases which

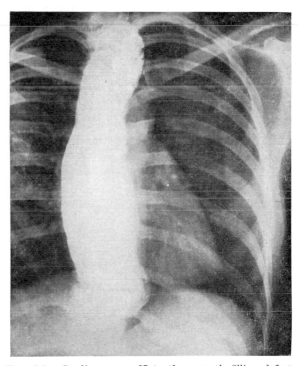

Fig. 4.6. Cardiospasm. Note the smooth filling defect at the lower end of the œsophagus, dilatation affecting the lower two-thirds of the gullet and the absence of the gastric air bubble.

distinguishes the condition from a local spasm associated with reflux œsophagitis, in which case the ulceration at the lower end is characteristic.

Treatment

The use of antispasmodic drugs has proved very disappointing except in extremely mild cases. Thorough dilatation by means of the Plummer hydrostatic bag should be tried in the first instance and is usually carried out at the time of confirming the diagnosis at œsophago-scopy. The use of the Plummer bag produces a symptomatic cure in about 70 per cent. of cases. If this method has proved unsuccessful after repetition, the patient is best treated by means of Heller's operation, which consists in dividing the muscle down to the mucous membrane at the œsophago-gastric junction and for a distance of one inch on either side of this junction. Heller's operation is most easily carried out through a left thoracotomy incision, but if it is essential to make a thorough examination of the abdominal contents, the operation can be undertaken from below after mobilization of the left lobe of the liver. The results of Heller's operation, if it is carried out meticulously, are excellent.

Sideropenic Dysphagia

This condition which was described by Paterson and Kelly, and usually associated with the names of Plummer and Vinson, has been regarded as dysphagia associated with anæmia, but recent work by Waldenström and Kjellberg has shown that although there is a deficiency of iron, anæmia is not always present, and for this reason they have suggested the term sideropenic dysphagia. The patients are almost always women and the condition runs an extremely chronic course. In untreated cases there is a tendency for carcinoma of the mouth or œsophagus to occur.

Signs and Symptoms

Dysphagia with solids is usually the presenting symptom and pain may be complained of in the neck. Epithelial changes occur, the tongue becoming sore and appearing smooth, and fissures may appear at the corner of the mouth. Koilonychia or spoon nails may be seen, the surface of the nail becoming concave and very often split. Pruritus of the vulva may be present. An achlorhydric type of gastritis may occur. The characteristic blood picture is hypochromic anæmia, but sometimes a typical anæmia is not present but the serum iron is deficient.

The pathological changes causing the dysphagia are not easy to evaluate, because few patients die from the condition unless cancer develops, but from those cases which have come to post mortem, and from biopsy material which has been examined, it seems that there is often a chronic inflammatory condition in the pharynx and cervical œsophagus, and hyper-keratinization is present. Beneath the epithelium are aggregations of lymphocytes and the muscular wall of the pharynx is thicker than usual.

Diagnosis

X-ray examination when carried out with care may show a fine filling defect just below the level of the cricoid cartilage, which is produced by a web of heaped up epithelium. Through the œsophagoscope this web appears as a fold which may extend round the lumen of the œsophagus, forming a circular membrane with an aperture in the centre.

Treatment

The iron deficiency must be corrected and in addition the entire vitamin B complex should be administered. Sometimes the underlying factor is atrophic gastritis which may be made worse by dysphagia. The treatment is often shortened by carrying out dilatation through the œsophagoscope. It is important to follow these patients up in order to make sure that malignant changes have not occurred.

Carcinoma of the Œsophagus

Carcinoma of the œsophagus is the most common form of new growth in this organ. The typical growth is a squamous celled carcinoma, although occasionally basal-celled carcinomata occur. An adeno-carcinoma extending upwards from the stomach is quite common, and very occasionally this variety may occur higher in the œsophagus in ectopic gastric mucous membrane. The condition is more common in men than in women excepting in the case of post-cricoid cancers which occur more frequently in women, often as a sequel to the Plummer-Vinson syndrome. Twenty-five per cent. of growths are situated in the hypopharynx and upper third of the œsophagus, 45 per cent. in the middle third and 30 per cent. in the lower third.

The serious consequences of cancer of the œsophagus are produced, to a large extent, by the anatomical relations, and the involvement of the lung or bronchus may cause the death of the patient before the growth has spread widely, but now that a considerable number of patients are subjected to a successful operation for the removal of the growth, it is becoming more evident that widespread metastases occur in this condition, just as they do in the case of growths in other parts of the alimentary canal. The extension of the growth is usually greater than would be thought by an inspection of the X-rays and it is particularly advanced in the submucous layer. The lung, bronchus or trachea may be directly involved, as may the great vessels, the pericardium or heart. Lymphatic spread occurs from the upper part of the œsophagus to the cervical lymphatic nodes, from the middle of the œsophagus to the tracheal lymph nodes, and from the lower part of the gullet the spread is to the lesser curvature of the stomach, the coeliac axis and the liver. Involvement of the recurrent laryngeal nerve may take place either by the growth itself or by a malignant node.

Diagnosis

The most constant symptom is dysphagia, which usually starts first with solids and becomes progressively worse until eventually the patient is unable to swallow his own saliva. Occasionally dysphagia is absent in the early stages and the complaint is one of fatigue and vague symptoms which may persist for some time until troubles with swallowing are noticed. In the case of growths arising in the stomach and extending upwards to the œsophagus, there may be a preliminary dysphagia due to spasm and this symptom may improve subsequently only to recur later, the remission sometimes giving rise to delay in diagnosis.

Physical examination may not show any abnormality other than loss of weight, but occasionally enlarged lymph nodes at the root of the neck may be felt, nodules may be palpable per rectum, or an examination of the abdomen may show an enlarged liver or a palpable gastric neoplasm. Changes in the voice may suggest involvement of the recurrent laryngeal nerve, and choking or coughing when fluids are taken gives rise to the suspicion that a fistula communicating with the air passages is present.

Radiological Examination

This should always be the first step in confirming the diagnosis, and in the thoracic part of the gullet the result of X-ray examination is very dependable. In the cervical œsophagus, however, a condition of spasm of the crico-pharyngeus will sometimes be reported as being malignant in nature, whereas a growth at the lower end of the œsophagus, or fundus of the stomach, may be concealed radiologically by an overlying spasm. For these reasons it is usually essential to confirm the diagnosis by direct inspection with the œsophago-scope when the typical ulcerative appearance of a neoplasm can be seen (Fig. 7).

Treatment

The choice of treatment depends upon the situation of the growth, the age and general condition of the patient, and the presence of any evidence of extension of the growth.

Irradiation. Treatment by irradiation has, in general, proved disappointing owing to

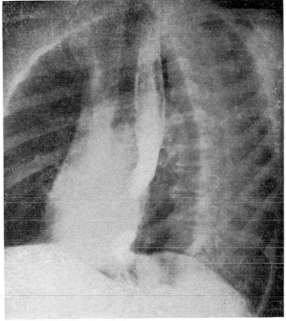

FIG. 4.7.   Carcinoma affecting the lower third of the œsophagus.

the inaccessibility of the greater part of the œsophagus. The hypopharynx and cervical œsophagus are irradiated more easily and unless the patient is very suitable for operation this method may be used with advantage in these sites.

Choice of Operation. A growth which is limited to the cervical œsophagus occurring in an otherwise fit patient, offers a reasonable hope for surgical excision. In addition it may be necessary to remove the larynx. The gullet is reconstituted by staged operations, making use of the skin of the neck to construct a skin tube. The foundation of this type of operation was laid by Trotter and various modifications and improvements in details have been made since.

If the growth is situated in the thoracic part of the œsophagus and is sufficiently far removed from the stomach, it is possible in many cases to resect a considerable part of the gullet and restore continuity by bringing up the mobilized stomach and anastomosing it to the œsophagus. These operations are conveniently carried out by a left abdomino-thoracic incision, supplemented in the case of a high growth by a second thoracotomy incision in about the fourth interspace. For the middle third of the œsophagus the approach from the right side is very attractive, and the arch of the aorta instead of being a hindrance to surgical excision, becomes a convenient barrier to protect the left pleura. The right-sided approach, however, has the great disadvantage that reconstitution of the gullet is sometimes more difficult, because the presence of the right lobe of the liver means that the patient's position has to be altered during an operation of great magnitude, and sometimes the necessary movements have a bad effect on the patient's general condition. For this reason the author has reverted to the left-sided approach.

If the growth is situated in the lower part of the œsophagus proper and there is no involvement of the stomach, the most satisfactory method is to make a left-sided approach as indicated above, dividing the costal margin. The incision should be made over the eighth rib or in the eighth interspace. Removal of the rib has the advantage that closing the chest is somewhat easier. On the other hand, if the thoracic cage seems reasonably mobile, an intercostal incision has the advantage that post-operative respiration may be more satisfactory. The diaphragm is divided in a radial manner down to the œsophageal hiatus and mobilization of the stomach carried out after first removing the spleen. The left gastric artery and the gastro-colic omentum have to be divided to achieve this mobilization. The fundus of the stomach is divided between clamps and the distal cut surface closed with a double row of sutures. The affected portion of the œsophagus and a margin of healthy tissue above it are now dissected free, after division of the left pulmonary ligament. Section of the vagi at the upper part of the area of dissection increases the mobility of the œsophagus. In dividing the œsophagus it is important to make a division of the muscular coats, so that first of all the mucous membrane is exposed rather like the inner tube of a motor-car tyre. Division of the mucous membrane is then carried out at the lower margin of this exposed portion so that when the anastomosis comes to be made there is no difficulty in including the mucous membrane in the stitches. A fresh opening is made in a convenient portion of the stomach and care taken to see that the size corresponds closely to the cross section of the cut œsophagus. The anastomosis is made by using interrupted mattress sutures of silk posteriorly, a continuous layer of catgut going right round the anastomosis and, finally, interrupted sutures introduced in a Lembert fashion over the front part of the suture line. These Lembert sutures have a tendency to cut out and it is sometimes better to turn back a flap of pleura and suture it over the anastomosis. Care must be taken to suture the stomach to the parietal pleura and when closing the diaphragm the latter must be attached very carefully to the stomach to avoid the possibility of herniation occurring. A large drainage tube

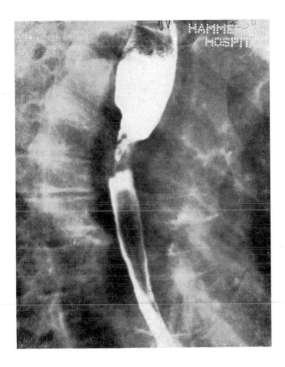

FIG. **4**.8. Carcinoma of the middle third of the œsophagus, which was found at operation to be firmly attached to the root of the lung and to the aorta.

FIG. **4**.9. The patient has been treated by a palliative short circuit, the stomach being brought up and anastomosed to the œsophagus above the arch of the aorta.

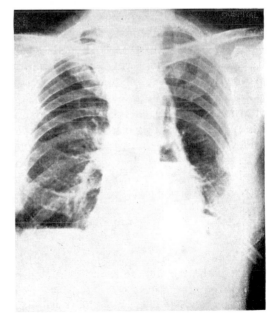

is introduced and led to a waterseal bottle and the chest closed.

If the growth involving the lower end of the œsophagus is invading the stomach, or if it is arising primarily in the stomach, it becomes essential to carry out a total gastrectomy and this can be best achieved by removing the stomach, spleen, tail of pancreas, and great omentum in one block as has been pointed out by Allison. Restoration of the continuity is brought about by using an undivided loop of small bowel if this will reach the lower end of the œsophagus. If an undivided loop will not reach, it becomes necessary to make a Roux anastomosis en Y. It is a good plan to see if a loop of bowel will come up to the proposed site of anastomosis at the beginning of the operation, before resection has been carried out, so that if it seems clear that a Roux loop is to be fashioned this may be done at the outset. By this means it is possible to ensure that the loop is viable before the time comes to use it in making the anastomosis.

A growth situated at the upper part of the thoracic gullet, or in the lower portion of the cervical œsophagus, presents a great problem from the point of view of surgical excision, and the only satisfactory radical operation is to mobilize the stomach through a left-sided thoraco-abdominal incision, resecting the whole of the thoracic œsophagus and anastomosing the mobilized stomach to the cervical œsophagus in the neck. This procedure is one of such magnitude that few patients will be found suitable for it and it may be preferable to use some palliative procedure such as the introduction of Souttar's tube. The use of a plastic tube, or a previously prepared skin tube, to bridge the gap caused by a local removal of a growth in this situation, presents an attractive alternative, but there are many technical difficulties associated with this method at the present time.

Palliative Procedures. The situation of the growth and the general condition of the patient may either separately or combined, make any attempt at radical excision unjustifiable, and in these patients a palliative procedure may be the proper one to adopt.

In the middle third of the œsophagus where a growth may be encountered, which is firmly adherent to the root of the lung or to the aorta, a palliative short circuit gives considerable relief. If preliminary inspection gives the impression that total removal is unlikely to be achieved, as much benefit may be given the patient by short-circuiting the obstruction as by carrying out a partial removal at the risk of a high immediate mortality (Figs. 8 and 9).

If a palliative short circuit operation is decided upon, the stomach is mobilized after division of the costal margin and diaphragm, and the spleen is removed. The thoracic œsophagus is freed as far as the growth itself. An intercostal incision is made in the fourth interspace after drawing tho scapula well forward. With the help of this incision the œsophagus is exposed above the arch of the aorta and a lateral anastomosis made between it and the fundus of the stomach. A palliative operation of this nature often enables the patient to survive some months in comfort and to die under less unpleasant circumstances than would otherwise be the case.

In those patients in whom it seems unjustifiable even to carry out a thoracotomy, the use of Souttar's tube should be considered. Souttar's tube consists of a close spiral of German silver wire made in a number of sizes and provided with a flange-like extension at the proximal end, which prevents the tube passing right through the strictured portion of the œsophagus. The introduction of the tube is effected through the large-sized œsophagoscope. Cautious dilatation is carried out and a tube of suitable size is introduced on a special introducer so that the flange rests at the upper level of the growth. The use of the Souttar's tube has obvious disadvantages in that it encourages the formation of a fistula and may be complicated by ulceration and hæmorrhage, and quite often the tube passes right through the stricture and down the alimentary tract. In spite of these disadvantages, however, the use of a tube enables the patient to regain reasonable powers of swallowing and often to resume normal activities. The possibilities of introducing a tube should be borne in mind in patients unsuitable for any more radical intervention.

Gastrostomy is not to be regarded as a satisfactory palliative procedure, but it must be carried out if the patient is quite unable to swallow fluids and relief cannot be obtained by other measures.

Whatever method of palliation has been employed considerable benefit is obtained by allowing the patient to sip diluted hydrogen peroxide solution, which helps to remove food debris and exerts a mild antiseptic action. Attention must also be given to the bowels, because many patients who are in a state of chronic starvation suffer from impacted fæces which may add considerably to their discomfort. Attention to these details not only helps to remove unnecessary pains and discomfort, but it has the great virtue that the patient feels he is continuing to receive treatment and has not been abandoned.

Diverticula of the Œsophagus

Pharyngo-œsophageal Diverticulum or Pharyngeal Pouch

This is a herniation of mucous membrane through a weak point, which lies between the oblique fibres of the inferior constrictor muscles

of the pharynx and the circular fibres which constitute the crico-
pharyngeal sphincter. This sphincter serves to prevent air entering the
œsophagus with each inspiration. Spasm of this sphincter is often the
underlying cause of a pharyngeal pouch. Negus has drawn attention
to this factor in the ætiology of the condition.

The hernia starts as a bulge and gradually forms an actual pouch
which becomes filled with food and mucus. As the result of this the
sac is dragged downwards and its orifice is rotated so that ultimately
the sac presents as a direct continuation of the pharynx. The opening
into the œsophagus is compressed anteriorly under the cricoid cartilage.
The symptoms are due in the first place to the underlying spasm and
later the sac itself causes symptoms by pressure on the œsophagus.
Other symptoms in a well formed sac are gurgling sounds on eating
and the regurgitation of food into the mouth at night, and sometimes
the inhalation of food. The symptoms tend to become progressively
worse and dysphagia may be marked, particularly towards the end of
a meal. The results of septic absorption are sometimes seen when the
condition has been present a long time, and occasionally cancer may
develop. Attacks of inflammation may occur from time to time.

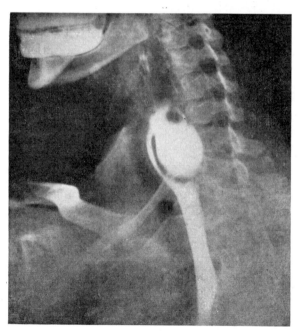

FIG. 4.10.   Pharyngeal pouch which was treated by
excision.

The diagnosis is
confirmed by a careful
X-ray examination
which shows the pouch
filling up and the
opaque material spil-
ling over from the
top (Fig. 10). This
feature serves to dis-
tinguish the condition
from the dilatation
which may occur with
a high stricture.

Treatment. In the
early stages of the
formation of a pouch
the underlying spasm
is treated by dilatation
and if anæmia is
present this must be
corrected. In more
advanced cases the
pouch itself may

require treatment. It is sometimes sufficient to wash the sac out periodically, and the patient may learn to do this by drinking copiously and holding his head in such a way that the fluid enters the sac.

Excision of the sac is a very satisfactory procedure provided it is done with meticulous care. Antibiotic cover must be given and any inflammatory changes in the sac allowed to settle down. The operation is best carried out in one stage and it is convenient to make an incision along the anterior border of the left sternomastoid muscle, extending from the angle of the jaw as far as the sternum. It may be necessary to divide the anterior part of the sternomastoid muscle close to its sternal insertion. The thyroid is retracted inwards and the carotid sheath outwards, and the inferior thyroid vessels are divided if they are in the way. When the retro-pharyngeal space has been identified it is a great help to pass a large œsophageal tube from the mouth. This usually enters the sac and serves to define it. The sac is held with stay sutures to prevent any unnecessary handling and is carefully freed from the surrounding parts until its origin from the pharyngo-œsophageal junction is clearly demonstrated. In carrying out this dissection it must be remembered that the greater part of the sac consists of mucous membrane only, but near its base there are thinned out muscle fibres derived from the constrictor muscles, and these should be carefully preserved so that after the sac has been excised the muscle can be folded over the suture line in the form of a protective cuff. It is sometimes difficult to know the precise level at which to excise the sac, too small an excision resulting in a recurrence and too large an excision causing a stricture. The œsophageal tube is of great assistance in showing the point at which excision should take place. By with-drawing it from the sac and then reintroducing it into the œsophagus proper, with the finger acting as a guide, it becomes much easier to remove the correct amount of pouch. The incision in the mucous membrane should be closed with a fine catgut suture and the muscles drawn over the suture line with fine interrupted silk sutures. To prevent recurrence it is wise to stitch the pharynx to the prevertebral fascia and so obliterate what would otherwise be a potential space. A soft drain is left near the suture line and the rest of the incision closed.

For a few days nothing is allowed by mouth other than sips of boiled water and penicillin solution, and a normal diet is not resumed until a fortnight after operation.

Diverticula of the Thoracic Œsophagus

Traction diverticula are caused by adhesion to the œsophagus of some neighbouring inflammatory condition such as a tuberculous lymph node. A pulsion diverticulum is produced by the herniation of the mucous membrane through the muscular wall, possibly as the result of congenital weakness. Traction-pulsion diverticula occur when the condition has started as the result of traction and these are encouraged to enlarge by the entry of food into the sac. This variety was drawn attention to by Barrett.

Symptoms

Very often the condition is discovered accidentally on X-ray examination, but sometimes dysphagia may be complained of. The diagnosis is usually obvious on X-ray examination, but the presence of some other lesion such as a carcinoma, must be borne in mind and œsophagoscopy is usually required to exclude this risk. If no symptoms are present and the condition has been discovered fortuitously, no treatment need be given. In other cases an associated spasm may require dilatation and, if symptoms are caused by attacks of inflammation or by the distended sac dragging downwards, it may be necessary to carry out a radical operation. If operation is necessary and the pouch is situated in the middle of the œsophagus, the right-sided thoracic approach is to be recommended. It may only be necessary to return the mucous membrane into the lumen of the œsophagus and to repair the defect in the overlying muscle with interrupted silk sutures. A large sac may require excision.

Œsophageal Varices

Œsophageal varices are the result of portal hypertension and the hæmorrhage which may occur from these varices accounts for more than half the deaths in patients who suffer from this condition. The hæmorrhage which occurs may be confused with bleeding from a peptic ulcer of the stomach or duodenum, but it is sometimes possible to differentiate the two types of hæmorrhage by taking a careful history. In the case of bleeding from œsophageal varices, the patient may have noticed a heavy feeling behind the sternum and soon after this bright red blood may be regurgitated without effort. Still later nausea may occur and the patient may then vomit dark red blood, together with gastric contents. Sometimes the hæmorrhage is occult and the symptoms produced are those of anæmia. Other evidence of portal hypertension may indicate the source of the hæmorrhage. X-ray examination shows a filling defect produced by the prominent veins and it is possible to differentiate this filling defect from the appearances associated with a growth, because in the case of varices variations in intrathoracic pressure and movements of the œsophagus alter the appearances of the filling defect. Confirmation may be obtained by carrying out an œsophagoscopic examination.

Treatment

Treatment may be required either for massive hæmorrhage or for the prevention of the repetition of such hæmorrhage, or again because the patient is suffering from a steady slight loss of blood. Immediate treatment may be carried out by applying pressure at the site of the hæmorrhage either by the use of a special bag which has been designed for this purpose (Burge), or, if this is not available, by using a Miller-Abbott tube, which is introduced to the proper distance and then distended. A blood transfusion must be given if required, but excessive transfusion encourages further bleeding. When the immediate danger has been overcome attempts should be made to decrease the risk of further hæmorrhage, and it is important to distinguish carefully intra-hepatic obstruction from extra-hepatic causes. The second type is more promising from a surgical point of view. The best operation which can be carried out in these cases is a matter of controversy, but the aim must be to reduce the portal blood flow. The most certain way of achieving this is by making a direct anastomosis between the portal vein and inferior vena cava. In all cases before operation is undertaken, adequate preparation on a suitable diet must be given, and the diet for these patients should be rich in carbohydrate and low in fat, and should not contain meat protein. Vegetable, milk and egg proteins should be given freely and it is important to give an adequate amount of vitamins and bile salts daily. If operation is not considered justifiable, it is wise to treat the patient as if he were suffering from reflux œsophagitis, on the assumption that a possible cause of gross hæmorrhage in these cases may be due to an ulceration of the œsophagus occurring in a patient who has varices.

Rare Conditions of the Œsophagus

Sarcoma

This tumour is extremely rare in the œsophagus and the history is often identical with that of carcinoma.

Melanotic Carcinoma

A case has been described by Jaleski and Waldo in which the primary lesion consisted of a polypoid mass in the œsophagus, with extensive metastases in the neighbouring lymph nodes and also in the liver and other organs.

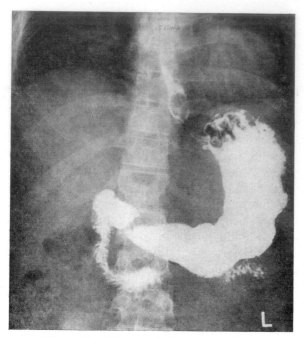

FIG. 4.11.   Fibroma of the œsophagus.

Simple Tumours

Simple tumours are very rare. They may arise from any of the coats comprising the œsophagus. Papillomata, myomata, leiomyomata and lipomata have all been described. Sometimes the history has resembled that of malignant disease and in other cases the tumour has been an incidental finding. Simple tumours occasionally undergo ulceration and produce hæmorrhage, and in other cases become pedunculated, and if they are situated near the upper end of the œsophagus they may be extruded from the mouth (Fig. 11).

Syphilis of the Œsophagus

In the past many examples of syphilis of the œsophagus were described, but it is doubtful if the diagnosis was accurate in many cases. Until comparatively recently the true nature of many simple conditions of the œsophagus has not been recognized. It is extremely rare to encounter a proved case of syphilis of the gullet at the present time.

Œsophageal Cysts

Congenital cysts may occur in the wall of the œsophagus and enlarge into the pleura, sometimes simulating the signs of an empyema.

Œsophageal Casts

This is a rare condition, possibly the result of some injury to the œsophagus although in the recorded cases a clear connection with an injury has not been proved. It is possible that the condition starts as a low-grade œsophagitis as suggested by Patterson, and as the result of this there is excessive epithelial growth and the mucosa separates from the cardiac end upwards and is eventually extruded in a tubular form. A similar condition has followed diphtheritic œsophagitis.

Scleroderma

Œsophageal symptoms may occur in the course of this condition and are produced by a thickening of the epithelium of the œsophagus, which may interfere with swallowing by the mechanical effect and by interfering with the proper propagation of peristalsis.

R. H. FRANKLIN

Bibliography

FRANKLIN, R. H. (1952) "Surgery of the Œsophagus." London, Edward Arnold & Co.
MACKENZIE, M. (1884) "Diseases of the Throat and Nose," Vol. II. London, Churchill.
TURNER, G. G. (1946) "Injuries and Diseases of the Œsophagus." London, Cassell & Co. Ltd.

References

Congenital Atresia of the Œsophagus:
LADD, W. E., and SWENSON, O. (1947) *Ann. Surg.* **125,** 23.
WILTON, T. N. P. (1951) *Anæsthesia* **6,** 30.

Endoscopic Examination
JACKSON, C. (1927) "Bronchoscopy and Esophagoscopy." Philadelphia, W. B. Saunders Co.
THOMSON, ST. CLAIR, and NEGUS, V. E. (1948) "Diseases of the Nose and Throat." London, Cassell & Co. Ltd.

Spontaneous Rupture of the Œsophagus
BARRETT, N. R. (1946) *Thorax* **1,** 48.
BARRETT, N. R. (1947) *Brit. J. Surg.* **35,** 216.

Reflux Œsophagitis
ALLISON, P. R. (1948) *Thorax* **3,** 20.
ALLISON, P. R., JOHNSTONE, A. S., and ROYCE, G. B. (1943). *J. Thorac. Surg.* **12,** 432.
BARRETT, N. R., and FRANKLIN, R. H. (1949) *Brit. J. Surg.* **37,** 194.
BARRETT, N. R. (1950) *Ibid.,* **38,** 175.

Cardiospasm
WOOLER, G. H. (1948) *Thorax* **3,** 53.

Diverticula of the Œsophagus
BARRETT, N. R. (1933) *Lancet* **i,** 1009.
DUNHILL, T. (1950) *Brit. J. Surg.* **37,** 404.
NEGUS, V. E. (1925) *J. Laryng.* **40,** 702.
NEGUS, V. E. (1950) *Brit. J Surg.* **38,** 129.

Sideropenic Dysphagia
WALDENSTRÖM, J., and KJELLBERG, S. R. (1939) *Acta radiol. Stockh.* **20,** 618.

Cancer of the Œsophagus
ALLISON, P. R., and BORRIE, J. (1949) *Brit. J. Surg.* **37,** 1.
LEWIS, I. (1946) *Brit. J. Surg.* **34,** 18.
SWEET, R. H. (1947) *J. Amer. med. Ass.* **135,** 485.
TANNER, N. C. (1947) *Overseas Postgrad. med. J.* **1,** 13.
TANNER, N. C. (1949) *J. int. Coll. Surg.* **12,** 409.

CHAPTER V

THE STOMACH AND DUODENUM

Congenital Pyloric Stenosis

INCREASING evidence is available that congenital pyloric stenosis is due to a fault in the gene. Numerous families are recorded of which more than one member is affected, and the concurrence in uniovular but not in binovular twins is fairly frequent. Gailey (1948) has put on record a family of four brothers. If a fault in the gene is truly responsible then a rise in incidence of pyloric stenosis may be expected as the result of the large proportion of survivors from the Rammstedt operation. The present incidence is 3 or 4 per 1,000 (Davison (1946)) and from the figures of Wood and Smellie (1951) it may be concluded that there is approximately 50 per cent. more risk of pyloric stenosis in a first born than in a later baby.

In diagnosis, clinical evidence is of importance, and no evidence is stronger than a palpable tumour, but where a tumour cannot be felt or where history is in any way unusual a barium meal examination is legitimate. It is very seldom necessary and can never supplant clinical evidence. The only definite radiological evidence is a persistent narrow line of barium in the pyloric canal (Teall, 1950).

In *treatment*, most surgeons advise operation in virtually every case. Replacement therapy is most important (Akin and Forbes, 1947) and some 24 hours of such a treatment may be necessary in babies under 6 lb. in weight. Intravenous hydrochloric acid (Hartmann, 1945) has not won much popularity and half strength saline is the usual medium at a rate not exceeding 100 ml. per pound body weight in the 24 hours. The stomach should always be emptied before operation but continued lavage should be avoided for it may wash out a dangerous amount of sodium. Chemotherapy is valuable as a method of treatment for, and as a prophylactic against, coincidental infection in other parts of the body, but it does not permit the clinician to be complacent. These babies should still be isolated and nursed with the most rigid precautions.

At *operation* there is still some dispute concerning anæsthesia. Local infiltration of the abdominal wall with 10 ml. of 1 per cent. procaine is entirely satisfactory and permits early feeding to be begun; its only inconvenience is the slightly increased difficulty of closure of the abdominal wound.

A transverse upper abdominal incision high under the costal arch permits of easier closure than a paramedian incision for the liver falls back into place when the abdomen is closed and prevents the protrusion of bowel.

The incision for division of the muscular coat of the pyloric canal should lie nearer the lesser curvature than the greater in a bloodless area there and should not be continued further distally than the pyloric vein. The forceps advised by Denis Browne, in the form of a sinus forceps with the blade slightly angled outwards near its tip is invaluable for stretching the muscular incision and Browne's paradoxical sign of completeness of the division of the muscle is valuable; the mucosa flattens out and ceases to bulge when gas passes through to the duodenum. After division, gas should be squeezed through from the stomach to make sure that the duodenal mucosa into which the tumour projects has not been opened. If a bubble of gas escapes, the perforation is closed by a single stitch which joins the proximal mucosal edge of the perforation to the whole thickness of the distal duodenum.

The mortality of operation has fallen substantially in the last ten years and there are reports of such figures as $2 \cdot 8$ per cent. (Akin *et al.*, 1947), 2 per cent. (Browne, 1952), $1 \cdot 3$ per cent. (Wood *et al.*, 1951), and $0 \cdot 89$ per cent. (Ladd *et al.*, 1946). The prognosis is worse in babies under 6 lb. in weight and in babies suffering from pre-operative or post-operative infection or other post-operative complications. The infective complications require an active search, for they are often overlooked. They include otitis media, conjunctivitis, thrush, omphalitis, upper respiratory infection, relaxed stool or frank enteritis, whitlow, skin sepsis, cystitis and wound infection. The other post-operative complications are continuing vomiting, usually due to incomplete division of the muscle or to the presence of some other obstructing element at a lower level, wound rupture, and peritonitis from a perforation of the duodenal mucosa which has not been detected at operation. Breast-fed babies do best for they usually remain free from infection. Levi (1941) treated 100 breast-fed children without a death, but had five deaths in 46 artificially fed babies.

Other Congenital Anomalies

Such congenital obstructions of the duodenum as *atresia*, *congenital bands* and *annular pancreas* may be mistaken for congenital pyloric stenosis and should always be sought if there is any doubt about the presence of a pyloric tumour. Babies who have incomplete duodenal obstruction from another cause sometimes develop a palpable hypertrophy of the pyloric canal.

Congenital gastric diverticula (Martin, 1936) are usually situated on the cardiac part of the posterior surface of the stomach near the lesser curvature, though occasionally they lie near the greater curvature or the fundus. They seldom give symptoms until adult life—belching, vomiting, tenderness, dysphagia, or bleeding. Perforation does not occur. In most cases any symptoms that are present are coincidental and related to some other pathological cause than the diverticulum. In a few cases, however, infection near the diverticulum from pressure on the stomach by the diverticulum may be a cause of digestive disability. The diverticulum is demonstrated either by X-ray or gastroscopy, and is sometimes particularly difficult to locate at operation. In the first place they should be sought by dividing the greater omentum and turning the stomach upwards and forwards (Casberg and Martin, 1948), but in some cases it is necessary to mobilize the spleen and cardia and to divide the lesser omentum close to the cardiac end of the lesser curvature. If it has been responsible for symptoms the diverticulum is excised and the defect in the stomach closed in layers. Simple invagination (Ferguson and Cameron, 1947) may be followed by recurrence (Bralow and Spellberg, 1948).

Duplication of the stomach (Ladd and Gross, 1940) may give rise to a cystic structure containing chocolate fluid and inseparable from the posterior wall of the stomach, though not in communication with the lumen of the stomach. Such a retrogastric cyst may produce obstruction of the stomach from external pressure (McCutchen, 1949). Duplication is probably responsible also for the much narrower *cardioduodenal duct*, a narrow passage in the posterior stomach wall (Høyer and Andresen, 1951).

Gastric Obstruction from Swallowing Corrosive Poison

Many cases have now been reported of corrosive stricture of the stomach in patients who have no associated corrosive burns of the mouth, pharynx or œsophagus (Strode and Dean, 1950; Paul, 1951). The antrum and pylorus is thick-walled and unyielding though not actually hard. The lumen is narrow, like that of the uterus and cervix (Moynihan, 1926). The stricture comes on rapidly, giving rise to obstruction some four weeks after the corrosive accident. Gastrectomy is probably the best treatment for corrosive stricture (Gray and Holmes, 1948) though it has seldom been performed; sometimes gastroenterostomy has been required (Strange *et al.*, 1951).

Volvulus of the Stomach

Volvulus of the stomach is rare but has a wide range of symptomatology. It may give rise to severe intermittent or transient distension;

it may persist in an acute phase with or without infarction of the colon or small intestine. It has been described in association with perigastric adhesions, extragastric tumour and diaphragmatic hernia. It may be mesenterico-axial, the pylorus folding to the left in front of or rarely behind the body, or it may be of organo-axial, the greater curvature folding upwards and forwards in front of the lesser, or it may involve the fundus. Melæna is present in 50 per cent. of all cases and in 100 per cent. of severe types with thrombosis (Mayo *et al.*, 1940). The initial treatment should be the passage of a broad bore stomach tube; the immediate escape of gas is an index of successful reduction. If relief is not obtained by a stomach tube laparotomy should be undertaken, the volvulus should be undone and recurrence should be prevented by the performance either of temporary gastrostomy to fix the stomach to the abdominal wall or of partial gastrectomy.

Giant Hypertrophic Gastritis

Gastric discomfort and even hæmatemesis may be associated with extravagant hypertrophy of the mucous folds. In the barium meal these folds may look like multiple polyps. At gastroscopy the folds are red and œdematous with superficial ulceration very like cancer, and indeed this appearance may be associated with an infiltrating submucous cancer (Matzner *et al.*, 1951). It is not known whether or not this appearance is truly inflammatory. Gastrectomy should be undertaken because of the difficulty of distinguishing the appearances, before or at operation, from cancer (Maimon *et al.*, 1947; Bourne, 1948; Grime and Whitehead, 1951). Sometimes total gastrectomy is required (Bartlett and Adams, 1950).

Prolapse of Redundant or Hypertrophied Gastric Mucosa

Prolapse of an antral fold of hypertrophied mucosa into the duodenum may give rise to bleeding or to antral or pyloric obstruction. The symptoms and the X-ray appearances may be difficult to distinguish from those of polyposis. At operation the antrum may be opened, the prolapsed fold excised, and the stomach wall closed again (MacKenzie *et al.*, 1946).

Eosinophilic Gastritis

This condition may affect adults of either sex. There is chronic pain unrelated to meals and sometimes attacks of acute pain with bleeding that may be massive. X-ray shows a narrow antrum. At gastroscopy there is a mammilated mucosa with narrowing of the antrum. There

may be eosinophilia during an acute attack—one argument for examining the blood picture in patients with acute dyspepsia or gastric
hæmorrhage (Vanek, 1949; Spencer *et al.*, 1950; Doniach and McKeown,
1951).

The Treatment of Peptic Ulceration

Increasingly often nowadays the treatment of chronic peptic
ulceration is surgical, and the surgical treatment of peptic ulceration
is increasingly safe.

The indications for operation differ a little in respect of gastric and
duodenal ulcers.

In gastric ulcer there are certain absolute indications and these
include the following:

1.   Hour-glass deformity or shortening, radiologically visible, of the
lesser curvature (Tanner, 1951); this indicates a substantial degree of
fibrosis and the virtual certainty of recurrent ulceration.

2.   Hæmorrhage repeated twice or oftener.

3.   Pain, not relieved by medical treatment in bed.

4.   An abnormal position of the ulcer, in the pyloric region or on
the greater curve or on the anterior wall—this always raises the
suspicion of malignancy.

5.   Large size of ulcer is also a reason for operation; some very large
ulcers, and perhaps even the largest of all, are benign even when they
are detected in older patients, but in general a large ulcer raises the
suspicion of malignancy.

6.   Continued activity of a gastric ulcer for more than six months
under medical treatment.

7.   Obvious signs of chronicity—fibrosis, for example—when the
ulcer is observed by gastroscope.

8.   Co-existent duodenal ulcer.

The indications for operation in duodenal ulcer are less clear cut.
The absolute indications include repeated bleeding, stenosis, pre-
stenotic diverticulum, associated gastric pain not relieved by medical
treatment in bed on milk drip, and repeated perforation. Many authorities would add to these: Glenn and Harrison (1950) for example, advise
resection after a single perforation of 3 to 4 months after closure of the
perforation.

Choice of Operation for Peptic Ulcer

The choice of operation for peptic ulcer is in general some form of
gastrectomy, though the form of gastrectomy varies to some extent
according to the site and character of the ulcer, and in a few cases some

operation other than gastrectomy is employed. The treatment of gastric ulcer involves the removal by gastrectomy of some two-thirds of the stomach. Even in the case of a high ulcer on the lesser curvature the ulcer is removed, and, if the ulcer is in fact a high one, a special operative technique is required. The treatment of choice for a duodenal ulcer is removal of three-quarters of the stomach.

Vagotomy is now reserved in most centres for the treatment of jejunal ulcer consequent upon one or more previous surgical interventions, though it may be applied also to young patients who have an anterior wall ulcer without stenosis, and, in these, must be accompanied by some form of gastric drainage, either a limited gastrectomy or gastro-jejunostomy. Vagotomy, together with some form of gastric drainage, has also been advised for high lesser curve ulcers (Dragstedt and Woodward, 1951), but most gastric surgeons prefer to perform high gastrectomy for this type of ulcer.

Gastro-enterostomy alone has largely been discredited as a method of treatment for peptic ulceration because of the incidence of jejunal ulceration. Even when it is performed in a patient who has pyloric stenosis and a low acidity, hyperacidity often develops again after the stomach is drained. It must still be considered, however, with or without vagotomy, as a most successful operation in many of the cases in which it has been performed and it should still have some application. It is probably the treatment of choice, for example, if pyloric stenosis is present in a patient over 50 who has no active ulcer, no pain, no hæmorrhage and a very low acid; in very aged and feeble patients with pyloric stenosis, and in younger patients with pyloric stenosis who are debilitated or who have concomitant disease, cardiac, pulmonary or renal (Maingot, 1948).

The Place of Vagotomy in the Treatment of Peptic Ulcer

Vagotomy is indicated to control the natural digestive or nocturnal secretion of hydrochloric acid, which usually, but by no means always, runs parallel with the histamine and insulin tests (Johnson, 1950).

Vagotomy was introduced by Latarjet in 1921; an abdominal form of the operation was developed by Wertheimer in 1922, but this early form of abdominal vagotomy was found nearly always to be incomplete because of branches which leave the vagi above the diaphragm and enter the abdomen separately from the main trunks. There are two available forms of the operation to-day—the trans-thoracic (Dragstedt, 1945), and the per-hiatal resection from below (Dragstedt, 1945; Orr and Johnson, 1947)

The vagotomy tide has on most surgical shores receded because of its "inconstant, variable and in most cases unpredictable" results (Walters *et al.*, 1947) and also because of its quite numerous and not infrequent complications.

1.   Gastric distension may be serious and progressive after vagotomy, partly from the loss of motility of the stomach and partly from contraction of the healing duodenal ulcer. Most patients suffer from retention for a time and 15 per cent. require a subsequent drainage operation.

2.   Vomiting occurs in some degree in 36 per cent. and is severe in 13 per cent. (Pollock, 1952).

3. Patients lose weight after vagotomy though certainly to a less extent than after gastrectomy.

4.   Dysphagia (Kipen and Stevens, 1949) is quite a frequent sequel and must be due partly to direct interference with the œsophageal musculature and partly to denervation; it is usually self-limiting (Wilcox, 1950).

5.   Paralytic ileus of the intestine sometimes follows operation and may be protracted.

6.   Diarrhœa of a mild type occurs in more than half of the patients in the first six months after a vagotomy and it is severe in about 16 per cent. (Pollock, 1952).

7.   The duodenal ulcer for which the operation is done persists or recurs in 10 per cent. of cases (Pollock, 1952). The duodenal ulcer bleeds or perforates very seldom (Daniels, 1950).

8.   Gastric ulcer (Orr and Johnson, 1949; Dragstedt *et al.*, 1949; Morrissey, 1950) may develop in patients who have previously suffered from duodenal ulcer alone, and the gastric ulcer is sometimes curiously painless (Kogel and Jantzen, 1949). Vagotomy should never be done in patients who have a gastric as well as a duodenal ulcer nor should it be done in patients who have a gastric ulcer alone.

9.   There is a decrease in pancreatic secretion which may have some part in the genesis of diarrhœa (Crider and Thomas, 1944).

10.   A diaphragmatic hernia has occurred in patients in whom the hiatus has been stretched during the operation, and not properly closed (Beal, 1948).

To avoid the retention which follows vagotomy the operation is sometimes supplemented by gastro-jejunostomy (Grimson *et al.*, 1947; Crile, 1951), pyloroplasty (Tanner, 1950), partial pylorectomy (Beattie, 1950) or even a standard subtotal gastrectomy (Colp, 1950).

Choice of Gastrectomy

There is as yet no unanimity about the relative suitability of the Billroth I operation on the one hand, and the Polya type of gastrectomy on the other. Indeed these operations cannot be reasonably compared. The Billroth I operation admittedly restores the upper enteric tract to some semblance of normality while the Polya operation distorts the normal anatomy very substantially. It is sometimes said that the dumping syndrome is less common after the Billroth I operation than after the Polya operation, but the patient most likely to develop dumping is the one who suffers from a large penetrating ulcer of the posterior wall of the duodenum, and it is in just this kind of patient that the Billroth I operation is difficult; the most likely dumpers are excluded from any Billroth I series. The Billroth I operation is essentially an operation for the expert. The permissible degree of tension between stomach and duodenum is difficult to gauge safely. In all but the most experienced hands obstruction at the anastomosis, injury to the bile duct and separation of the suture line are more common after the Billroth I operation than after the operation of Polya type. The apprentice who is learning gastrectomy is wisest to adhere to one single operative technique applicable to all types of ulcer. The Billroth I operation is not applicable to all types of ulcer; it cannot be performed safely for deep posterior wall ulcers of the duodenum nor can it usually be performed for large penetrating ulcers of the posterior wall of the stomach.

The Technique of the Polya Operation

The patient is prepared for operation with careful attention to replacement of water and electrolytes, and of protein by the frequent administration of fluid meals with amino-acids if these are required, and to clearance of a distended stomach by tube aspiration.

Either a paramedian or a transverse incision may be employed. The abdomen is opened and the upper abdominal organs are palpated for verification of the diagnosis. The greater omentum is then divided. The gastro-colic ligament is picked up well to the left of the midline and divided between ligatures from there to the duodenum. In most centres this omentum is divided distal to the gastro-epiploic vessels though this seems to have no advantage over separate division of the branches of the gastro-epiploic artery between that vessel and the greater curvature. The right gastro-epiploic artery is divided where it emerges below the pylorus. The pylorus and duodenum are then gently elevated forwards from the pancreas by gauze dissection as far as the line of the gastro-duodenal artery. Attention is now turned to the lesser omentum. An

opening is made in this above the pylorus and the right gastric vessels
are ligated. If the duodenal ulcer is a large or penetrating one, it is
sometimes convenient at this point to divide the antrum between
crushing clamps and to use the distal crushing clamp as a lever while
the duodenum is separated forward from the pancreas. Its separation
is in any case effected with division of the small vessels passing to the
first part of the duodenum from the main gastro-duodenal trunk, and
from the superior pancreatico-duodenal artery. For the division of
these vessels fine hæmostats should be used and fine silk, and each tiny
vessel should be taken individually. This part of the operation is easy
in cases of gastric ulcer (or carcinoma of the stomach) but exceedingly
difficult if there is a large penetrating posterior wall ulcer. If it can be
effected, the duodenum is divided beyond the level of the ulcer and the
duodenal stump is closed.

There are many ways of closing the duodenal stump. The duodenum
can be divided between clamps, and the distal clamp can then be over-
run by a through-and-through suture. Alternatively, instead of a
crushing clamp, immediately distal to the point of section an occlusion
clamp can be applied rather farther away and a running suture inserted
to close the cut end. If this is done, the clamp is removed on completion
of the suture and the closed duodenal stump is invaginated by sero-
muscular stitches. A row of interrupted silk may be used for this, or,
if the duodenum is narrow, a purse-string stitch. A convenient method
of closure is to put a sero-muscular stitch at the upper corner of the
stump, taking up posterior wall, upper border and anterior wall in that
order. A similar stitch can then be inserted to invaginate the lower
end of the closed stump. This avoids the difficulty of invaginating a
corner after inserting a row of sero-muscular stitches from above downwards. A few more sero-muscular sutures complete the invagination
and the closed stump may then be sewn to the fibrous tissue on the
surface of the pancreas.

If penetration of a posterior wall ulcer makes difficult the separation
of duodenum from pancreas, the duodenum may be circumcised around
the ulcer to leave the ulcer clear, and divided beyond the right edge
of the ulcer, or the ulcer may conveniently be left and the duodenum
divided between the left edge of the ulcer and the pylorus (Eastman
and Cole, 1949). If the ulcer is left, the anterior edge of the duodenum
may be sutured to the right edge of the ulcer and the ulcer extruded as
it were from the duodenal stump, the sero-muscular coat of the anterior
wall being doubled over the ulcer (Nissen, 1945). In any event, the
entire mucosa of the antrum must be removed; if it remains, a jejunal
ulcer is almost inevitable. In cases of extreme difficulty the Bancroft

manœuvre may be employed (Bancroft, 1932). A circular incision is made through the sero-muscular coat of the antrum short of the pylorus, the mucosa of the antrum being left intact at that point. The muscular coat is then stripped by gauze and scissor dissection from the underlying mucosa as far as the pyloric ring. The mucosal tube is then divided between ligatures and the ligated stump of pyloric mucosa is buried by drawing together the muscular walls of the stump of the antrum over it. Stitches are inserted from within so that the muscle surfaces of the antrum are brought together, and finally serous coat of one wall is sutured to serous coat of the other. If this measure is adopted, dissection should proceed as far as the pyloric muscle but no farther. Another important technical point is that the sero-muscular tube of antrum cannot be invaginated; its open base is wider than its pyloric apex.

Tanner (1951) suggests that the beginner may in case of difficulty leave the antrum and remove it later as a second stage. In the rare ulcers of the second part of the duodenum no attempt should be made to remove the ulcer.

In preparation of the duodenum for closure, the bile ducts may be put to hazard, and, if there is any doubt of their integrity, the common bile duct should be opened and a probe passed into the duodenum to assist in their identification and to prove their continuing patency.

If closure of the duodenal stump offers particular difficulty, it is advised that a tube be inserted in it and the stump closed round it by a purse-string suture, the tube being brought out to form a temporary duodenal fistula (Whipple).

Attention is now turned to the curvatures. The division of the gastro-colic ligament, which was previously effected only to a point just to the left of the midline, is carried round the greater curvature with ligation of the main gastro-epiploic vessels and is carried up the gastro-splenic ligament to the level of the upper pole of the spleen. At this point it is wise to keep close to the greater curvature in case the short gastric veins are divided too close to the splenic pedicle; when this is done there is sometimes bleeding from the splenic pedicle which requires splenectomy for its control. The lesser omentum is then divided along the lesser curvature on a straight line from pylorus to cardia and the left gastric vessels are divided. It is convenient to divide these twice, in the first place close to the origin of the left gastric artery from the coeliac axis after raising the stomach forwards and identifying the artery behind it, and next by dividing the vessels again where they reach the lesser curvature. This double division allows the lesser curvature to lengthen and gives a more convenient stomach for the purpose of anastomosis.

For anastomosis, a loop of jejunum is chosen, not too far from and not too close to the ligament of Treitz. There is diversity of opinion between a short loop and a long loop reconstitution, but there seems to be no particular advantage in making the loop too short; if this is done there is a narrower opening between posterior abdominal wall and stomach for small intestine to herniate through. A convenient length of jejunum should in any case be taken to avoid tension. Some operators insist on carrying this loop always in the same direction, from lesser to greater curvature, but it is usually convenient to allow the loop to pass in whichever direction leaves it lying more naturally. It is also said that a Hofmeister valve should be fashioned by closing the upper part of the opening in the stomach and using only the lower part of that opening for anastomosis, but is is our experience that there is no difference in the incidence of dumping in those cases which have such a valve made and in those cases in which the whole breadth of stomach is employed. There is also some argument still about the relative advantages of the retro-colic and the ante-colic operation. Argument about this is unprofitable, for there seems little difference in the results.

Special difficulty in dealing with the stomach may be met with in cases of high gastric ulcer. In general, such an ulcer should be removed together with the body of the stomach and antrum. This entails a high division of the lesser curve near the œsophagus, but the greater curve need not be so radically dealt with. A point can be chosen on the greater curve vertically below the right edge of the oesophagus or even further to the right on the greater curvature, and two clamps are placed directly across the organ to reach the mid-point between the curvatures. This part of the stomach is then divided between the clamps, and two other curved clamps may be applied across the remainder of the stomach to reach the lesser curvature near the oesophagus. The remainder of the stomach is then divided between these two clamps and the distal portion is removed. The upper part of the stomach remnant is then closed by a running stitch around the clamp, and invaginated, and the lower part of the organ is used for anastomosis to the jejunum. Alternatively a Schumaker clamp may be employed to control the upper part of the opening in the stomach near the œsophagus, or indeed the required portion of the stomach, and the whole lesser curvature may be excised by cutting with scissors without the use of clamps at all (Tanner, 1949).

The Billroth I Operation

In the Billroth I operation the same technique of removal of stomach is employed, but the upper part of the open end of the stomach is closed by one of the methods already described, and invaginated, and the lower part of the opening in the stomach is used for anastomosis to the duodenum. Careful attention should be paid to the junction of the closed portion of the stomach and the lower part which is used for anastomosis, and a circular sero-muscular stitch through lesser curvature, edges of anastomosis and upper border of duodenum is the safest method of preventing leakage at this point.

The Complications of Gastrectomy

(1) **Perforation of the duodenal stump** is the immediate complication of gastrectomy most to be feared. It usually gives rise to sudden and alarming peritonitis within seven to eight days of operation, though it has occurred quite commonly up to fourteen days after operation and indeed at any time up to five and a half months (Goodall *et al.*, 1951). In most cases it is due to distension of the afferent loop of jejunum and consequent rupture of the line of closure. In a few cases it seems to be due to perforation of an ulcer of the duodenum not removed by the gastrectomy. The treatment of this complication when it develops is the insertion of a drain in the perforation of the stump and the closure of the stump round that drain.

(2) **Internal hernia** may occur through the opening left behind the stomach, an opening whose boundaries are posterior abdominal wall, lesser curvature, anastomosis, afferent jejunal loop and ligament of Treitz. The signs are those of post-operative obstruction with a gas shadow of the distended herniated bowel on X-ray and perhaps a palpable abdominal swelling (Hublin, 1951).

(3) **Pancreatitis and pancreatic injuries** may follow gastrectomy (Warren, 1951). A main duct injury should be seen at operation if it occurs, but sometimes an accessory duct of Santorini draining high into the duodenum may be injured, to give rise to discharge of a few hundred ml. of a clear fluid after operation. There is always an anatomical connection between the duct of Santorini and the main duct, and such a fistula heals as soon as the drainage tube is withdrawn.

(4) **Leakage from the suture line** between stomach and jejunum or between stomach and duodenum may give rise to early post-operative peritonitis. It is probably always due to a fault in technique.

(5) A mild degree of **diarrhœa** is not uncommon after gastrectomy, but in the case of severe and persistent diarrhœa suspicion arises whether anastomosis has not been performed between stomach and ileum instead of between stomach and jejunum. This apparently elementary error is less unlikely than it sounds; when it has occurred there has usually been some anomaly of rotation whereby the colon has lain

behind the superior mesenteric vessels instead of the duodenum
(Moretz, 1949).

(6) The **dumping syndrome** is the complication of gastrectomy which
has attracted most interest during the last few years. The symptoms
are post-prandial. Within 30 minutes of a meal there is abdominal
discomfort, nausea, palpitation and a general surface sensation of hot
and cold. Consequent upon this there is weakness, fatigue and drowsiness which may persist for 1½ to 3 hours. Certain vasomotor changes
accompany this sensation. Tachycardia, a high respiration rate, pallor
and sweating rather suggest an adrenaline-like effect. The normal
flushing and rise of skin temperature which follow the taking of food
are absent until the attack of dumping passes off.

Dumping occurs most often after a Polya type of gastrectomy, but
it occurs also after a Billroth I operation and even after vagotomy.
Dumping is not always improved by converting a Polya gastrectomy
into a Billroth I. A few duodenal ulcer patients give records of
symptoms similar to those which occur in dumping as having accompanied their original dyspepsia before any operation at all has been
undertaken. The dumping syndrome is most common after gastrectomy
performed for large penetrating duodenal ulcer, a fact which may
explain its more frequent occurrence after the Polya type operation
than after the Billroth I. The type of gastrectomy done does not affect
its incidence much; the formation of a valve does nothing to affect its
incidence. It can be said, however, that the more extensive the
gastrectomy the more severe the dumping and its severity is greatest
after total gastrectomy.

Seventy-five per cent. of patients have some dumping, and 12·5 per
cent. severe dumping still after 6 months; 47·5 per cent. of patients
have some dumping and 7·1 per cent. severe dumping after 18 months
(Goligher and Riley, 1952).

The cause of dumping is not known. A few of these patients (Gilbert
and Dunlop, 1947) can be shown to have hypoglycæmia after food, but
not all of them show this and those who do show it are sometimes free
from symptoms at the height of the hypoglycæmia which occurs very
early after food (Muir, 1949). Distension of the jejunum, either of the
proximal or of the distal loop, can be shown to be present in a number
of patients who dump and in these patients the symptoms can be
reproduced in their entirety by passing a swallowed mercury bag into
the jejunum (Butler and Capper, 1951; Goligher and Riley, 1952).
Brain and Stammers (1951) blame malabsorption of fat for the
syndrome; pancreatic secretion is lessened after gastrectomy (Mimpriss
and Birt, 1948) and food enters the jejunum before bile and pancreatic

juice can mix with it. Some of the patients also show potassium deficiency.

(7) **Gastro-Jejunal ulcer** is quite rare now that subtotal gastrectomy is the standard operation for duodenal ulcer though it still does occasionally occur. This complication can be virtually abolished by performing a very high gastrectomy and leaving only a tiny remnant of stomach, but so extensive a gastrectomy carries a relatively high mortality and it is doubtful whether the frequency of gastro-jejunal ulcer after a less extreme operation justifies the extra risk. Gastro-jejunal ulcer is probably best treated by a further gastrectomy if the original gastrectomy has been inadequate and by transthoracic vagotomy if an extensive segment of stomach has been already removed.

Of the complications of gastro-jejunal ulcer, the most important recent advance has been in the treatment of **gastro-colic fistula.** It has been clearly shown (Pfeiffer and Kent, 1939) that the deterioration in the patient's condition which is so serious once a gastro-colic fistula is present is unquestionably due to the entrance of the contents of the colon into the small intestine and the consequent chemical or bacterial enteritis which results. The diarrhœa and emaciation of a gastro-colic fistula can be relieved completely by temporary colostomy in the ascending colon proximal to the fistula and later operation can be undertaken to treat the responsible jejunal ulcer.

(8) Two forms of **jejuno-gastric intussusception** may occur after gastrectomy (Aleman, 1948). The intussusception may be acute with swelling of the inverted bowel and hæmatemesis or it may be chronic and intermittent with vomiting and the demonstration of the sausage-shaped filling defect in the stomach by X-ray. The filling defect shows concentric or fan-shaped streaking from the valvulæ of the inverted bowel loop. Most intussusceptions are retrograde, the efferent loop telescoped backwards into the stomach, though a few are descending, the afferent loop passing through the stoma. Very rarely there is a combined form in which both loops return into the lumen of the stomach.

Massive Hæmorrhage from Peptic Ulcer

One of the most gratifying recent advances in gastroenterology has been the increased opportunity which surgeons have had for treating hæmatemesis and melæna by operation. It is now generally agreed that if a bleeding patient in or beyond middle age is known to have a chronic peptic ulcer the following cases justify operative interference : (1) previous massive hæmorrhage; (2) hæmorrhage continuing when the patient comes in for treatment in hospital; (3) associated severe pain continuing under treatment; (4) associated pyloric stenosis, and, of course, (5) associated perforation. Even in a younger person it is wise to intervene if two or more of these indications are present together. In general the operation to be performed for a duodenal or gastric ulcer in cases of massive hæmorrhage is subtotal gastrectomy together with removal of the ulcer.

Gastrectomy for Cancer of the Stomach

In most centres the standard operative procedure for the treatment of cancer of the stomach is subtotal gastrectomy together with the removal of the lesser omentum, the whole of the greater omentum and the first inch of the duodenum. The general procedure does not differ greatly from the technique of the subtotal gastrectomy already described except that the lesser omentum is divided close to the liver and the greater omentum is stripped from the transverse colon.

In growths of the fundus, cardia and upper part of the body total gastrectomy is required and that operation is also necessary for extensive infiltrating tumours affecting the greater part of the body of the stomach. In these higher growths the spleen is usually removed together with the stomach. For high growths of the stomach an abdomino-thoracic or thoracic approach is desirable, the spleen is removed with the stomach and reconstitution is by some form of œsophago-jejun-ostomy such as is described elsewhere in the treatment of carcinoma of the lower third of the œsophagus.

Subtotal gastrectomy is, of course, far from an ideal cancer operation for the lymphatic drainage field is hardly touched and it is not surprising that, over all cases, the five-year survival rate in England still does not exceed 7 per cent. (Harnett, 1952). The operability rate has, however, increased and gastrectomy of some kind now is done for more than a half of all cases of cancer of the stomach who come to operation. The five-year survival rate of those who come to resection is 22 to 35 per cent. (State *et al.*, 1947; Pack and McNeer, 1947).

In some growths an attempt has been made to extend the scope of gastrectomy and a total gastrectomy is advised by the most radical surgeons now as a routine treatment for cancer of the stomach (Morton, 1942; Lahey and Marshall, 1944; Longmire, 1947; Lockwood, 1950). It is argued that a much wider lymphatic removal is accomplished by performing a total operation and by removing *en masse* the first inch of duodenum together with the lesser and greater omentum, the spleen, the tail of the pancreas and even in some centres the posterior peritoneum of the lesser sac. There is no question that an operation of this kind is not only desirable but is in fact technically easier than lesser operations for high growths in the region of the cardia and fundus. The tissue to be removed can be mobilized on a pedicle at whose base are the left gastric and splenic arteries. The argument against the adoption of so radical an operation as a routine procedure (Walters *et al.*, 1948; Fletcher, 1951; Thomas *et al.*, 1951) is that even this operation makes no attack on the suprapancreatic glands. The glands in the hilum of the spleen, whose removal it ensures, are affected early only in high growths. Moreover, the mortality of total gastrectomy is at best of the order of 20 to 30 per cent.—twice as high as the immediate mortality for partial gastrectomy in cancer of the stomach.

Palliative Operations for Cancer of the Stomach

Where there is no hope of cure, in a patient who has, for example, hepatic metastasis, *partial gastrectomy* if it is technically possible, is the best palliative operation for carcinoma of the stomach. There is little risk after it of gastric symptoms returning. Where partial gastrectomy is not possible the available alternatives are gastroenterostomy, gastric exclusion and jejunostomy. In those cases in which *gastroenterostomy* is performed, extension of disease is liable later to block the stoma. *Exclusion*, with division of the stomach proximal to the growth, closure of the distal open end, and implantation of the proximal open end into the jejunum is theoretically a desirable operation and it ensures greater continuing comfort than a gastroenterostomy does. It is often technically extremely difficult, however, to close the distal stump over a bulky polypoid tumour. The secret of the exclusion operation is to mobilize both curvatures to a very high level and to transect the stomach high. *Jejunostomy* is performed only as a last resort in patients who are *in extremis* as a result of malignant gastric obstruction.

IAN AIRD

References

Congenital Pyloric Stenosis:
AKIN, J. T., and FORBES, G. B. (1947) *Surgery*, **21**, 512.
BROWNE, D. (1952) *Proc. R. Soc. Med.* **44**, 1055.
DAVISON, G. (1946) *Arch. Dis. Childh.* **21**, 223.
GAILEY, A. A. H. (1948) *Brit. med. J.* **i**, 100.
HARTMANN, A. F. (1945) Brennemann's "Practice of Pediatrics," Vol. **1** Hagerstown Md.
LADD, W. E., PICKETT, L. K., and WARE, P. F. (1946) *J. Amer. med. Ass.*, **131**, 647.
LEVI, D. (1941) *Brit. med. J.* **i**, 963.
TEALL, C. G. (1950) "Modern Trends in Pediatrics." London, Butterworth & Co. Ltd.
WOOD, E. C., and SMELLIE, J. M. (1951) *Lancet* **ii**, 3.

Other Congenital Anomalies:
BRALOW, S. P., and SPELLBERG, M. A. (1948) *Gastroenterology* **11,** 59.
CASBERG, M. A., and MARTIN, W. P. (1948) *Amer. J. Surg.* **76,** 172.
FERGUSON, L. R., and CAMERON, C. S. (1947) *Surg. Gynec. Obstet.* **84,** 292.
HØYER, A., and ANDRESEN J. (1951) *Oslo City Hospit.* **1,** 225.
LADD, W. E., and GROSS, R. E. (1940) *Surg. Gynec. Obstet.* **70,** 295.
MCCUTCHEN, G. T. (1949) *Ann. Surg.* **129,** 826.
MARTIN, L. (1936) *Ann. int. Med.* **10,** 447.

Gastric Obstruction from Swallowing Corrosive Poison:
GRAY, H. K., and HOLMES, C. L. (1948) *Surg. Clin. N. Amer.* **28,** 1041.
MOYNIHAN (1926) "Abdominal Operations," 4th edit., Vol. **I,** p. 342. London.
PAUL, M. (1951) *Lancet* ii, 1064.
STRANGE, D. C., FINNERAN, J. C., SHUMACKER, H. B., and BOWMAN, D. E. (1951) *Arch. Surg.* **62,** 350.
STRODE, E. C., and DEAN, M. L. (1950) *Ann. Surg.* **131,** 801.

Volvulus of the Stomach:
MAYO, C. W., MILLER, J. M., and STALKER, L. K. (1940) *Coll. Pap. Mayo Clin.* **32,** 321.

Giant Hypertrophic Gastritis:
BARTLETT, J. P., and ADAMS, W. E. (1950) *Arch. Surg.* **60,** 543.
BOURNE, W. A. (1948) *Proc. R. Soc. Med.* **41,** 43.
GRIME, R. T., and WHITEHEAD, R. (1951) *Brit. J. Surg.* **39,** 1.
MAIMON, S. N., BARTLETT, J. P., HUMPHREYS, E. M., and PALMER, W. L. (1947) *Gastroenterology* **8,** 397.
MATZNER, M. J., RAAB, A. P., and SPEAR, P. W. (1951) *Gastroenterology* **18,** 296.

Prolapse of Redundant or Hypertrophied Gastric Mucosa:
MACKENZIE, W. C., MACLEOD, J. W., and BOUCHARD, J. L. (1946) *Canad. med. Ass. J.* **54,** 553.

Eosinophilic Gastritis:
DONIACH, I., and MCKEOWN, R. C. (1951) *Brit. J. Surg.* **39,** 247.
SPENCER, J. R., COMFORT, M. W., and DAHLIN, D. C. (1950) *Gastroenterology* **15,** 505.
VANEK, J. (1949) *Amer. J. Path.* **25,** 397.

The Treatment of Peptic Ulceration:
GLENN, F., and HARRISON, C. S. (1950) *Ann. Surg.* **132,** 36.
TANNER, N. C. (1951) *Edinb. med. J.* **58,** 261.

Choice of Operation for Peptic Ulcer:
DRAGSTEDT, L. R., and WOODWARD, E. R. (1951) *J. Amer. med. Ass.* **145,** 795.
MAINGOT, R. (1948) *Ann. R. Coll. Surg.* **3,** 248.

The Place of Vagotomy in the Treatment of Peptic Ulcer:
BEAL, J. M. (1948) *Surgery* **24,** 625.
BEATTIE, A. D. (1950) *Lancet* i, 525.
COLP, R. (1950) *Surg. Gynec. Obstet.* **91,** 306.
CRIDER, J. O., and THOMAS, J. E. (1944) *Amer. J. Physiol.* **141,** 930.
CRILE, G. (1951), *Surg. Gynec. Obstet.* **92,** 309.
DANIELS, H. A. (1950) *Lancet* i, 398.
DRAGSTEDT, L. R. (1945), *Ann. Surg.* **122,** 973.
DRAGSTEDT, L. R., CAMP, E. H., and FRITZ, J. M. (1949) *Ann. Surg.* **130,** 843.
GRIMSON, K. S., BAYLIN, G. J., TAYLOR, H. M., HESSER, F. H., and RUNDLES R. W. (1947) *Arch. Surg.* **55,** 175.
JOHNSON, H. D. (1950) *Ann. R. Coll. Surg.* **8,** 160.
KIPEN, C. S., and STEVENS, G. A. (1949) *Arch. Surg.* **59,** 814.
KOGEL, A. L., and JANTZEN, J. (1949) *Gastroenterology* **12,** 993.

LATARJET, M. A. (1921) *Bull. Acad. Méd. Paris* **87,** 681.
MORRISSEY, D. M. (1950) *Brit. med. J.* **ii,** 651.
ORR, I. M., and JOHNSON, H. D. (1947) *Lancet* **ii,** 84.
ORR, I. M., and JOHNSON, H. D. (1949) *Brit. med. J.* **ll,** 1910.
POLLOCK, A. V. (1952) *Lancet* **ii,** 795.
TANNER, N. C. (1950) *Postgrad. M.J.* **26,** 575.
WALTERS, W., NEIBLING, H. A., BRADLEY, W. F., SMALL, J. T., and WILSON,
    J. W. (1947) *Arch. Surg.* **55,** 151.
WILCOX, R. S. (1950) *Amer. J. Surg.* **79,** 843.

The Technique of the Polya Operation:
BANCROFT, F. W. (1932) *Amer. J. Surg.* **16,** 223.
EASTMAN, W. H., and COLE, W. H. (1949) *Arch. Surg.* **59,** 768.
NISSEN, R. (1945) "Duodenal and Jejunal Peptic Ulcer," p. 50. New York,
    Grune and Stratton.
TANNER, N. C. (1949) *Postgrad. med. J.* **26,** 575.
TANNER, N. C. (1951) *Edinb. Med. J.* **58,** 285.

Complications of Gastrectomy:
GOODALL, R. E., HINDMAN, R., and HEIMLICH (1951) *Surgery* **30,** 701.
HUBLIN, H. (1951) *Acta. Chirurg.* **101,** 230.
MORETZ, W. H. (1949) *Ann. Surg.* **130,** 124.
WARREN, K. W. (1951) *Surgery* **29,** 643.

The Dumping Syndrome:
BRAIN, R. H. F., and STAMMERS, F. A. R. (1951) *Lancet* **1,** 1137.
BUTLER, T. J., and CAPPER, W. M. (1951) *Brit. med. J.* **i,** 1177.
GILBERT, J. A. L., and DUNLOP, D. M. (1947) *Brit. med. J.* **ii,** 330.
GOLIGHER, J. C., and RILEY, T. R. (1952) *Lancet* **i,** 631.
MIMPRISS, T. W., and BIRT, ST. J. M. C. (1948) *Brit. med. J.* **ii,** 1095.
MUIR, A. (1949) *Brit. J. Surg.* **37,** 165.

Gastro-Jejunal Ulceration:
PFEIFFER, D. B., and KENT, E. M. (1939) *Ann. Surg.* **110,** 659.

Jejunal-Gastric Intussusception:
ALEMAN, S. (1948) *Acta radiol.* **29,** 383.

Gastrectomy for Cancer of the Stomach:
FLETCHER, A. G. (1951) *Surgery* **30,** 403.
HARNETT, W. L. (1952) "The Survey of Cancer in London."
LAHEY, F. H., and MARSHALL, S. F. (1944) *Ann. Surg.* **119,** 300.
LOCKWOOD, J. S. (1950) *Surgery* **27,** 527.
LONGMIRE, W. P. (1947) *Surg. Gynec. Obstet.* **84,** 21.
MORTON, II, C. B. (1942) *Arch. Surg.* **44,** 72.
PACK, G. T., and McNEER, G. (1947) *J. Amer. med. Ass.* **135,** 267.
STATE, D., MOORE, G., and WANSGENTEEN, O. H. (1947) *J. Amer. med. Ass.* **136,**
    262.
THOMAS, W. D., WAUGH J. M., and DOCKERTY, M. B. (1951) *Arch. Surg.* **62,** 847.
WALTERS, W., GRAY, H. K., PRIESTLY, J. T., and WAUGH, J. M. (1948) *Proc.
    Mayo Clin.* **23,** 554.

CHAPTER VI

ACUTE INTESTINAL OBSTRUCTIONS

In recent years considerable progress has been made in the treatment of acute intestinal obstructions of all varieties. The basis has been a much more accurate appreciation of pathology and, in particular, of the lethal factors which must be countered if good results are to be obtained.

Pathology and Lethal Factors. The Small Intestine

Simple occlusion of the small intestine leads to collapse of the bowel distal to the occlusion and, proximally, a growing dilatation with liquid and gas and a rising intra-luminal tension. Peristalsis becomes first exaggerated, then violent and incoordinated, finally inhibited by gross stretching of the bowel wall, in which interference with the local circulation is also important, the high intra-luminal tension causing venous obstruction and capillary stasis, thus decreased absorption and increased transudation of fluid into the lumen and tissue-spaces of the intestinal wall.

There has for some years been general agreement that in high small bowel occlusions death occurs from dehydration and hypochlorhæmia due to the rapid loss of water and salt in the vomit. About low small bowel occlusions there has been more argument, for whilst some have claimed that here, too, dehydration is the sole factor of importance, others have stressed certain clinical differences between high and low occlusions and expressed the opinion that some other factor must be present too, such as toxic absorption from the distended bowel.

Now it is true that there are differences between the patient with a high occlusion and one with a low. Few now believe, however, that a factor of real importance is toxæmia from the absorption of a poisonous substance from the intestinal lumen, for despite all the experimental work devoted to the subject, no one has yet succeeded in demonstrating this elusive toxin in the lumen of the bowel, in the portal or systemic blood or the thoracic duct of experimental animals. It is probable that in low as in high occlusions the important lethal factors are dehydration and chemical imbalance, and that minor differences in the clinical manifestations are due to minor differences in the exact nature of the electrolytic loss and in the rate of loss.

Intestinal Strangulations

Intestinal strangulations are customarily divided into long, medium and short loop strangulations. The first two are seen mainly in mesenteric vascular occlusions, which may be arterial or venous and thrombotic or embolic in type. Life is in danger from the sudden withdrawal of fluid from the circulation into the hæmorrhagic infarct. If the patient survives this phase, the bowel may become gangrenous and perforate, leading to peritonitis.

A short loop strangulation occurs very frequently in a strangulated external hernia, which has proved the most common variety of acute intestinal obstruction in most published series. It can also occur in a strangulated internal hernia, diaphragmatic, retroperitoneal or trans-mesenteric, or from pressure on the bowel by an intraperitoneal band, inflammatory or congenital. In a strangulation of this type, firstly it must be remembered that apart from the strangulated loop itself a condition of simple occlusion exists in the bowel above, with all the changes already described. Secondly, it is possible that toxic absorption plays some part in the pathology of strangulating obstructions, for it has been shown that the products of septic autolysis of an intestinal loop are intensely toxic, but the point is perhaps of more academic than practical importance, for the picture is dominated by a third factor, the threat of gangrene, perforation and peritonitis, and this naturally has a profound effect upon treatment.

Closed Loop Obstructions

Obstruction of a closed loop without strangulation occurs clinically in acute obstructive appendicitis, occlusion of the large bowel if the ileocæcal sphincter is competent, and certain rarities such as occlusion of the base of a Meckel's diverticulum. In the pathology, three phases can be recognized, a phase of mounting intraluminal tension, with reflex interference with peristalsis over a wide area, hence colic, vomiting and constipation, a phase of "toxæmia" due probably to dehydration and chemical imbalance, and a phase of perforation and peritonitis.

Functional Obstructions

An area of intestinal spasm can act as a simple occlusion, but most functional obstructions are paralytic. True paralytic ileus without peritonitis is rare, but may be neurogenic in origin, caused by multiple fractures or any severe trauma, for instance, or by painful renal conditions, or it may occur in certain toxic states, such as pneumonia or uræmia. Uncontrolled dilatation of the flaccid bowel wall may perpetuate a paralytic obstruction by gross stretching of the intestinal muscle and by its effect upon the local circulation.

The so-called paralytic ileus of general peritonitis is seldom truly paralytic, for the obstruction is organic at least in part, multiple sites of adhesion, œdema and kinking providing a mechanical element.

Obstruction of the Large Intestine

Acute simple occlusion of the large intestine is nearly always caused by a carcinoma and this is most commonly situated in the left colon or pelvi-rectal junction. Complete occlusion is precipitated by fæcal impaction above the malignant stricture and made permanent by local œdema. The outstanding pathological feature is the rapid dilatation of the proximal large bowel with gas, most of which is swallowed air. If the ileocæcal valve is incompetent, the rising intraluminal tension is rapidly transmitted to the lower ileum, in which all the changes typical of a low small bowel occlusion occur. If the ileocæcal valve is competent, it shuts off the ileum from the rising tension while still allowing it to empty into the cæcum as each wave of peristalsis arrives. This type of obstruction is really a closed loop obstruction, in which the tension rises rapidly to a level far higher than that occurring in any simple occlusion of the small bowel. Vascular changes in the bowel wall ultimately leading to ulceration and finally perforation are not uncommon and may occur anywhere above the obstruction, but most frequently in the cæcum.

Strangulating obstructions of the large intestine are uncommon. Apart from strangulation in a hernia or by a band, volvulus of a redundant colonic loop, usually of the pelvic colon, may lead to rapid extreme dilatation of the loop and complete obliteration of its blood supply with ultimate gangrene and perforation.

Diagnosis

The classic clinical features of acute intestinal obstruction are well known. It is highly desirable to-day to decide not only whether or not obstruction is present but, if so, at what site and whether intestinal strangulation is also present. Various manifestations provide evidence helping to distinguish between a simple and a strangulating obstruction. The latter is suggested by the presence of a constant pain, apart from the waves of colic, by local tenderness, rebound tenderness, guarding or rigidity of abdominal muscles or an abdominal mass. Later fever, leucocytosis and signs of established peritonitis demonstrate not a strangulating obstruction but the late results of a neglected strangulation. In the early stages, even in the absence of all suggestive signs, it is not possible to exclude a strangulating obstruction with absolute certainty, and this fact naturally has an important bearing upon treatment.

In the last decade, the use of plain X-ray films as an aid to diagnosis has become universal. Positive radiological evidence is obtainable 4 to 8 hours after the onset of complete obstruction and if films of good quality are available they will distinguish with reasonable certainty a small from a large bowel obstruction and, in the latter, demonstrate the site with a fair degree of accuracy. Certain special obstructions, such as a volvulus, can be clearly shown radiologically. A barium enema, correctly employed, sometimes helps to confirm the site of a large bowel obstruction.

The conventional double enema should not be used as a diagnostic measure until after plain X-rays have been taken, for otherwise fluid levels may appear in the films and prove difficult to interpret.

Treatment

Twenty years ago, a diagnosis of acute intestinal obstruction meant immediate operation. To-day it must be accepted that in many cases the risk to the patient of immediate operation is greater than that of delay while the secondary effects of obstruction are overcome. Three possible lines of treatment will be considered by the surgeon:

1. Immediate operation.
2. Delayed operation, the patient being prepared with intravenous fluids and gastro-intestinal suction.
3. No operation, the so-called conservative plan of treatment.

Ideally, all strangulating obstructions should be treated by early operation, all simple occlusions of the small bowel by delayed operation, operation even being avoided altogether if the relief of distension by suction also relieves the obstruction, and all functional obstructions without operation. Obstructions of the large bowel present an individual problem which will be discussed later.

In practice it is found that diagnosis is not sufficiently accurate to allow a clear-cut plan of this kind to govern treatment. It is difficult, indeed it is sometimes quite impossible, to exclude a strangulating obstruction with certainty and this weighs the scales heavily against too great reliance being placed upon a prolonged period of conservative treatment in organic obstructions. Even in cases where obstruction has been present for several days, the surgeon has been surprised on occasion by eventually opening the abdomen and finding a coil of non-viable intestine, a chastening experience.

If obstructive symptoms have been present for less than 24 hours, early operation should be undertaken; if for more than 24 hours, the surgeon has to balance the risk of intervening while the patient is in a state of gross chemical instability against the risk of allowing vascular damage to the bowel to occur. He can but ask himself which is the lesser risk. If it is decided that operation is to be delayed while suction and intravenous fluids are used to improve the general condition, it follows that frequent re-examination, clinical and radiological, is essential.

In temporizing with intravenous fluids and gastro-intestinal suction it does sometimes happen that an obstruction, due in part to adhesion, distension, œdema and kinking, is itself relieved, with the appearance of gas in the large bowel in check X-rays and with no renewal of distension or colic if the suction tube is clipped off. Now there is a big difference between setting out to prepare a patient for operation and accepting gratefully the unexpected relief of the condition without surgery, and setting out with the avowed intention of curing the obstruction by suction and with the intention of intervening only if it is shown that this cannot be achieved. The writer holds the view that if operation is delayed in order to improve the condition of the patient with intravenous fluids and suction, operation should follow as soon as this object has been achieved and the patient made fit for surgery. This must not be held to be a criticism of the principle of gastro-intestinal decompression as an essential part of the treatment of all acute obstructions, but of its misuse. The use of suction is a most valuable therapeutic measure. *Its misuse may be an equally lethal one.*

The actual mechanism of intubation may not be easy. If early operation is intended, partial decompression with a duodenal tube is sufficient. If it is hoped to deflate a grossly dilated proximal intestine, a tube such as the Miller-Abbott must be used. In theory this piece of apparatus is ideal, but many surgeons have been rather disappointed to find that the more distended the patient and the more highly desirable it seems to decompress the small bowel, the more difficult it is to persuade the tube to pass the pylorus. A little mercury in the balloon may help, or stiffening the tube with wire, but sometimes one has to retire defeated and be satisfied with a duodenal tube. In such a case, it may well be considered right to pass a Miller-Abbott tube again when the abdomen is open and for the surgeon to help it through the pylorus so that the small bowel may be properly deflated.

How much Water and Salt?

There is no biochemical test which can estimate accurately how much water and salt a dehydrated patient needs, and clinical signs offer evidence just as valuable as laboratory investigations. Assuming that complete obstruction is present and the patient presents signs of marked dehydration, he requires some 8 litres of fluid intravenously in 24 hours in order to correct dehydration in this period. If this were all given as physiological saline, too much salt would be given. Alternate bottles of physiological saline and 5 per cent. dextrose strikes about the right balance. After the first 24 hours, the patient's needs can be calculated from the fluid balance chart shown below.

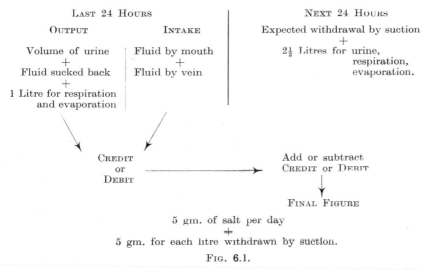

Last 24 Hours		Next 24 Hours
Output	Intake	Expected withdrawal by suction
		+
Volume of urine	Fluid by mouth	2½ Litres for urine,
+	+	respiration,
Fluid sucked back	Fluid by vein	evaporation.
+		
1 Litre for respiration and evaporation		

Credit or Debit ⟶ Add or subtract Credit or Debit

Final Figure

5 gm. of salt per day
+
5 gm. for each litre withdrawn by suction.

Fig. 6.1.

The number of litres of fluid to be given in 24 hours multiplied by 12 gives approximately the speed at which the drip should run, in drops per minute.

Operative Technique

Certain general principles in the surgical treatment of acute obstructions will bear repetition.

1. Operate at the right moment, accepting neither unreasonable delay with avoidable hazard to the blood supply of the bowel, nor unreasonable haste in dealing with the very sick patient whose general condition can be greatly improved pre-operatively with less risk than that of operating without preparation.

2. Whatever therapeutic use is made of gastro-intestinal suction, the stomach must be empty when the anæsthetic is given. Induction with pentothal is rapidly followed by the insertion of a cuffed intra-tracheal tube. Modern relaxants are valuable in operating upon the obstructed patient, but without precautions the risk, always considerable, of aspiration of stomach contents is increased by their use.

3. Make an incision in the right place and large enough to carry out the essential steps of the operation without preventable difficulties due to inadequate access.

4. Distended coils of intestine must be handled gently and the mesentery not pulled upon. Evisceration is not in itself harmful

provided that the weight of the heavy, water-logged bowel is not supported by the mesentery and that loss of heat and fluid by evaporation is prevented. Certainly, if a deeply placed obstruction is difficult to expose, it is far better to allow the dilated coils to prolapse out of the wound, where they are at once covered by warm moist packs and supported by an assistant, than to rely upon heavy retraction and packing off with gauze squares with, even so, an inadequate exposure.

Post-operative Treatment

Gastro-intestinal suction and intravenous fluids must continue until it is clear that the function of the intestine is once more adequate to prevent flaccid dilatation and to allow normal absorption. Morphine is a valuable drug in the early post-operative period and is better given in small repeated doses than in full therapeutic doses at irregular intervals. Even if the intestine is slow to resume its function, little is to be gained by the use of aperients and enemata, though the latter will, of course, be most successful if the small intestine has regained its tone and the large intestine is distended with gas. Certainly the wrong way to treat a case post-operatively is to withdraw the suction too soon and then treat the resultant abdominal distension and constipation by purgatives, enemata, pituitrin and the like without bothering to consider whether it is the small or large bowel which is dilated.

If for any reason gastro-intestinal suction and therefore intravenous fluids must continue for several days or more, the problem of maintaining fluid and electrolytic balance becomes more complicated. The reader is referred to Chapter I.

Individual Varieties of Acute Obstruction

Strangulated Hernia

There is little to arouse controversy in the management of these cases. Should the intestine, when released, prove to be non-viable, resection and anastomosis for the small intestine and exteriorization for the large intestine are the accepted methods. When considering whether or not to resect, one should remember the quite extraordinary powers of recovery possessed by the intestine. Attention is, of course, paid to the colour of the bowel, the state of the peritoneal coat, the presence or absence of peristalsis, the state of the mesentery and presence or absence of pulsation in the vessels, and the reaction to warming in hot moist squares, as has often been described, but it is probably true that if, after this, there is any doubt about viability, the gut will probably recover if returned to the abdomen, though possibly with the later development of a stricture.

Acute Obstruction of the Large Bowel due to Carcinoma

During the last 10 to 15 years, the advocates of exploration for all cases of carcinoma of the large bowel with acute obstruction have been fighting a losing battle. A few protagonists of this school still argue that exploration eliminates completely the risk of misdiagnosing a strangulating obstruction, that sometimes an immediate one-stage resection can be performed, and that even if this is not possible, a valuable assessment of operability can be made and a colostomy then performed. These arguments will not bear examination. It is true that if a strangulating obstruction is a possibility laparotomy must be undertaken, but it is to-day very rare for there to be any doubt upon this point, particularly if plain X-ray films of good quality are available. One-stage resection is often possible but very rarely advisable, for although the immediate hazards are not perhaps quite as formidable as some would make out, a very real risk exists that for technical reasons, such as the distension of the bowel and consequent shortening of the mesentery, the resection, and in particular the lymphatic clearance, may fall short of that strictly desirable. Assessment of operability in the presence of acute obstruction is notoriously most unreliable, for a growth which is fixed and irremovable may be half its size and reasonably mobile once local œdema and inflammation have subsided as a result of diversion of the fæcal stream by a properly placed colostomy. Moreover, an attempt to estimate local fixity is not without its dangers, for it has occasionally happened that an exploratory hand has ruptured the œdematous, softened, distended bowel just above the growth, and this accident is almost invariably fatal.

For these reasons it is generally accepted that acute obstruction due to a carcinoma of the large bowel should usually be treated by operative decompression without a full exploration of the abdomen. The great majority of obstructing carcinomas lie in the pelvic colon or pelvi-rectal region, and a transverse colostomy through the right rectus should be performed. For obstruction at the splenic flexure or in the left half of the transverse colon, the first part of the ascending colon should be mobilized and a similar defunctioning colostomy performed. This is better than a cæcostomy, which does not completely divert the fæcal stream and is an inadequate preliminary to resection. Obstruction by a growth of the cæcum or right colon is less common. This is the one type of case in which one-stage resection is often indicated. Alternatively, ileo-transverse colostomy may be employed to short-circuit the obstructing growth and serve as a first stage, resection being performed later, though it should be remembered that if the growth completely obstructs, say, the hepatic flexure and the ileocæcal valve is competent, ileotransverse colostomy still leaves an unrelieved closed-loop obstruction. For this reason, in cases of this kind in which the cæcum is greatly distended, anastomosis of the ileum to the transverse colon, if preferred to immediate resection, should be supplemented by cæcostomy.

Mesenteric Infarction

It is no longer considered that resection must always be carried out for mesenteric infarction. There was a time when a competitive element seemed to be creeping into the case reports of resections of more and more of the small intestine, 18 and 19 feet of bowel being excised for superior mesenteric occlusion. Almost invariably patients undergoing a lengthy resection of this kind perished. To-day it is generally agreed that unless there is actual gangrene, blood transfusion, suction, morphine, antibiotics, and anti-coagulants give a better chance of survival than resection.

Obstruction by Bands and Adhesions

Intraperitoneal bands and adhesions, whether congenital or inflammatory in origin, may cause or contribute to acute intestinal obstruction in a variety of ways, and the obstruction may be a simple occlusion or strangulating in type, or it may start as one and end as the other. Treatment of a patient seen during the first 24 hours after the onset of obstruction is early operation. If obstruction has been present for several days, gross distension, dehydration and chemical imbalance but without signs of strangulation may make it safer to delay operation than to intervene at once. Intravenous fluids and gastro-intestinal suction should be employed to improve the local and general condition, but unless unmistakable evidence demonstrates that obstruction is no longer present, laparotomy should follow as soon as sufficient improvement has taken place, for relief of an occlusion by suction alone does not occur sufficiently often to compensate for the occasional case in which an unduly delayed operation has revealed a non-viable loop of intestine.

Paralytic Ileus

Little is to be gained by exploring the abdomen in a case of paralytic ileus, except for the purpose of eliminating a cause of general peritonitis, such as a perforated appendix. This apart, therapy has three aims:

(i) To treat the cause of the paralytic ileus.

(ii) To empty the paralysed, dilated bowel by suction and to keep it empty, so that the paralysis does not become perpetuated by the effects of uncontrolled stretching of the flaccid bowel wall and the coincident vascular engorgement.

(iii) To correct dehydration, hypoproteinaemia and chemical imbalance by intravenous fluids, continued until the recovery of intestinal motility and absorption.

As has already been stated, the most common variety of paralytic ileus encountered is that caused by a widespread peritonitis, though even here the obstruction is in part mechanical, due to adhesion, œdema and kinking of the bowel. The three elements in treatment are well illustrated; the cause of the ileus, peritonitis, is treated by surgical elimination of any local cause and by antibiotics whilst gastro-intestinal suction and intravenous fluids have contributed enormously to the recent considerable drop in fatality rates. Further discussion is unnecessary, but the reader is referred to Chapter XII on Peritonitis and Chapter I on Fluid Replacement in the Surgical Patient.

Apart from intestinal obstructions in infancy and childhood (*vide infra*), other varieties of acute obstruction will not be individually considered, for the aim is not to repeat well-known facts to be found in any standard textbook, but to comment upon aspects of surgical treatment of particular importance or demonstrating some change in thought or technique during the last 10 or 15 years. It may be said in conclusion that the following three principles appear to emerge as a result of developments during this period:

(i) Gastro-intestinal suction has not altered the necessity for immediate intervention if it is suspected that a strangulating obstruction is present or may be present.

(ii) If a strangulating obstruction can be excluded with reasonable certainty, pre-operative correction of dehydration and electrolytic imbalance and decompression of the upper gastro-intestinal tract by suction greatly improve the prognosis.

(iii) The progress of this decompression requires the closest scrutiny, both clinical and radiological, and whilst one may be gratified to find occasionally that spontaneous relief of the obstruction has occurred, there are considerable hazards in setting out with the avowed intention of curing an obstruction without surgery. It is better to set out with the intention of operating when the maximum benefit has been reaped from suction and intravenous fluids and, at any rate, it must be regarded as a considerable misdemeanour to allow a patient to die of organic obstruction without a scar upon his belly.

RODNEY SMITH

CHAPTER VII

INTESTINAL OBSTRUCTIONS IN INFANCY AND CHILDHOOD

INTESTINAL obstruction in the new-born baby and infant has its own problems and requires individual consideration. Various errors of development can give rise to neo-natal obstruction and may be conveniently grouped together under the following headings:

(i) Atresia and stenosis of the intestine.
(ii) Errors of rotation.
(iii) Meconium ileus.
(iv) Malformations of anus and rectum.

To these may be added, as a cause of obstruction in the infant or young child:

(v) Obstruction due to Meckel's diverticulum.
(vi) Intussusception.
(vii) Acute obstruction in Hirschprung's disease.

Atresia and Stenosis of the Intestine

Between the fifth and tenth week of fœtal life, epithelial proliferation leads to a temporary obliteration of the intestinal lumen, followed by recanalization, which is usually complete by the twelfth week. If this process of recanalization is arrested, atresia or stenosis is the result, and this may take the form of a complete or incomplete membrane across the bowel, or there may be an absolute lack of continuity with a blind end above and below, with or without a fibrous band connecting the two. Atresia or stenosis may be present at one or more than one site.

The bowel below a complete atresia is empty, save for a little mucus, and is no more than some 5 mm. in diameter. The blind proximal bowel is often grossly dilated and the thinned wall is in great danger of undergoing avascular necrosis, with spontaneous perforation.

Signs and Symptoms

A baby with intestinal atresia or a stenosis of any severity vomits from the day of birth and the vomit contains bile, for it is very rare for the obstruction to be situated above the papilla of Vater. Abdominal distension is common, but its degree depends upon the site and duration of obstruction. There is often visible peristalsis. Absolute constipation is not the rule and although the stools are usually dry and scanty, sometimes they resemble normal meconium.

94

Investigations

Plain X-rays will usually show the greatly distended proximal bowel and fluid levels in the erect film (Fig. 1). It is seldom necessary to employ contrast radiography with barium.

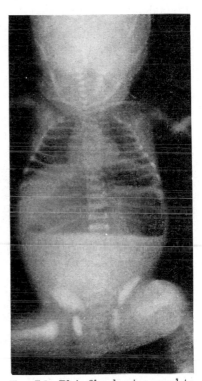

Farber's Test. This may provide evidence in the doubtful case. Amniotic fluid contains squamous epithelial cells desquamated from the skin of the foetus. The foetus *in utero* swallows this fluid and the meconium therefore contains many of these cells. If a swab is taken from the centre of the meconium stool and a smear on a glass slide is stained appropriately, it is possible to say with certainty whether or not these epithelial cells are present. Complete absence means atresia at some point; presence proves that the intestinal tract is patent right through but, of course, does not rule out areas of stenosis.

Treatment

A mild degree of stenosis is quite compatible with survival and need not be treated surgically in the first few days of life. The baby will, however, gain weight but slowly and recurrent

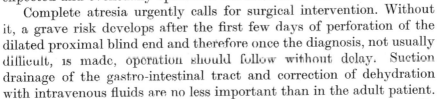

FIG. 7.1. Plain film showing complete obstruction of the jejunum due to atresia in a newborn baby.

vomiting is likely. When mixed feeding begins, further trouble is to be expected and eventually operation will have to be undertaken.

Complete atresia urgently calls for surgical intervention. Without it, a grave risk develops after the first few days of perforation of the dilated proximal blind end and therefore once the diagnosis, not usually difficult, is made, operation should follow without delay. Suction drainage of the gastro-intestinal tract and correction of dehydration with intravenous fluids are no less important than in the adult patient.

Ether anaesthesia is very satisfactory for tiny babies and generally preferable to local anaesthesia. The abdomen is opened through a right paramedian incision. The dilated proximal and collapsed distal bowel are easily found and the former must be handled with care, for rupture of the greatly thinned wall may easily occur. The whole of the alimentary tract must be examined to exclude other areas of atresia or coincident anomalies of rotation.

Jejunal and Ileal Atresia

The proximal and distal bowel are now joined by lateral anastomosis. This is technically difficult on account of the great disparity in size, the former being 3-4 cm. and the latter often 3-4 mm. in diameter. It helps a little to empty the dilated loop by aspiration and to inflate the collapsed and empty distal loop with air or saline. Ladd and Gross recommend employing two layers for the actual anastomosis, but often this is not possible and a single layer of catgut, employing an inverting Connell stitch anteriorly, must suffice.

Duodenal Atresia

Atresia above the level of the papilla of Vater is rare. Gastro-jejunostomy or, occasionally, duodeno-jejunostomy, should be performed. Atresia of the duodenum distal to the papilla of Vater usually results in considerable dilatation of the proximal duodenum and duodeno-jejunostomy is the procedure of choice.

Post-operative Treatment

Gastro-intestinal suction must continue and reliance must be placed upon parenteral feeding for several days. In order to aid in opening up the contracted lower bowel, Ladd and Gross recommend saline enemata two or three times daily.

The Results of Treatment

In 1941, Ladd and Gross recorded 7 recoveries out of 52 atresias operated upon. The prognosis is a little better to-day, but the mortality is still over 50 per cent.

Errors of Rotation

From the sixth to the tenth week of intra-uterine life, the length of the alimentary tract increases faster than does the capacity of the body cavity and part of the midgut is temporarily extruded into the base of the umbilical cord. From the tenth week onwards the body cavity increases relatively in size and the intestine returns into the abdomen. As it does so, rotation in an anti-clockwise direction takes place, carrying the transverse colon across in front of the duodenum and mesentery of the small bowel and bringing the cæcum first up into the upper abdomen, then across to the right hypochondrium under the liver and finally downwards into the right iliac fossa, after which the cæcum and ascending colon acquire peritoneal attachments to the posterior abdominal wall and the mesentery of the small bowel acquires a linear attachment from the duodeno-jejunal flexure to the Ileocæcal region.

Mal-rotation may cause intestinal obstruction in various ways:

(*a*) Incomplete rotation often leaves the cæcum just below the pylorus and this anomaly is nearly always accompanied by the presence of abnormal peritoneal bands running from the cæcum to the posterior abdominal wall, across the duodenum, which is compressed and obstructed.

(*b*) If rotation is incomplete, the mesentery of the midgut loop often has a very narrow attachment around the superior mesenteric vessels, and rotation of the whole loop around this duodeno-colic isthmus is possible, leading to the so-called "volvulus neonatorum". Frequently volvulus of the midgut loop and duodenal compression by a peritoneal band are present coincidently.

(*c*) A rare anomaly is reversed rotation, the intestine returning to the peritoneal cavity with the distal midgut behind the proximal. Instead of the duodenum running behind the transverse colon, the transverse colon lies in a tunnel deep to the superior mesenteric vessels and is likely to become compressed at this point.

(*d*) A normally placed cæcum which has not acquired its peritoneal attachment to the posterior abdominal wall, being abnormally mobile may itself undergo volvulus. It does not follow that it will do so in infancy or childhood. Indeed, most patients are adults. The condition will not be further discussed here.

Signs and Symptoms

Obstruction from mal-rotation usually presents as an acute obstruction of the duodenum, with the rapid onset of vomiting, dehydration and circulatory failure. The obstruction being a very high one, distension is minimal unless volvulus is present, and even then the duodenal obstruction usually dominates the picture and should lead to operation before there has been time for distension to become marked. Similarly, although infarction of the whole midgut loop may occur in volvulus neonatorum, surgical intervention will probably be undertaken before this has had time to occur.

The rare obstruction of a transverse colon abnormally placed behind the superior mesenteric vessels leads to the less dramatic onset of large bowel occlusion with more distension and less dehydration and collapse.

Plain X-rays may aid in diagnosis. It is unlikely that contrast radiography with barium will be thought necessary.

Treatment

Laparotomy must follow as soon as the diagnosis is made. Ether anæsthesia and a long right paramedian incision are usually employed. If nothing but coils of small intestine present, with no visible colon, a midgut volvulus is present, the twist being nearly always in a clockwise direction. If no volvulus is present, or alternatively after it has been untwisted, the cæcum should be sought and it will usually be found lying under the pylorus, with stout peritoneal bands running from it to the posterior abdominal wall below the liver. Division of these bands allows the cæcum to fall away, downwards and to the left, and relieves the compression of the duodenum.

Obstruction of the posteriorly placed transverse colon can be relieved by anastomosis of the bowel proximal to the obstruction to the pelvic colon, or by colostomy preparatory to short-circuit. The writer has not encountered a case of this kind.

One final word on intestinal obstruction due to mal-rotation; the dramatic onset of complete obstruction is not invariable. In a certain percentage of cases intermittent partial obstruction occurs instead and sometimes leads to chronic ill-health and malnutrition, resembling cœliac disease. The possibility of a mechanical cause should be borne in mind in the older child presenting in this way.

Meconium Ileus

Intestinal obstruction in the newborn may sometimes occur from the impaction of inspissated meconium. The association between meconium ileus and fibrocystic disease of the pancreas is now well established, and it is clear that absence of pancreatic ferments from the bowel leaves the meconium of a putty-like consistency which can easily clog up the intestine with its sheer bulk and hardness. Symptoms usually occur in the first days of life, but very occasionally the infant struggles on for a week or two or even a month or two. The writer operated upon one exceptional case of meconium ileus, ending fatally, in a baby of six months, post-mortem examination revealing a typical fibrocystic disease of the pancreas. If an obstruction of this type leads to exploration of the abdomen, the surgeon may occasionally find that a hard mass of putty-like meconium impacted at the ileocæcal valve can be squeezed through into the large bowel, while enterotomy and direct removal of the obstructing material has sometimes been carried out. Whatever treatment is adopted, the outlook is poor.

Malformations of Anus and Rectum

Imperforate anus or rectal stenosis, with or without an associated fistula between the bowel and the urogenital tract or the exterior, not uncommonly causes intestinal obstruction. Diagnosis is not difficult to make, the infant failing to pass meconium and, if untreated, becoming progressively distended, local examination disclosing the cause. If the anus is imperforate, radiological examination must precede surgery. Films should be taken with the baby inverted and a coin taped upon the anal dimple. The gas in the large bowel rises into the blind rectal

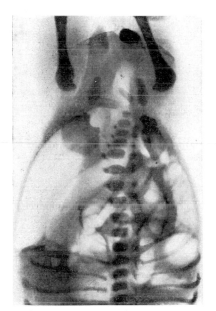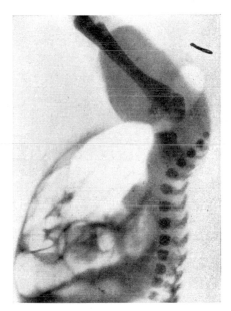

Fig. 7.2A and B.   Imperforate anus. The blind rectal stump separated from the exterior by a mere thin partition.

stump and it can be seen at once how near the exterior the bowel lies (Figs. 2 and 3). If a thin membrane only is the sole cause of obstruction, it can be incised and the condition very simply solved thereby. If the bowel lies an inch or so above the anal dimple, perineal exploration allows it to be brought down and stitched to the anal margin. If the bowel lies high in the false pelvis, it is just possible for a combined abdominal and perineal operation to bring it down, but it is usually thought that acute obstruction should be cured by a temporary colostomy in the hope that a definitive operation and closure of the colostomy will be possible when the child is older.

Obstruction Due to a Meckel's Diverticulum

A Meckel's diverticulum may lead to acute intestinal obstruction in a variety of ways. Although a congenital anomaly, it does not follow that symptoms necessarily occur in infancy or even childhood. Quite often the diverticulum remains unsuspected for years and first gives rise to symptoms in adult life. A patient of the writer preserved his diverticulum for 39 years but finally made good use of it, for an acute volvulus laid him low just six hours before his military unit was to figure as the initial wave carrying out the assault across the river

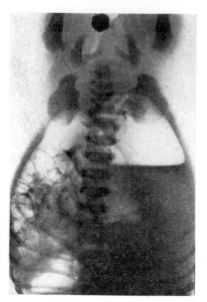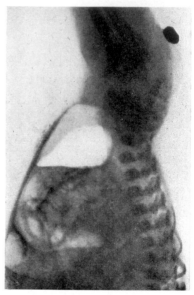

Fig. 7.3a and b.   Imperforate anus with a blind colonic stump ending high in the false pelvis.

Sangro in Italy in the recent war. In spite of some understandable scepticism on the part of his unit Medical Officer, he underwent a successful resection of gangrenous bowel sufficiently early to survive, in which he was more fortunate than many of his mates.

Intestinal obstruction may be caused in the following ways:

(*a*) A band, congenital or inflammatory in origin, associated with the diverticulum, may ensnare the bowel and cause occlusion or strangulation.

(*b*) An inverted diverticulum may form the apex of an intussusception.

(*c*) Torsion of the diverticulum may lead to infarction, or the twist may take up the coil of ileum bearing it and lead to an acute volvulus of the small bowel.

(*d*) Peptic ulceration, scarring and fibrosis may lead to a stricture, across the base of the diverticulum or even sufficient to obstruct the ileum.

(*e*) The mere size of the diverticulum or a tumour of it may, if sufficiently large, occasionally compress and obstruct the bowel.

(*f*) Perforation of the diverticulum, leading to diffuse peritonitis, may result in paralytic ileus.

Treatment is identical with that of similar lesions not associated with a Meckel's diverticulum, save that the diverticulum itself requires removal, care being taken when closing the base that the ileum is not narrowed.

Intussusception

The classic features of idiopathic intussusception are too well known to need repetition. Certain aspects of diagnosis and treatment are, however, worth mention.

(*a*) An early vomit is an extremely common symptom.

(*b*) Passage of blood per rectum is not an early symptom and indicates considerable engorgement and vascular embarrassment of the intussusceptum. The aim of treatment should be to intervene if possible before this stage is reached.

(*c*) In any case of suspected intussusception, prolonged careful examination of the abdomen is essential, for the tell-tale lump, classically "hardening under the hand", may only be detected as the plain muscle of the bowel contracts.

(*d*) Dance's sign, emptiness of the right iliac fossa, is unreliable.

(*e*) In spite of claims to the contrary, most authorities do not feel that hydrostatic reduction with a barium enema, under radiological control, is as certain or as safe as a properly performed operation.

(*f*) An irreducible intussusception means a high mortality under any form of treatment. Resection and anastomosis probably offers as good a chance of survival as any other. Operations based upon the establishment of a temporary enterostomy are not satisfactory as a rule, for an infant or young child tolerates very badly the inevitable loss from the fistula of fluid and electrolytes.

Acute Obstruction in Hirschprung's Disease

Acute obstructive episodes are not uncommon in Hirschprung's disease. It is now accepted that in this condition, not to be confused with the minor colonic inertias of childhood, the underlying pathology is an absence of ganglion cells in a segment of bowel at or about the pelvi-rectal junction which, failing to relax with the peristaltic wave, remains spastic and acts as an organic obstruction, leading to dilatation and hypertrophy of the large bowel and persistent severe constipation, only curable by excision of the abnormal segment of intestine.

Acute obstruction with extreme colonic distension may provide an emergency of no little danger. Diagnosis is not difficult and treatment should follow four stages:

(*a*) Deflation of the dilated colon by the passage of a rectal tube up through the spastic segment into the bowel beyond;

(*b*) The establishment of proximal drainage of the bowel by a transverse colostomy, which will prevent any further acute obstructive episodes and prepare the bowel for the third stage, the definitive operation.

(*c*) Resection of the abnormal segment by rectosigmoidectomy.

(*d*) Closure of the colostomy.

RODNEY SMITH

CHAPTER VIII

ULCERATIVE COLITIS

THE ætiology of ulcerative colitis remains obscure, but increased knowledge of its pathological changes and sequelæ together with an earlier recognition of the limitations of present medical treatment have greatly increased the frequency of surgical intervention. The disease may be divided arbitrarily into three clinical types: the mild chronic, the severe chronic, and the acute toxic varieties. The first properly remains a medical problem and its disability, while recurrent, is usually slight. The second and third destroy the patient or produce chronic invalidism with a poor expectation of life. To them surgery can at present offer more than other forms of treatment and, once their severity is recognized, surgery should be early rather than late. It is difficult to know the true frequency of these clinical types, but it is said that some 20 per cent. of all cases require surgery (Cattell and Sachs, 1948; Bacon and Trimpi, 1950) and that 5 per cent. are of the acute toxic variety (Crile and Thomas, 1951).

Indications for Surgery

Surgery is indicated as a life-saving measure, where permanent and severe organic changes such as pseudo polyposis have occurred in the bowel wall, for complications such as stricture, fistula, arthritis or skin ulceration, and where it is impossible for the patient to lead a normal or useful life without it.

Appendicostomy

This operation is now seldom performed, but it might be justifiable if surgery were advised and the patient refused an ileostomy.

Ileostomy

While this can rightly be regarded as a life-saving measure, the sudden loss of fluid and electrolytes which ensues may turn the scales against a severly toxic patient and everything possible must be done, by ensuring a proper balance and the use of antibiotics, that the patient is brought to the optimum condition before operation is performed. It is recognized that almost all ileostomies are permanent and the patient must be given confidence that in the future they will be able to lead a useful life. In some hospitals ileostomy clubs have been formed where patients gather to discuss the difficulties which can be overcome and give confidence to prospective members.

There are now surgical advocates of a more extensive primary procedure, but ileostomy alone is in general use as the first operation for ulcerative colitis. The use of a Rubzen or similar bag (Counsell and Goligher, 1952) and adhesive skin fixation greatly reduces the patient's discomfort from cutaneous excoriation and the terminal ileostomy stoma should be placed some 2 inches to the right and below the umbilicus through a small right transrectal incision. A lower stoma or one placed further to the right may cause the bag to ride up on sitting or make fixation to the skin more difficult. A loop colostomy is unsuitable for a Rubzen bag.

Some surgeons close and infold the distal end of the divided ileum. Gabriel (1952) advises its division just proximal to the ileocæcal valve so that its closure may be flush with the cæcum and a subsequent colectomy made easier. Others exteriorize the divided lower end through a separate stab incision above and lateral to the ileostomy stoma, claiming that the risk of stump leakage is avoided and that it is available for irrigation of the colon. Appendicectomy may be performed and Brooke (1951) advises closure below the cæcum of the "para-ileal" peritoneal gutter. In the closure of the incision the divided mesentery of the ileum is sutured to the peritoneum, thus limiting prolapse. One or two inches of ileum should project beyond the skin and tight suturing of the parietes around the bowel must be avoided: small transverse cuts may be made in the posterior wall of the rectus sheath where it is in contact with the bowel. It is usual to drain the ileum for the first few post-operative days by means of a soft rubber tube or a small Pauls Tube. The application of an immediate skin graft or skin flap from the abdominal wall to the projecting bowel has been advocated as a convenience to the patient but is not in general use.

Mortality and Complications of Ileostomy

Published series at the present time suggest an operative mortality of 5 to 10 per cent. but in general it is probably higher. Death may result from a combination of toxæmia and fluid imbalance or intraperitoneal perforation of an ileal ulcer, often at the junction of bowel and abdominal wall. Colic and mild obstructive symptoms are very common and may be relieved by the careful passage of a soft rubber catheter and gentle irrigation with saline. In spite of the Rubzen bag, excoriation may prove very troublesome until the ileal actions are less frequent and a "fluid absorber" such as "Isogel" may assist. Stenosis of the stoma should be prevented by regular digital dilatation.

Involvement of the Ileum in Ulcerative Colitis

In a reported series of 103 cases of ulcerative colitis from the Mayo Clinic the terminal ileum was also involved in 28 per cent. (McCreedy *et al.*, 1949). Intermittent solitary ulcers are rarely present in the jejunum. Involvement of the ileum is not a terminal event but may be present at an early stage of the disease in association with a right sided ulcerative colitis. Radiological evidence of this was present in 10 out of 19 cases examined for this purpose at the Mayo Clinic. Brooke, (1951) suggests that right sided ulcerative colitis with ileal involvement may be a different type of the disease and that fat balance tests, a macrocytic anæmia, abnormality of serum protein and glossitis may suggest its presence. Ileal involvement may account for failure after ileostomy. When discovered at operation some surgeons advise the resection of the diseased ileum down to the ileocæcal valve: others that ileostomy should only be performed if it can be placed well above the affected area.

The Results of Ileostomy and Subsequent Treatment

Ileostomy usually produces a great improvement in chronic ulcerative colitis as evidenced by gain in weight, absence of pyrexia and in some cases a return to a wage earning existence. Unfortunately the diseased bowel remains and its changes appear to be permanent. Exacerbations may occur with bowel hæmorrhage and the onset of arthritis. It is true that in a few cases with minimal bowel changes the ileostomy has been closed but many of these have required ileostomy again (Cattell and Sachs, 1948). For these reasons many surgeons have in the past advised that a total colectomy should follow an ileostomy. This view has been greatly strengthened by the recognition of the association between chronic ulcerative colitis and carcinoma of the colon. Shands, Dockerty and Bargen (1952) recently reviewed a series of 73 cases of adenocarcinoma of the large bowel associated with chronic ulcerative colitis. The average duration of symptoms before carcinoma developed was $15 \cdot 3$ years. In 64 cases a change of symptoms heralded the onset of the growth: in nine there was none. In $52 \cdot 5$ per cent. there were present multiple foci of malignancy. Similar results have been reported by other writers and it is now recognized that in colons removed for ulcerative colitis a careful search not uncommonly reveals flat infiltrated areas of early carcinoma. It is obvious that in ulcerative colitis the bowel symptoms will make the early diagnosis of colonic cancer difficult and that the prognosis is likely to be poor. In the 73 cases described by Shands, Dockerty and Bargen only two patients survived five years from the recognition of the growth.

Total or Subtotal Colectomy

This is either performed as a routine procedure once the patient's condition has been improved by ileostomy or because progress after ileostomy has been unsatisfactory. As already stated, there is strong evidence in support of a routine colectomy in all cases requiring ileostomy. The operation is best performed in one stage through a long left paramedian incision and a small transverse incision on the right side including the stoma of the ileal stump if this has been exteriorized, but the extent of the operation must necessarily depend on the condition of the patient and the surgeon's judgment. The distal level of the resection may be the upper end of the rectum which is closed and covered over with pelvic peritoneum or the middle of the sigmoid which is exteriorized through the lower end of the abdominal incision or through a stab incision in the left iliac fossa. The mortality of this operation is probably between 5 and 10 per cent.

Primary Colectomy and Ileostomy

Resection of the greater part of the colon at the same time as the ileostomy is now recommended in a number of surgical centres (Ripstein *et al.*, 1952; Bacon and Trimpi, 1950; Crile and Thomas, 1951, and others). In favour of this proceeding it is pointed out that primary resection of the colon eliminates both toxic absorption and blood and protein loss while the performance of ileostomy alone adds the loss of fluid and electrolytes to these factors. Ripstein *et al.* report one stage resection and ileostomy in 72 patients with only three deaths, and it would seem that this operation is likely to be performed more widely in the future.

The Treatment of the Rectum in Ulcerative Colitis.   Ileorectal and Ileo-anal Anastomosis

With very rare exceptions, which few surgeons have ever encountered, the rectum is always involved in ulcerative colitis, but the degree of involvement may vary from a somewhat granular mucosa to gross ulceration, stricture formation and fistulæ. The view expressed by the majority of writers at the present time is that where ulcerative colitis is sufficiently severe to require ileostomy, it should usually be followed by colectomy and the subsequent removal of the rectum, since the chance of a successful restoration of bowel continuity is small and there are dangers in leaving the rectal stump (Gabriel, 1952; Bacon and Trimpi, 1950). Ripstein *et al.* (1952) list the indications for rectal removal as discharge and bleeding, strictures, anorectal fistulæ, polyposis and malignancy and evidence of toxic absorption such as arthritis, fever and failure to gain weight. They consider that its removal is indicated in the majority of cases.

Removal of the rectum and lower sigmoid may be performed by any method of combined resection or if only the rectal stump has been left after colectomy, by perineal resection alone.

When rectal changes are minimal and the patient has made a good recovery from ileostomy and colectomy it is not surprising that some surgeons still consider an attempt at bowel restoration to be justified. Anastomosis of the terminal ileum to the distal sigmoid by a crush anastomosis has been described by Devine and Devine (1948) but this method would seem to have the disadvantage of retaining some of the sigmoid colon, and if an attempt is to be made to restore bowel continuity the wisest course would seem to be an anterior resection of the rectum leaving a rectal stump at least 3 inches in length to which the distal ileum is anastomosed. This operation has the advantage that it removes a considerable part of the rectum while retaining sufficient to act as an emergency reservoir and ensure continence. It has the disadvantages that the reservoir is small and bowel actions frequent, perhaps twice nightly. Further, the rectal stump may develop further signs of disease and fistula, stricture and hæmorrhage follow. Irritation of the perianal skin by the ileal contents can be most troublesome.

Attempts to remove the rectum completely and perform an anastomosis between the ileum and the anal canal have been made by several surgeons. Best (1952) in an interesting review of twelve cases in which the operation was performed for ulcerative colitis by Ravitch, Wanganstern and Best states that in 50 per cent. it proved a failure and ileostomy became necessary. Apart from any difficulty with the fluid ileal contents, it is now generally accepted that it is impossible to preserve normal continence when all the rectal mucosa has been removed (Gaston, 1950; Goligher, 1951).

Because of the failures and the need to resort again to ileostomy many surgeons feel that attempts to preserve rectal function in chronic ulcerative colitis are unjustified. This is perhaps an extreme view, but if such operations are to be attempted the patient must be selected with the greatest care and the surgeon must be aware of the difficulties to be expected.

Segmental Colitis

In certain cases radiological evidence suggests that the disease is limited to one area of the colon, and success is said to have sometimes followed resection of the affected area. Gabriel (1952), however,

believes that the disease always spreads and that such cases require the
same treatment as any other case of ulcerative colitis.

Vagotomy

It is difficult to believe that vagotomy can alter the organic changes
already present in the bowel wall at the stage when surgical assistance
is sought in the treatment of ulcerative colitis. Eddy (1951) in a review
of 42 patients upon whom this operation had been performed considered
that the best results were obtained in severe cases with a short history
and that when the disease had been present for five years or more,
permanent changes in the colon made improvement unlikely. Few
surgical centres consider the operation to be of any value, but like
psychiatry and hypnosis it will no doubt continue to achieve the
occasional "cure" in this curious psychosomatic disease.

ACTH and Cortisone

The use of these drugs, of which ACTH is considered superior to
Cortisone, can hardly be considered a surgical measure, but since they
may produce a remission in the disease they may be of value in the
pre-operative preparation of a difficult patient. Reports state that the
majority of patients develop a sense of well being, a decrease in the
number of stools, a great increase in appetite with a gain in weight and
an improvement in anæmia (Halsted *et al.*, 1951). The treatment does
not effect a cure but is a most potent weapon for producing a remission
(Rehfuss, 1951). A number of complications attend its use. ACTH
inhibits the proliferation of fibroblasts and retards healing. It is not
surprising that perforation of a gastric or duodenal ulcer may occur
under treatment and Tullin, Kern and Almy (1952) report three cases
of peritonitis occurring in seventeen cases of ulcerative colitis treated
by ACTH. Because of the danger Crile and Thomas (1951) advise that
ACTH should only be used in the immediate pre-operative period to
improve the patient's condition.

Chronic ulcerative colitis is typically a disease of young and mid-
adult life. It is chastening to reflect that when medical measures fail,
modern surgery can seldom do more than persuade these patients that
life with a permanent ileostomy is still to be enjoyed and demand from
them the sacrifice of their large bowel from ileum to anus. It is true
that it is a successful form of treatment for a crippling and dangerous
disease: that surgery, and at present only surgery, can return many of
these patients from chronic invalidism to an economic life, and that
the majority of patients can adapt themselves and conquer the difficul-

ties of an ileostomy. Nevertheless, its very finality is a little depressing, and it is to be hoped that future treatment will lessen its need or at least permit more restorative measures than are at present possible.

E. G. MUIR

References:

BACON, H. E., and TRIMPI, H. D. (1950) *J. Amer. med. Ass.* **137,** 929.

BEST, R. R. (1952) *J. Amer. med. Ass.* **150,** 637.

BROOKE, B. N. (1951) *Ann. R. Coll. Surg. Engl.* **8,** 440.

BROOKE, B. N. (1951) *Lancet* **ii,** 462.

CATTELL, R. B., and SACHS, E. (1948) *J. Amer. med. Ass.* **137,** 929.

COUNSELL, P. B., and GOLIGHER, J. C. (1952) *Lancet* **ii,** 1045.

CRILE, G., and THOMAS, C. Y. (1951) *Gastroenterology* **19,** 58.

DEVINE, H., and DEVINE, J. (1948) *Brit. med. J.* **ii,** 127.

EDDY, F. D. (1951) *Surgery* **29,** 11.

GABRIEL, W. B. (1952) *Brit. med. Jour.* **i,** 881.

GASTON, E. A. (1950) *Surg. Gynec. Obstet.* **87,** 780.

GOLIGHER, J. C. (1951) *Ann. R. Coll. Surg. Engl.* **8,** 421.

HALSTED, J. A., ADAMS, W. S., SLOAN, S., WALTERS, R. L., and BASSETT, S. H. (1951) *Gastroenterology* **10,** 698.

McCREADY, F. J., BARGEN, J. A., DOCKERTY, M. B., and WAUGH, J. M. (1949) *New Engl. J. Med.* **240,** 119.

REHFUSS, M. (1951) *Gastroenterology* **19,** 730.

RIPSTEIN, C. B., MILLER, G. G., and GARDNER, C. M. (1952) *Ann. Surg.* **135,** 14.

SHANDS, W. C., DOCKERTY, M. B., and BARGEN, J. A. (1952) *Surg. Gynec. Obstet.* **94,** 302.

TULLIN, M., KERN, F., and ALMY, T. P. (1952) *J. Amer. med. Ass.* **150,** 559.

CHAPTER IX

CARCINOMA OF THE COLON

CANCER of the large bowel is responsible for the deaths of some 15,000 to 20,000 patients annually in England and Wales. As far as is at present known, two conditions predispose to its occurrence, chronic ulcerative colitis and familial intestinal polyposis. The former is considered in the chapter on ulcerative colitis; the latter, through the work of Lockhart-Mummery (1925) and Dukes (1939, 1952) has been carefully studied.

Familial Intestinal Polyposis

The result of this gene mutation is never present at birth but develops in childhood or early adult life as scattered patches of epithelial hyperplasia in the mucous membrane of the colon and rectum. In a group of 41 families investigated by Dukes (1952) there were 156 cases of polyposis and the average age at onset of symptoms was 20 years. Of these 156 cases, 114 had developed cancer of the large bowel, usually about 15 years after the first onset of symptoms. Polyposis affects males and females equally: either may transmit: as a rule in a polyposis family only half the children are likely to inherit the abnormality: only those who have inherited can transmit: the severity of the disease and the liability to cancer varies, being greater in those families in which the polyposis develops early in life (Dukes, 1952).

Treatment

The majority of patients seek advice for bleeding, diarrhœa or because they are aware of the family disease. Mild cases may require no more than sigmoidoscopic diathermy to those polypi within reach and regular supervision for the remainder of their life. In more severe cases, if the rectum can be brought under control by diathermy and cleared of polypi, the whole colon may be excised and the ileum anastomosed to the rectal stump. The surgical ideal would be the excision of all large bowel mucosa and an ileo-anal anastomosis, but the results of this operation are often unsatisfactory as regards function. The development of cancer is often multifocal and its appearance is usually regarded as an indication for at least a total colectomy.

The average age of death in the series of polyposis studied by Dukes was $41 \cdot 6$ years as compared with an average age of death from rectal cancer in other cases of $67 \cdot 9$ years.

Cancer of the Colon

An increased knowledge of the essentials in preparing a patient for major surgery, with the sulphonamides and antibiotics, has greatly reduced the mortality of planned operations on the large bowel. It is probable that this is now not more than 5 per cent. but, as an unfortunate contrast, the surgery of acute intestinal obstruction from a colonic growth still carries a high mortality. Newell (1951) reported a series of 490 cases of colonic cancer at the Association of Surgeons Meeting in 1951 in which 59 per cent. were undiagnosed until obstruction had occurred and the mortality in this group was as high as 38 per cent.

Treatment: Acute Obstruction

The treatment of acute obstruction is considered more fully elsewhere. In colonic cancer it is much more common with growths in the left rather than the right colon (87 per cent. Morgan, 1952). The site of the growth may often be localized by a plain X-ray film of the abdomen. While surgical opinion may vary in subacute obstruction, there is unanimity of opinion that in fully developed acute intestinal obstruction, believed due to a carcinoma of the colon, laparotomy is unwise and bowel decompression alone should be performed. A Miller-Abbott tube will decompress small bowel but unless it passes the ileo-caecal valve it will not relieve the closed loop of obstructed colon between a competent ileocaecal valve and a constricting growth. A right transverse colostomy, performed just distal to the hepatic flexure, is the most useful proceeding for an obstructing growth of the left colon for it permits future surgery in a clear field and probably on a clean bowel from which the faecal stream has been diverted.

A caecostomy may be used if the growth is in the right or transverse colon and the patient's condition unsuitable for exploration. Caecostomy has received considerable criticism but it can still be a life saving measure and its presence does not seriously interfere with future surgery. Further it is better to do a caecostomy than make an ill-judged transverse colostomy in close proximity to a growth.

Before discussing planned surgery of the large bowel consideration must be given to the not infrequent situation in which the surgeon is confronted with an operable growth in an unprepared patient. Laparotomy may have been properly performed for early obstructive symptoms or for some other suspected condition.

If the growth is in the left colon a right transverse colostomy should be performed with a view to subsequent resection.

In the splenic flexure or transverse colon a Paul Mikulicz extra-peritoneal resection is an excellent solution in a fit patient. A right transverse colostomy may be used only if the growth is well over to the left side, there is a long transverse colon and the colostomy will not interfere with the subsequent resection.

If an unsuspected growth is found in the middle of the transverse colon it may be treated by a Paul Mikulicz resection if the patient is fit, or a cæcostomy if unfit.

If the growth is in the right colon or hepatic flexure there is a choice between a one stage resection with ileal drainage (*vide infra*), an ileo-transverse colostomy performed at least 12 in. from the ileocæcal valve and well away from the growth or a cæcostomy. The first has many advantages (Muir, 1947) but the decision in all these unexpected cases must depend on the patient's fitness and the surgeon's experience and choice.

Non-obstructed Cases: Pre-operative Treatment

The patient must be prepared for the operation. The condition of the cardiovascular system, lungs and kidneys must be known and improved if possible. Calorie and vitamin intake, fluid balance and blood picture must be satisfactory. The large bowel should be completely decompressed and as sterile as modern therapy can make it. For five days before operation phthalyl sulphathiazole is given in regular doses and for two days either aureomycin or streptomycin in addition. Large doses of Vitamin C and B complex are also desirable. If locally acting sulphonamides or antibiotics have been used for more than five days, Vitamin K should also be given (Morgan, 1952).

Purgation must be avoided but a mild aperient such as Petrolagar or Milk of Magnesia is used regularly for four or five days before operation up to the last 48 hours. Daily colonic lavage for three or four pre-operative days should assist in giving a clean and empty bowel. Some surgeons prefer to have a Miller-Abbott tube passed to the lower ileum as a pre-operative measure.

The Operation

The incision must give adequate access. For the right side it may be oblique, paramedian or transrectal: on the left side access to the splenic flexure makes a long vertical incision desirable.

All surgeons agree that fixity of a growth to spleen, stomach or other structures does not necessarily render it inoperable for part or the whole of the adjacent organs may be excised *en bloc*, the adhesions may be inflammatory and even if malignant it need not mean widespread metastases.

The lymphatic drainage of the colon is intimately associated with its vascular supply and the extent of each resection depends on these factors.

Right Colon

A right hemicolectomy is performed with removal of the last six inches of ileum. The ileocolic and right colic arteries are ligated at their origin from the superior mesenteric artery. If the hepatic flexure is involved the right half of the transverse colon must also be removed with ligation of the right branch of the middle colic artery at its origin.

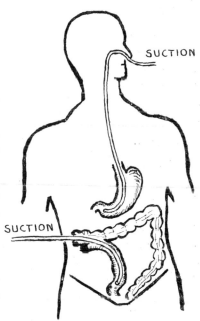

Continuity may be restored by an end-to-end, end-to-side or side-to-side anastomosis between ileum and transverse colon. At the present time the first is the most popular proceeding. If there is any evidence of small bowel obstruction a side-to-side or end-to-side anastomosis may be made and a soft rubber tube or catheter introduced through the colon and up the lumen of the ileum for some six inches. This is brought out through a separate stab drain in the abdominal wall and acts as an ileostomy drain. It is easily removed in 7 to 10 days, and if the colon has been infolded around it there is seldom any leakage (Muir, 1947) (see Fig. 1).

FIG. 9.1.—Combined gastric and ileal suction drainage after Rt. hemicolectomy. (*By kind permission of the Editor, "Proceedings of the Royal Society of Medicine".*)

Transverse, Descending Colon and Proximal Part of the Sigmoid Loop

Growths in these situations may be treated by primary resection and end-to-end anastomosis, by a Paul Mikulicz extraperitoneal resection or by a preliminary right transverse colostomy followed by a resection and end-to-end anastomosis. The first is the ideal but is admissible only when there is no obstruction and effective pre-operative treatment has been carried out. The second is particularly indicated when the patient's condition is poor, the operation unexpected or some minor degree of obstruction present. A desire to perform it must never lead to the ineffective removal of diseased tissue. The third is indicated in the same conditions as those requiring a Paul Mikulicz resection but particularly when such part of the sigmoid is involved which would make a Paul Mikulicz impossible or ineffective.

Growths in the transverse colon will require mobilization of both the hepatic and splenic flexures unless the mesocolon is very long. As a rule ligation of the middle colic artery or of both its branches near their origin will be required for an adequate removal of the lymph drainage system.

Growths at the splenic flexure require the ligation of the left branch of the middle colic artery and, in the descending colon, the ligation of the left colic artery at their origins. A growth in the proximal part of the sigmoid loop requires the ligation of both the left colic and the first sigmoid at their origins from the inferior mesenteric artery (*vide infra*). This may render it unsuitable for a Paul Mikulicz operation. The splenic flexure will usually require mobilization.

Sigmoid and Rectosigmoid Colon

A growth in a long sigmoid loop may be suitable for a Paul Mikulicz operation, but there is a danger that this procedure may lead to ineffective removal of the lymph drainage system, and it is best treated by an end-to-end anastomosis with ligation of the sigmoid arteries at their origin from the inferior mesenteric artery. As the site of the growth nears the rectosigmoid region its lymph drainage becomes more intimately associated with the inferior mesenteric artery. Growths in the distal sigmoid and rectosigmoid regions require the ligation and removal of the inferior mesenteric artery and its associated lymph glands from immediately below the left colic or first sigmoid arteries. In fact the operation required is an anterior, intraperitoneal resection of the upper rectum, the rectosigmoid and the distal half of the sigmoid loop. Continuity is restored by end-to-end anastomosis of the sigmoid and the rectal stump. Anything less than this is likely to be ineffective and anything more must be an abdominoperineal. It is a point of interest that some who oppose an anterior resection for a rectosigmoid growth on the grounds that it is an ineffective operation are yet content to perform wedge resections of the sigmoid loop.

Ligation of the inferior mesenteric artery at its origin from the aorta is advocated by several writers. Ault, Castro and Smith (1952) state that its ligation proximal to the left colic branch allows the removal of an additional 2 in. of gland bearing vascular pedicle and they believe that the function of the marginal arteries of the colon is sufficiently good to prevent necrosis. Grinnell and Hiatt (1952) described 41 resections in which the inferior mesenteric artery had been ligated at the aorta. Of these 18 were resections with anastomosis, 16 abdomino-perineal and 7 abdomino-anal pull through operations. There were three deaths but in only one was the fatality due to necrosis and that in a pull-through operation. They hold that simple wedge resection of the sigmoid without excision of the inferior mesenteric artery and its lymphatics is inadequate and should be discontinued. Some may feel that this is an extreme view but it is probably true that more ineffective resections of the lymphatic field are performed in the sigmoid than in any other part of the colon. Unfortunately this is by far the most common part of the colon to be affected by carcinoma.

Post-Operative Care

This is similar to that required for all major abdominal operations: gastric suction and fluid requirements given intravenously until peristalsis has returned, and the use of antibiotics to prevent infection. It is now recognized that in post-operative surgical cases there is an increased potassium loss, higher than can be explained by tissue wastage and above the normal K/N ratio. The clinical signs of a K deficit are inhibitory effects on cardiac, voluntary and smooth muscle associated with a fall in the peripheral circulation and paralytic ileus. Its effects are more likely to become apparent when it is necessary to prolong unduly the period of intravenous fluids and in such cases potassium chloride in the strength of 0·2 per cent. may be added to the glucose saline. In no case should the strength of potassium chloride exceed 0·4 per cent. (Elman *et al.*, 1952).

In order to avoid distension in the large bowel a flatus tube is passed a few inches into the rectum three times daily after the first 48 hours and when flatus has been passed glycerine suppositories are used to encourage bowel action. After the first five or six days liquid paraffin, petrolagar or other mild aperients may be used.

Mortality

If cases of colonic cancer with acute intestinal obstruction are excluded the mortality of resections is low—probably not more than 5 per cent. Once acute obstruction is present the general mortality is almost certainly not less than 20 to 25 per cent.

Prognosis

As with cancer in other sites this depends mainly on the lymphatic involvement at the time of resection and the histology of the growth. When no glands are involved over 60 per cent. are alive five years after the operation and nearly 60 per cent. are alive ten years after. When the glands are involved only 21 per cent. survive five years (Colcock, 1951).

The sharp difference in prognosis between the late and early case, and the really terrifying rise in mortality once acute obstruction has supervened, make it essential that elderly patients with vague bowel symptoms should always be investigated.

E. G. MUIR

References

AULT, G. W., CASTRO, A. F., and SMITH, R. S. (1952) *Surg. Gynec. Obstet.* **94,** 223.
COLCOCK, B. P. (1951) "Surgical Practice of the Lahey Clinic." Philadelphia and London, W. B. Saunders.
DUKES, C. E. (1939) *Lancet* **ii,** 586.
DUKES, C. E. (1952) *Ann. R. Coll. Surg. Engl.* **10,** 293.
ELMAN, R., SHATZ, B. A., KEATING, R. E., and WEICHSELBAUM, T. E. (1952) *Ann. Surg.* **136,** 3.
GRINNELL, R. S., and HIATT, R. B. (1952) *Surg. Gynec. Obstet.* **94,** 526.
LOCKHART-MUMMERY, J. P. (1925) *Lancet* **i,** 427.
MORGAN, C. N. (1952) *Ann. R. Coll. Surg. Engl.* **10,** 305.
MUIR, E. G. (1947) *Proc. R. Soc. Med.* **40,** 831.
NEWELL, R. L. (1951. Quoted by Morgan, C. N. (1952).

CHAPTER X

CARCINOMA OF THE RECTUM

DURING the past decade, interest in the treatment of rectal cancer has been evinced mainly in two directions: the place of radical restorative resection and the effectiveness of the standard combined excision especially for low rectal growths.

The lymphatic drainage of that part of the rectum above the peritoneal reflection is almost entirely in an upward direction through the inferior mesenteric chain of glands. Below that level the lymph drainage is upwards but is also laterally to the internal iliac and other lymph glands on the side wall of the pelvis. These glands are not removed in the standard combined excision and Deddish (1950) has found evidence suggesting that in low rectal growths they are involved much more commonly than was supposed, for it was at one time thought that lateral spread in rectal cancer was only likely when the glands above were blocked by growth.

Dukes (1944) found venous involvement in 17 per cent. of rectal cancer and Sunderland (1949) an even higher incidence, 27·6 per cent. In the latter's series there was a definite relationship to the site of the growth, 42·6 per cent. within 6 cm. of the anus, 22·2 per cent. between 6-12 cm. and 3·5 per cent. when the growth was more than 13 cm. from the anus.

The lower rectum is much more intimately related to structures such as intrapelvic fat, fascia, muscle, other pelvic organs and the associated lymphatics than is the upper rectum in its peritoneal envelope. This fact, its lymphatic drainage and the increased frequency of venous involvement would suggest a worse prognosis and a higher local recurrence rate after combined excision for low rectal growths. This is confirmed by experience (Gilchrist and David, 1947; Waugh and Kirklin, 1949; Guernsey et al., 1951) and it is accepted by all that the proper treatment of a carcinoma in the lower rectum is the removal of the bowel, intrapelvic fat, fascia, levatores ani muscles and ischiorectal fat en bloc. The side walls of the pelvis should be stripped of fat and lymph glands and other intrapelvic organs in relationship to the growth such as the posterior vaginal wall, should be excised if practical (Knight et al., 1952; Sauer and Bacon, 1952).

These objects can only be achieved by a somewhat extended combined excision: restorative resection cannot be justified for growths in this site. The position regarding the upper rectum and rectosigmoid is

117

somewhat different. The work of Dukes (1944) and others has shown that downward lymphatic spread in the inferior mesenteric and superior hæmorrhoidal lymph paths is rare and that such spread above 5 cm. is almost confined to advanced or highly malignant growths. Since the peritonealized upper rectum has no lateral lymphatic spread it would seem that the pathological requirements of an efficient operation would be obtained if the bowel were divided more than 5 cm. below the distal level of the growth, thus permitting a radical restorative operation.

All recent work has stressed the importance of the upper lymphatic spread in rectal cancer and the removal of the para-aortic glands from the duodenum downwards is advocated by several writers. The standard site of ligature of the inferior mesenteric artery, the same both for combined operations and restorative resections, is immediately below the first sigmoid artery but recent writers have advocated ligation at the aorta in order to remove still more of the inferior mesenteric lymphatic chain.

Note

At the present time there are two operations in general use in the treatment of rectal cancer. A combined excision, whether it be abdomino-perineal, perineo-abdominal or synchronous combined, has stood the test of time and with its modifications or extensions is likely to remain the standard operation for the majority of cases. Radical restorative resection is in a sense still on trial, but many believe that it has an important part in the treatment of this disease.

The Selection of Cases for a Radical Restorative Resection

This subject has received considerable attention (Bacon, 1945; d'Allaine, 1950; Muir, 1948, 1952; Morgan and Lloyd Davies, 1950). The following would seem to be the accepted criteria:

1. The lower edge of the growth must not be less than 10 cm. from the anus and 2 in. above the lowest peritoneal reflection in the Pouch of Douglas. Growths discovered on sigmoidoscopy or just palpable on full digital rectal examination 2 in. to 3 in. above the cervix or vesicles are usually suitable, but the final decision can only be made on laparotomy.

2. Advanced growths with extrarectal spread are unsuitable and require a combined excision.

3. Growths shown on biopsy to be of high malignancy are more likely to spread widely and many hold that such cases should always be treated by a combined excision.

4. Restorative operations may be of great difficulty in an obese subject with a narrow pelvis. Even if the growth is otherwise suitable such cases may require a combined excision.

5. The rectal stump to be retained should be of sufficient size to allow proper function (Goligher, 1951) and its mucous membrane should be free of adenomata, or such adenomata should have been removed.
6. The sigmoid colon must reach the rectal stump without tension and with a good blood supply. Much can be done by mobilization of the descending colon and occasionally the splenic flexure.

It is probable that 20 per cent. to 25 per cent. of operable rectal growths are suitable for this operation.

Palliative Restorative Resection

The presence of hepatic metastases with a removable growth strongly favours a restorative resection rather than a permanent colostomy, with or without a combined excision, and the essential criteria may be somewhat relaxed in such cases. An anastomosis performed without a sufficient margin below a growth may, however, lend to local recurrence before the patient's death.

Methods of Radical Restorative Resection

There are a number of different operations but that in common use is abdominal resection and anastomosis, known as an anterior resection. For growths of the rectosigmoid and distal sigmoid loop (for which it should be used much more frequently) the rectum is divided at the level of the peritoneal reflection in the Pouch of Douglas and the anastomosis is intraperitoneal. For growths of the upper rectum the bowel is freed as fully as in a combined resection and the anastomosis performed at the lowest possible level.

A right transverse colostomy should be performed as a preliminary in all cases with evidence of obstruction, or at the conclusion of the operation if there is any doubt regarding the viability of the bowel. The antibiotic drugs are making its routine use much less common at the present time.

The Disadvantages of Radical Restorative Resection

There are a number of experienced surgeons who are strongly opposed to this operation. Their criticisms are on two main grounds Firstly, that its use in the hands of enthusiasts will lead to ineffective operations for malignant disease and, secondly, that there is a definite risk of local recurrence at the suture line. As regards the first, it may be a valid criticism but it is not a ground for condemning the operation. The second is undoubtedly correct and its occurrence is a matter of great surgical and pathological interest.

Recurrence in the Rectosigmoid Anastomosis

Local recurrence in the soft tissues of the pelvis can and does occur after combined excision for rectal cancer, particularly when it has been performed for a low growth (Gilchrist and David, 1947). A similar recurrence might take place after a restorative resection, particularly if it had been wrongly performed for a low growth and involve the anastomosis. This could be attributed to ill-judged surgery. Unfortunately a number of cases have now been recorded where recurrence has taken place in or near the anastomotic line and where extrarectal recurrence could be almost certainly excluded (Lloyd Davies, 1948; Muir, 1948, 1952; Long *et al.*, 1950; Goligher *et al.*, 1951). It is thought that these cases are due either to the stimulus of repair in the anastomotic line causing a fresh growth to arise in pre-cancerous bowel or to inplantation of cancer cells from the original growth on the raw surfaces of the anastomosis at the time of resection. Present opinion mainly favours the latter and attempts to prevent its occurrence by washing out the rectal stump during the operation after a clamp has been applied below the growth are now advised.

It will be obvious that if local recurrence at the suture line through implantation of cancer cells takes place in the operation of restorative resection it cannot be uncommon for it to occur in other anastomotic operations on the alimentary tract. Its recognition in restorative resection is not due to some peculiar fault of that operation, but to the fact that the anastomotic line can be felt and seen after the operation. Cole (1952) in a recent article urging care in the handling of a bowel growth where divided surfaces were to be exposed and sutured, considered that, of 55 cases of large bowel resection, recurrence at the suture line took place in 16 per cent. and that in 10 per cent. it might be attributed to implantation.

The Results of Restorative Resection

Dixon (1948) has published the largest series of these cases and he obtained a five-year survival rate of $67 \cdot 7$ per cent. with restorative resection as against $44 \cdot 8$ per cent. with combined excision. In a sense this is an unfair comparison for restorative resection would only be employed for the high growths and these have a better prognosis. The risk of an anastomotic recurrence, which could not take place with a combined excision, must be set against the retention of normal bowel function and the avoidance of a colostomy. It would appear that at present the anastomotic recurrence rate is in the region of 10 per cent.

E. G. Muir

References:

BACON, H. E. (1945) *Surg. Gynec. Obstet.* **81,** 113.
COLE, W. H. (1952) *Arch. Surg.* **65,** 204.
D'ALLAINE, F. (1950) *Proc. R. Soc. Med.* **43,** 697.
DEDDISH, M. R. (1950) *Proc. R. Soc. Med.* **43,** 1075.
DIXON, C. F. (1948) *Ann. Surg.* **128,** 425.
DUKES, C. E. (1944) *Proc. R. Soc. Med.* **37,** 131.
GILCHRIST, R. K., and DAVID, V. C. (1947) *Ann. Surg.* **126,** 421.
GOLIGHER, J. C. (1951) *Ann. R. Coll. Surg. Engl.* **8,** 421.
GOLIGHER, J. C., DUKES, C. E., and BUSSEY, H. J. R. (1951) *Brit. J. Surg.* **39,** 199.
GUERNSEY, D. E., WAUGH, J. M., and DOCKERTY, M. B. (1951) *Surg. Gynec. Obstet.*
    92, 529.
KNIGHT, C. D., WAUGH, J. M., and DOCKERTY, M. B. (1952) *Surg. Gynec. Obstet.*
    95, 220.
LLOYD DAVIES, O. V. (1948) *Proc. R. Soc. Med.* **41,** 822.
LONG, J. W., MAYO, C. W., DOCKERTY, M. B., and JUDD, E. S. (1950) *Proc. Mayo
    Clin.* **25,** 169.
MORGAN, C. N., and LLOYD DAVIES, O. V. (1950) *Proc. R. Soc. Med.* **43,** 701.
MUIR, E. G. (1948) *Brit. med. J.* **ii,** 286.
            (1952) "Surgical Progress," 1952. London, Butterworth & Co. Ltd.
SAUER, I., and BACON, H. E. (1952) *Surg. Gynec. Obstet.* **95,** 229.
SUNDERLAND, D. A. (1949) *Cancer* **2,** 429.
WAUGH, J. M., and KIRKLIN, J. W. (1949) *Ann. Surg.* **129,** 22.

CHAPTER XI

DIVERTICULITIS COLI

CLASSICAL descriptions of this disease have existed for many years, but it is since the beginning of the century, associated with the spread of radiology, that it has attracted increasing surgical attention. The frequency of its precursor, diverticulosis, cannot be accurately known, though it is common to find evidence of this condition in autopsies on the older age groups. One in ten persons over 40 have diverticula of the colon (Babington, 1948). Pemberton, Black and Maino (1947) reported that, of 47,000 radiological examinations of the colon performed at the Mayo Clinic diverticulosis was discovered in 8·5 per cent.: that in 600 (15 per cent.) of these there was diverticulitis of the sigmoid colon, and that 144 or 24 per cent. required surgical treatment. The average age of this group was 53·6 years but, though uncommon, diverticulitis is certainly not unknown in the younger age groups. Though it may be widespread it is typically a disease of the sigmoid, and this part of the colon was affected in 198 out of 202 cases treated surgically by Mayo and Blunt (1950). Isolated diverticula in the cæcum and elsewhere, while they may require surgery, are probably of congenital origin and not part of the disease considered here.

All writers agree that the great majority of cases of diverticulitis should receive medical treatment, and surgery is indicated for perforation, abscess and peritonitis, obstructive symptoms, fistulæ, recurrent attacks and where diagnosis is doubtful. = complications,

The Diagnosis of Diverticulitis

Both carcinoma of the colon and diverticulitis are most common in the sigmoid. There is no evidence that patients suffering from diverticulitis are more liable to develop cancer, but since the same age groups are commonly affected it is natural that they should occasionally co-exist. Since the great majority of patients with diverticulitis will receive conservative treatment, accurate diagnosis is of great importance. The usual history is of recurrent attacks of lower abdominal pain and tenderness associated with constipation, malaise and perhaps a little pyrexia. A barium enema and a sigmoidoscopy should demonstrate the diverticulitis and exclude the possibility of a growth in the upper rectum or rectosigmoid region. In the more severe cases requiring surgery the history may be short: Pemberton *et al.* (1947) found that 12 per cent. of a surgical series were operated upon within one month and 31 per cent. within six months of the onset of the disease. Evidence of inflammation, such as tenderness, fever and leucocytosis was present in 79 per cent., obstructive symptoms in 30 per cent., diarrhœa in 19 per cent., the passage of blood in 8 per cent., and in 36 per cent. a mass was palpable either on abdominal or rectal examination. In 42 per cent. a fistula was present, but this figure is exceptional and no doubt may be explained by the fact that a number of these patients had undergone preliminary operations elsewhere. A barium enema typically demonstrates the diverticula and an area of spasm, "saw-toothing" and narrowed lumen in the sigmoid colon. The appearance is not that of the "filling defect" of a carcinoma, but in some cases diagnosis may be difficult and may be assisted by repeating the enema after the use of antispasmodics such as Banthine. An early growth of the rectosigmoid region may be missed and the patient's symptoms attributed to a proved diverticulitis of the sigmoid loop. The upper rectum and rectosigmoid are difficult areas for the radiologist and for this reason sigmoidoscopy should never be omitted. The orifices of diverticula may be seen, or fixation of the bowel and an intrapelvic mass may prevent the full passage of the instrument. None of these findings exclude neoplasm. A fixed mass in the pelvis may be either diverticulitis or carcinoma, but a large fixed mass in a fit patient with some pyrexia is more likely to be the former. Pemberton *et al.* (1947) state that after a barium enema diverticulitis could be diagnosed in 66 per cent., an obstructing lesion in 22 per cent., an obstructing lesion of questionable malignant nature in 3 per cent., and a fistula of the sigmoid only in 8 per cent. They consider that in 25 per cent. of cases carcinoma could not be excluded by clinical methods of examination, and it is well known that even at operation it may not be possible for the surgeon to distinguish between carcinoma and diverticulitis.

The passage of blood occurs in a small proportion of patients with diverticulitis and may be due to ulceration or erosion of a small vessel in a diverticulum, to granulation tissue or possibly to mucosal congestion in proximity to an inflammatory mass. Bacon and Sherman (1950) report bleeding in 18 per cent. of these cases. It is probably wise to regard such cases as suspected carcinoma until this can be excluded.

Experience suggests that in the great majority diverticulitis can be diagnosed and neoplasm excluded with confidence. In some it is difficult and in a few it is quite impossible. If any doubt exists surgical treatment is indicated with removal of the affected area.

Perforation, Abscess and Peritonitis

This occurred in 35 per cent. of a series treated surgically by Morton (1946), commonly as a localized abscess, and in over 25 per cent. in that of Mayo and Blunt (1950). Where there is evidence of spreading peritonitis immediate laparotomy is required. A perforated diverticulum has occasionally been excised or the perforation oversewn, but in many cases it is not possible to do more than wrap or wall off the area of bowel in omentum and drain the pelvis. The majority of writers advocate a transverse colostomy at the same time. This should be performed on the right side so that it will interfere as little as possible with any mobilization of the left colon which may subsequently be necessary. The after treatment of these cases will be that usually adopted for peritonitis, gastric suction and intravenous fluids until bowel activity has returned and the use of antibiotics.

When a localized abscess is present drainage is required. While Grieg (1950) considers a colostomy seldom necessary it is a safety measure which many advise. The mortality of perforation and peritonitis in diverticulitis has been reported as surprisingly high, 33 per cent. (Morton, 1946), 35·5 per cent. (Babington, 1948). At the present time the mortality rate of these complications is almost certainly much lower, but many of these patients are elderly and are poor surgical risks.

When operation, performed for an acute inflammatory complication in diverticulitis, reveals a single perforated diverticulum or only a short length of sigmoid involved, it is natural that the surgeon should sometimes hope to avoid a colostomy. Pemberton *et al.* (1947) discussing the after results of closure of a perforation or excision of a diverticulum, concluded that they were unsatisfactory and unpredictable, while Morton (1946) found post-operative complications in 50 per cent.

Obstruction

Surgery was performed for obstructive symptoms in over a third of the cases reported by Mayo and Blunt (1950). Full acute obstruction is not common in diverticulitis, unless small bowel is involved in an inflammatory mass, and the obstructive symptoms frequently settle down with rest, oil enemata and antibiotics though recurrence is common. These symptoms are usually associated with an inflammatory mass in the pelvis and right transverse colostomy, as a preliminary to resection, is generally advised.

Fistulæ

These may form between the sigmoid and the bladder (vesico-colic), between the sigmoid and the skin (sigmoidocutaneous) and between the sigmoid and the small bowel (entero-colic): the first is the most common.

Vesico-colic fistula is a complication of diverticulitis which is much more common in men, since in the male the sigmoid loop lies in close contact with the bladder. In a series of 32 patients described by Mayfield and Waugh (1949) 28 were men. The symptoms are those of a urinary infection, often with pneumaturia and the passage of fæces in the urine. Cystoscopy may clearly show the fistulous track or a localized area of cystitis and in some cases a barium enema will enter the bladder. The complication is a serious one and rightly regarded as an indication for surgery, but patients are occasionally found with a vesico-colic fistula living with minimal disability. The most satisfactory treatment for vesico-colic fistula is resection of the affected segment of the colon though colostomy alone usually produces great improvement and should be the first step towards a resection.

A fæcal fistula between the sigmoid and the skin (sigmoidocutaneous) usually occurs after an operation for an acute inflammatory complication of diverticulitis such as abscess or peritonitis. Some of these heal spontaneously in time, particularly if a proximal colostomy is performed. They are best treated by resection preceded by colostomy.

Entero-colic fistula is uncommon but was present in five out of 198 cases of sigmoid diverticulitis treated surgically by Mayo and Blunt (1950). It requires the same treatment.

Recurrent Diverticulitis

Repeated inflammatory "episodes" in diverticulitis, not sufficiently severe to warrant emergency surgery, without fistulæ but producing recurrent invalidism and ill-health, present a problem on which there can be no universal rule. Much must depend on the patient. A good surgical risk whose living is threatened by his disability should receive radical surgery: a stout, elderly lady with chronic bronchitis should persevere with medical measures. Radiological evidence of extensive disease; barium, not in a diverticulum, seen after evacuation outside the normal bowel outline and suggesting a pericolic abscess, are indications that conservative treatment is not likely to be successful. It is an individual problem and in assessing the case due consideration must be given to the fact that it is not a malignant disease, that future complications may make surgery more difficult, that colostomy once performed may be permanent and that the antibiotics have done much to lessen the risks of radical surgery in this condition.

Colostomy

Colostomy, performed in a normal proximal area of colon usually leads to a considerable improvement in the inflammatory changes in diverticulitis. A right transverse colostomy is the most useful and is usually performed for the complications already discussed or as a preliminary to resection. While of great benefit, it does not bring the inflammatory changes of diverticulitis to an abrupt halt. Of 27 patients in whom colostomy alone had been performed and where sufficient time had elapsed to evaluate the results, 2 patients still had vesico-colic fistulas and residual symptoms, 19, including 2 other vesico-colic fistulas, considered themselves cured, and 6 patients eventually died of complications from diverticulitis (Pemberton *et al.*, 1947).

Evidence suggests that the closure of a colostomy, without resection of the affected bowel, is not devoid of risk even when a considerable time has elapsed. Of 29 patients treated in this way and subsequently followed up, 9 were well and 20 had serious recurrent symptoms (Pemberton *et al.*, 1947).

A colostomy alone is a valuable measure in diverticulitis and the diversion of the fæcal stream leads to a cessation of symptoms in some two-thirds of the cases. In the remaining third residual symptoms persist or death eventually occurs from the complications of the disease and the mortality is between 20 to 25 per cent. When a colostomy is used and subsequently closed without resection of the diverticulitis, two-thirds of the patients suffer from serious recurrent symptoms.

Resection in Diverticulitis

For many years this was regarded as a hazardous proceeding for the extensive area of sigmoid involved made restoration of continuity difficult and the inflamed bowel, fibrosed and laden with fat was unpleasant to handle. In the past resection tended to be reserved for those patients whose symptoms continued after colostomy and bowel anastomosis was seldom attempted. The present aim is the resection of the affected bowel and the restoration of continuity.

When colostomy has been required for complications in diverticulitis it is considered wise to wait some six months before attempting resection, thus allowing the inflammatory process time to subside. If colostomy has not already been required it should be used as a preliminary to resection if there is evidence of obstruction, fistulæ or an intrapelvic mass. In cases not so affected primary resection and anastomosis may be considered. The proper requirements preliminary to such an operation on large bowel are that it should be empty and clean, that its contents should be as sterile as possible, that the patient's state of nourishment, blood and fluid balance should be satisfactory and potential infection should be avoided by chemotherapy. At the present time these conditions should be obtainable in many patients.

Resection in diverticulitis is best performed through a long left paramedian or transrectal incision stretching from the pubes to well above the umbilicus. This is necessary in case the splenic flexure requires mobilization. The affected sigmoid is usually adherent and may require separation from the bladder, small intestine and almost every other organ in its neighbourhood. It may be "frozen" to the side walls of the pelvis and adherent to the ureter: in such cases the separation may be easier if ureteric catheters have been passed (Lloyd Davies, 1952). Though it may be involved in the mass, it is rare for the rectum to be directly affected in diverticulitis and the lowest limit of the bowel resection can usually be made in the rectosigmoid region. The upper limit depends on the extent of bowel involved: it may be easy to restore continuity by end to end anastomosis between the left iliac colon and the rectosigmoid: it may be necessary to mobilize and bring down the splenic flexure and in some cases with a short transverse colon it may be impossible to restore the continuity of the large bowel. In such cases a "transplant" of terminal ileum with its blood supply preserved has sometimes been used successfully to bridge the gap. Preoperative X-rays will give an assessment of the length of large bowel available and the difficulties to be expected. After continuity has been restored the anastomotic site may be extraperitonealized with the peritoneum in the lateral peritoneal gutter and drainage made to the site. If doubt exists about the security of the anastomosis a right transverse colostomy is performed at the conclusion of the operation. As an alternative to end-to-end anastomosis an exteriorization operation may be performed.

The advances in chemotherapy have greatly reduced the mortality of resection in this disease. Pemberton *et al.* (1947) comparing a series of cases treated before and after 1940 found a decrease in the mortality rate from 16 per cent. to 2·7 per cent., and, at the same time, an increase in the resectability rate from 60 per cent. to 77 per cent.

When urgent surgery is required in diverticulitis, drainage and a right transverse colostomy are usually performed. After some months, when diversion of the fæcal stream has produced improvement in the local inflammatory condition, resection of the affected sigmoid with restoration of continuity should be performed in all patients who can be regarded as reasonable risks, followed by closure of the colostomy. When recurrent diverticulitis is a cause of ill-health in an otherwise fit patient careful pre-operative treatment may allow a primary resection and anastomosis; in other cases a preliminary colostomy should be followed by resection-anastomosis at a later date. The after results of resection are claimed to be extremely good and it is indeed the only treatment that holds out a good chance of permanent cure.

E. G. MUIR

References

BABINGTON, S. H. (1948) *J. int. Coll. Surg.* **11,** 504.
BACON, H. E., and SHERMAN, L. F. (1950) *Amer. J. Surg.* **80,** 3.
GRIEG, G. W. V. (1950) *Proc. R. Soc. Med.* **43,** 1068.
LLOYD DAVIES, O. V. (1952). Awaiting publication.
MAYFIELD, L. H., and WAUGH, J. M. (1949) *Ann. Surg.* **130,** 186.
MAYO, C. W., and BLUNT, C. P. (1950) *Surg. Clin. N. Amer.* **30,** 1005.
MORTON, J. J. (1946) *Ann. Surg.* **124,** 725.
PEMBERTON, J. DE J., BLACK, B. M., and MAINO, C. R. (1947) *Surg. Gynec. Obstet.* **85,** 523.

CHAPTER XII

GENERAL PERITONITIS

THE last twenty years have witnessed a reduction in the mortality of general peritonitis from the region of 25 per cent. to less than 10 per cent. The condition, however, remains one of the gravest of acute abdominal emergencies and the current mortality still presents a challenge to further improvement in which all the resources of modern surgery must play their part. One of the prime functions of the surgeon is to let out pus but in the treatment of general infection of the peritoneal cavity, this is neither entirely possible nor adequate owing to its complex anatomical arrangement and to an absorbing area approximately equivalent to the whole surface area of the skin. General peritonitis kills by bacterial toxaemia and from biochemical changes associated with small bowel obstruction and it is attention to these factors, as well as to actual operative details, which has so greatly improved the outlook in this condition.

Mortality from General Peritonitis

	Year	No. of Cases	Mortality
Hunter	1927	62	17·7%
Reid, Poer and Merrell	1936	280	33%
Grey Turner	1938	96	29·2%
Young and Russell	1939	332	19-24%
Corry, Brewer and Nicol	1939	26	11·5%
Vaughan Hudson and Rodney Smith	1942	24	8·3%
Gardiner	1942	47	2·1%
Crile	1946	50	2%
Moloney, Russell and Wilson	1950	97	6·2%
Gilmour and Lowdon	1952	35	11·4%
Wright, Schreiber, Metzger and Parker	1952	235	7·69%

Natural History of General Peritonitis

In the vast proportion of cases, general peritonitis is due to perforation of a hollow viscus due either to disease, trauma or operative surgery. Less commonly, infection may enter through the genital passages or via the blood stream as in so called primary peritonitis such as streptococcal, pneumococcal and gonococcal peritonitis. Leakage of normal body fluids into the peritoneal cavity, such as blood, urine, bile, gastric juice or pancreatic juice, even though initially sterile, will inevitably result in infection of the inflammatory exudate with intestinal organisms and a secondary peritonitis will result. In many instances the body defences are able to localize these infections but on other occasions the normal mechanisms are overwhelmed and a general peritoneal infection ensues.

The natural history of general peritonitis is one with which everyone is familiar, though many of its features are masked or complicated by modern treatment. The onset of general peritonitis, whether gradual or sudden, is characterized by generalized abdominal pain which is practically always associated with vomiting. Signs of peritonism are manifest and the pulse and temperature start to rise. It is sometimes taught that abdominal pain and a temperature of over 102° F. in the first 24 hours is seldom due to an intra-peritoneal lesion but in children especially, a fulminating acute appendicitis with general peritonitis can, nevertheless, give rise to a high temperature at an early stage. Less frequently, diarrhœa or urinary symptoms may result from the peritoneal irritation and confuse the diagnosis. Within the first 24 hours the peritoneal cavity is bathed in a thin, turbid pus and an inhibitory ileus, essentially a beneficent defence mechanism, results in a silent abdomen. This is one of the most significant physical signs in the diagnosis of general peritonitis. Hyperæmia and œdema of the bowel wall and of the serous and subserous layers of the peritoneal cavity occurs as in other inflammatory conditions with the outpouring of a fibrinous, buttery exudate which glues together the paralysed loops of bowel. At this stage the initial rigidity or guarding of the abdominal wall, gives way to progressive distension. The small bowel dilates with gas and fluid, vomiting increases and the frequent effortless regurgitation of yellow fluid soon becomes brown and fæcular. The soggy and dilated loops of gut, heavy with fluid, have lost their power to contract either from over distension or perhaps from paralysis of Auerbach and Meissner's plexus and are now the site of a true paralytic ileus. X-ray pictures taken in the erect position will show dilated loops and fluid levels indistinguishable from those found in mechanical obstruction. Loss of electrolytes and fluid from vomiting causes a coincident reduction in blood volume and hæmo-concentration, while exudation from the peritoneal surface and into the gut results in a reduction of the total circulating protein, especially of albumen. Estimation of the plasma protein at this juncture will, however, give normal figures, since the fall is masked by the hæmo-concentration. Secondary oliguria and nitrogen retention adds still further to the biochemical disturbance. In his final hours, the anxious and exhausted patient lies motionless. The vomiting becomes less for he is too weary. The classical Hippocratic facies with sunken grey features and bright eyes, the cold clammy skin, the falling temperature and the rapid running pulse betoken the fatal peripheral circulatory failure. Overwhelmed by toxæmia, from bacterial absorption and biochemical upset, the patient succumbs to his disease.

Less dramatic, but no less fatal, is post-operative peritonitis. Insidious in onset the initial physical signs are often absent. Indeed a vague uneasiness that the patient is not doing as well as one would like and failure of the pulse and temperature to fall in the normal way may be the only suggestive signs. Vomiting and distension may only occur shortly before death. Such patients may come to post mortem without peritonitis even having been suspected as a cause of death. The patient who survives the early days of his infection runs the risk of residual abscesses in the usual situations, but more lethal is the combination of localized infection often in multiple pockets with mechanical ileus. This condition is possibly more frequent than in former days, for more survive the initial peritonitis and there are, therefore, more patients in whom residual abscesses may form. This combination of infection and mechanical obstruction presents a dilemma where one would prefer to treat a localized infection conservatively in the hope that it will be dealt with by the defences of the body, but where surgical measures may be demanded to relieve the mechanical obstruction. It is in these cases that the use of the Miller-Abbott tube can be most profitably employed.

Treatment

As in a steeplechase the treatment of general peritonitis involves a number of obstacles, each of which must be successfully cleared in order to complete the course. These consist of:

1. Pre-operative preparation.
2. The actual operation.
3. Control of infection.
4. Fluid and electrolyte balance.
5. General post-operative management.

Pre-operative Preparation

There are few occasions when a diagnosis of general peritonitis is in doubt and in those where doubt exists, the old adage of "look and see" is still the right policy. Temporization in such cases with antibiotics and supportive measures is not only unwise but negligent. There are certain exceptions where conservative treatment is advised, at least temporarily, but even with these, differences of opinion with regard to non-operative treatment exist. These exceptions are:

1. General peritonitis resulting from pelvic infections in women.
2. Appendix abscesses which are well localized.
3. Acute pancreatitis where the diagnosis is established with certainty.
4. Some cases of perforated peptic ulcer in poor risk patients.
5. Moribund patients where operation would obviously be fatal.

These patients should be treated along the general lines to be discussed later, with the proviso that if they do not improve rapidly on palliative measures, operation should be reconsidered. The history of the patient will usually offer a reasonable clue as to the origin of the infection, but where no obvious cause is manifest, one should not too lightly assume that the infection is primary or blood borne, for this is exceedingly rare in practice. Such primary peritonitis may, no doubt, be treated conservatively provided that this condition is diagnosed, but one can never be entirely sure that it is indeed primary. Once having decided upon operation, there is no reason for delay unless the patient is exhausted, collapsed or very toxic. Under these conditions two or three hours for resuscitation is time well spent when intravenous fluids can be administered, the stomach can be aspirated and the patient rested with morphine. One of the most important parts of the pre-operative preparation is the passage of a large stomach tube immediately prior to the induction of the anæsthetic in all patients who have vomited or who felt nauseated. Although this may seem a somewhat barbarous action on an ill patient, it is in fact life saving in preventing the inhalation of regurgitated vomit during the induction of anæsthesia. Even this may not be entirely adequate to remove solid food particles and as a further safeguard, an inflatable cuff should be used round the intratracheal tube.

The Operation

Regarding the choice of anæsthetic, the skill and experience of the anæsthetist are of more importance than the actual anæsthetic agent used, provided a smooth induction and complete relaxation are ensured for the operation. The reason for operation in cases of general peritonitis is to remove the cause, and in doubtful cases to make sure of the diagnosis. Where the cause is unequivocally the appendix, a McBurney incision will suffice but in all other cases a generous paramedian incision is required, above or below the umbilicus depending on the suspected site of the primary lesion and a para-umbilical incision in doubtful cases which can be extended later up or down as required. As soon as the peritoneum is opened, a swab of the pus should be taken for culture and for determination of the antibiotic sensitivities of the organisms for future use. In the early hours of the infection such pus may often be found to be sterile, and if so an easier convalescence and better prognosis can be predicted. The free pus in the peritoneal cavity should now be sucked out. During this procedure some indication will be given of the site of the primary lesion for there it is usual to find the fibrinous exudate most noticeable. The peritoneal cavity is rapidly and gently explored without exteriorization of more bowel than is absolutely necessary. Once discovered, the site of the primary lesion is carefully walled off with packs. Perforations are closed and infected and gangrenous viscera are dealt with in the accepted manner, limiting oneself, however, to the strict essentials necessary for the patient's recovery. Pelvic infection, if not previously diagnosed and discovered at operation, is best left except for the occasional removal of an advanced pyosalpinx or leaking tubo-ovarian abscess if this is practicable, provided there is no evidence of the condition being tuberculous, for it is in these that post-operative sinuses and fistulæ may develop. A final toilet of the peritoneum is then carried out, removing free food particles, fæcoliths and pus by gentle mopping and suction especially from the pelvis and Rutherford Morrison's pouch. Despite antibiotics, abdominal incisions in cases of general peritonitis are liable to infection with subsequent breakdown or wound dehiscence and especial care should be exercised in closure, using many interrupted sutures in addition to the continuous layers. Catgut is preferable to non-absorbable sutures but where the latter, for example nylon, are used, these should be interrupted rather than continuous stitches. Where the primary source of infection is not readily found during the first few minutes of the examination, it is expedient to enlarge the incision and to work methodically through the viscera, paying especial attention to the lesser curvature of the stomach for small leaking ulcers, and working successively through all the loops of the large and small bowel for perforations which might have been due to foreign bodies, diverticula, growths, etc. If, after an adequate and orderly examination of all the peritoneal contents no primary lesion can be discovered, the peritoneal cavity is sucked out and the abdomen closed in the usual way.

Drainage

Drainage of the peritoneal cavity is performed less frequently than formerly for it is now recognized that in most cases the peritoneum can well look after itself provided no continuous leak occurs. It was shown many years ago that it was impossible to drain the peritoneal cavity for longer than four to six hours, for the drain rapidly becomes walled off in its own track. Exceptions exist, however, and drainage should be provided in the following circumstances:

1. Localized abscess, e.g. appendiceal, pelvic and sub-phrenic abscesses.
2. Where there is doubt about a suture line remaining intact.
3. Where there is excessive oozing of blood following the intra-abdominal manipulations.

Except in the case of localized abscesses, such drains should generally be removed within two to four days, the track so formed allowing for the discharge of any accumulation of pus which might occur at a later date. Compared with intraperitoneal drainage, drainage of the abdominal wall should be performed more often to minimize the effect of infection of the abdominal incision, especially in obese patients. A soft corrugated rubber or Penrose drain should be inserted into the superficial layers of the wound and brought out through one end of the incision.

Control of Infection

The discovery of the sulphonamides opened a new chapter in the treatment of general peritonitis and many early communications indicated the great improvement in results using either parenteral or intraperitoneal sulphonamides or both. Indeed, some observers maintain that the results of sulphonamide therapy have not been surpassed by antibiotics. The clinical assessment of the value of chemotherapeutic drugs and of the antibiotics is exceedingly difficult, for this treatment was introduced very much at the same time as the use of gastric suction and intravenous fluid therapy and the mortality of general peritonitis has fallen continuously ever since. Both treatments are obviously of paramount importance but which has caused the greatest reduction in mortality it is hard to say. On the other hand, a great deal of work has been done on experimental peritonitis treated with nothing except antibiotics and this gives some indication of the relative value of these different drugs. The subject is complicated by the frequent production of new preparations which are extolled before the proper clinical use of the last has been evaluated. In 1936, Domagk demonstrated the value of sulphonamides in peritoneal infection in mice and the original work of Whitby (1938) investigating new forms of sulphonamide proved the value of sulphapyridine in experimental pneumococcal peritonitis in mice. In 1936 Corry, Brewer and Nicol reported a mortality of 11·5 per cent. in 26 cases of general peritonitis treated with Soluseptasine (Sulphasolucine) and Proseptasine (Benzyl Sulphanilamide) given in relatively small doses intramuscularly. In 1942 Hudson and

Smith considered that intraperitoneal sulphanilamide was an extremely valuable method and one preferable to oral administration. They reported a fall in mortality of general peritonitis and peritoneal contamination from 55·5 per cent. to 8·3 per cent. Gardiner in 1944 also advised intraperitoneal sulphapyridine in that this method gave a slow absorption and a 75-100 times greater local concentration than when given orally. The pendulum has, however, swung away in recent years from the use of intraperitoneal sulphonamides despite these good authorities for it has been shown that the drug is not well absorbed from the inflamed peritoneal cavity and that it is inactive in the presence of pus. The less soluble forms may cake and act as foreign bodies and there is a real danger of adhesions due to the drug. Occasional cases of infection have been reported due to the powder itself which should, of course, be sterilized. One further reason for giving up intraperitoneal sulphonamide is that the improved mortality has been maintained when the drug is given orally or by injection so that these remain the standard methods of administration. The advent of antibiotics at this time diverted the limelight from chemotherapy and indeed continues to do so, but it must not be forgotten that the great improvement in mortality in general peritonitis did originate with the sulphonamides. Crile in 1946 showed a mortality of 2 per cent. in 50 cases of general peritonitis due to appendicitis treated with penicillin. The fact that penicillin can be destroyed by Bact. coli, the commonest organism isolated in general peritonitis, does not detract from its usefulness. Penicillin in the large doses in which it is given may well be bacteriostatic for Bact. coli as well as for the gram positive organisms found in peritonitis, for example Streptococcus faecalis. In addition, the lower mortality is due in some degree to the reduction by penicillin of the chest complications which so often occur with general peritonitis. If sulphonamides and penicillin are of proved, if limited value, streptomycin, as might be expected from its wider bacterial spectrum, is likely to be still more effective, and this has been confirmed by experimental work. Murphy and Ravdin in 1946 and Yeager and his associates in 1949, both producing experimental appendicitis and general peritonitis by a standard technique in dogs showed a 60 per cent. survival of dogs treated with streptomycin alone as against a 70-80 per cent. mortality in the control series. Streptomycin is excreted more slowly than penicillin and may attain a higher concentration in the peritoneal fluid than in the blood which is obviously a very valuable attribute in this condition. It is impossible at the present time to assess the value of chloramphenicol, aureomycin and terramycin in the treatment of general peritonitis. Aureomycin has been favourably reported on by Wright *et al.* (1951) who in 250 cases of general peritonitis noted an overall mortality of 7·69 per cent. and an "antibiotic" mortality of 3·04 per cent., the latter figure referring to those cases where no factor outside the control of the antibiotic was a cause of death. An unpleasant complication of the present preparations of aureomycin for intravenous use is the high incidence of thrombo-phlebitis. Pulaski, Artz and Reiss have used terramycin successfully in 52 out of 56 cases of peritonitis due to appendicitis and penetrating gun-shot wounds of the abdomen. Chloromycetin has not been used extensively in the treatment of general peritonitis for it is not easily given parenterally, and the slight but definite risk of aplastic anæmia following its prolonged use contra-indicates it if other effective preparations are available. One has only to consider the variety of organisms which may be found in cases of general peritonitis to realize that their sensitivities to chemotherapy and antibiotics vary not only for different strains but that any one strain may rapidly become resistant. Under such circumstances at the present stage of knowledge no one agent is likely to be effective in all cases or if effective at the start to remain so for long. For this reason a blunderbuss treatment is rational and one commonly prescribed at the present time consists of a combination of the following drugs:

Sulphamezathine (Sulphadimidine B.P.) 1 gm. of the soluble solution is given by injection immediately after operation and repeated at six to eight hourly intervals until the patient can take the drug by mouth when it is continued at the same dosage.

Penicillin, $\frac{1}{2}$-1 megaunit twice a day by injection.

Streptomycin, $\frac{1}{2}$ gm. twice a day by injection.

This course is started at once in all cases of general peritonitis since the exhibition of these drugs is most valuable in the early stages of the disease and should continue for a period of five days. In certain cases after they are discontinued, the temperature may rise and the local signs of residual infection become manifest, the general effects of the infection having been temporarily masked. Although these must be watched for, it is of no disadvantage for the most dangerous period of the peritoneal infection has been tided over and the management of such residual abscesses presents little of the hazard and urgency compared with generalized peritonitis. It is highly likely that with the introduction of new antibiotics, the plan of treatment outlined above will become outmoded before many years have passed, but while others are being proved, this plan is giving a good measure of success. The incidence of residual abscesses is probably higher since the introduction of chemotherapy since more of the seriously ill patients are saved to develop this complication. Where such abscesses are diagnosed in the post-operative period and the general condition of the patient is not giving rise to anxiety, further chemotherapy and antibiotics are not usually advised. Such abscesses are well walled off and the drugs are not able to penetrate or affect the purulent collection already present. If given, chemotherapy tends to delay their discharge and prolong the illness. The patients should be watched carefully until a fall of temperature indicates the evacuation of the abscess or until local signs call for further surgery.

Fluid and Electrolyte Balance

The maintenance of a normal biochemical background for the patient, despite all the changes resulting from bacterial toxæmia and paralytic ileus is the goal to which one aspires but it is one whose complexities are only just beginning to be unravelled, let alone treated. The fluid requirements of the body, the normal metabolic reaction of the patient undergoing surgery or trauma, the shifts of ions between the cells and fluids of the body, the selective secretory activities of the kidney, the relative losses of certain known ions from the secretions of the body are but a few of the factors, many of which can be determined only with considerable difficulty which must be considered before rational intravenous therapy can be instituted. The writing of an elegant prescription in the old days was a simple pastime compared with the prescribing of the water, electrolytes and protein to be administered to a patient who is desperately ill with general peritonitis. It is emphasized that correction of deficits of water, sodium, potassium, chlorides, protein and calories which are the basic substances we have available for intravenous use, should not be thought of as separate items but collectively as part of a general scheme to correct a disordered metabolism. The use of these substances is probably responsible for saving more lives than any others, but even to-day, many patients suffering from general peritonitis will recover without their aid. A watchful eye during the first 24 post-operative hours in the less seriously ill patients will generally determine whether oral or rectal administration of fluids will be sufficient for the patient's recovery. Before attempting to correct deficiencies due to disease or inadequate treatment, it is essential to be acquainted, in terms of biochemistry, with the normal response of the body, to disease, trauma typified by surgery and to starvation which usually accompanies major surgery. Moore and his associates (1951), by detailed analysis of such cases, have advanced and correlated much of the information pertaining to this new dimension in surgical care.

Much of the matter presented below is taken from their monograph in which, however, the authors are at pains to emphasize that the complicated metabolic balances there described are to discover basic constants so that effective care can be given without carrying out a research project on each patient. Before proceeding, it may be useful to define some of the terms in current use and to give the normal figures found in the relevant laboratory investigations. It is more useful to work with milliequivalents per litre than milligrammes per 100 ml. for the former gives at once the relative losses and gains of acid and basic ions. To convert mgm. per 100 ml. to mEq. per litre the following formula should be used:

$$\frac{\text{Mgm. per 100 ml.} \times 10 \times \text{valency of element}}{\text{Atomic weight of element}} = \text{m.Eq. per litre.}$$

Thus 1 m.Eq. of sodium is 23 mgm. of potassium 39 mgm. and of chloride, as sodium chloride, is 58·5 mgm. per litre of fluid.

Normal Blood Figures:

	Mgm. *per* 100 *ml.*	m.Eq. *per litre*
Blood Urea	20-40	
Sodium	310-350	135-150
Potassium	16-20	4·0-5·0
Chloride expressed as NaCl . .	560-615	96-105
Alkali Reserve	53-70 vols. per 100 ml.	24-31
Plasma Protein	6·3-8·0 gm. per 100 ml.	

After any trauma, disease or operation, whether great or small, a metabolic response of varying degree will occur, consisting of the following changes:

1. A temporary elevation of temperature and pulse.
2. A retention of sodium chloride and water.
3. A loss of nitrogen.
4. A loss of potassium.

In an uncomplicated convalescence, provided no extra-renal loss of ions is occurring in the immediate post-operative days, these alterations from normal usually adjust themselves within 2-5 days and in themselves need no treatment. Generally speaking, it is only when the illness if prolonged beyond three days or when complications occur, that special measures need to be taken to replace the lost ions. In general peritonitis such extra-renal losses may occur immediately post-operatively from vomiting, gastric suction, from secretion into the intestinal canal and later from excessive diarrhœa, resulting in undue loss of sodium, potassium and chloride, when the blood figures for these electrolytes may fall well below the normal. For this reason the immediate control of the electrolyte and fluid balance is necessary in patients suffering from general peritonitis, and this should continue throughout the whole period of treatment. Such control is most satisfactorily maintained under ideal conditions when the clinician can call on the help and collaboration of his biochemical colleagues. The estimation of blood electrolytes gives the most accurate information available as to what is happening to the metabolism of the patient, but the interpretation of the results and their translation into intravenous therapy is not always an easy matter. Such biochemical information should be closely correlated with the clinical condition of the patient, for it is possible for the blood figures on occasion to remain normal in the early stages of the disease and yet fail to indicate the total loss of various ions from the body, particularly potassium. Much useful information may be gained from an accurately kept fluid balance chart by which one may estimate what losses are occurring and approximately what ions and fluid should be replaced. Especially where no biochemical facilities are available such observations will be of inestimable value in the management of these cases (see tables below). Potassium loss is not easily detectable clinically though lassitude, and muscle weakness may be noticed and there may be characteristic changes in the electro-cardiogram both with deficiency and intoxication. In addition the Fantus test (1936) for estimating urinary chlorides is a useful approximation which may help in regulating therapy provided that its limitations are recognized. A urinary chloride excretion of 5 grammes or more per litre generally signifies that the patient is not salt deficient provided that he is not being infused with saline at the time. In practice, however, there are few patients with general peritonitis who are likely to escape such an infusion which lessens the clinical value of the test considerably. Unfortunately, too, the test does not necessarily reflect the level of Sodium in the body and, as has been pointed out by Taylor (1951) the use of the test may lead to errors in the hands of inexperienced persons. A urinary chloride below 3 grammes per litre is, however, as a general rule a red light which should call for active steps and a full blood chemistry if it is at all feasible.

Extra-renal Potassium Losses

Gastric Juice
High free acid: $0 \cdot 5$-$20 \cdot 0$ m.Eq. per litre.
Low free acid: $15 \cdot 0$-$35 \cdot 0$ m.Eq. per litre.

Bile
> 3·0-15·0 m.Eq. per litre.

Miller-Abbott Tube Drainage (Non-obstructed bowel)
> 2·0-12.0 m.Eq. per litre.

Ileostomy
> 5·0-15·0 m.Eq. per litre (may be higher during period of ileostomy diarrhœa).

Diarrhœal Stools
> 15-70 m.Eq. per day (the larger figure in profuse diarrhœa).

Formed Fœces
> 10 m.Eq. per day or less.

Purulent Discharge
> 10-40 m.Eq. per day, the larger figure in extensive burns.

Extra-renal Sodium Losses

Gastric Juice
> High free acid: 5-25 m.Eq. per litre.
> Low free acid: 20-120 m.Eq. per litre (note the extreme values sometimes found in anacidic gastric juice).

Bile
> 130-165 m.Eq. per litre.
> 40-75 m.Eq. per litre (higher in the profuse discharge).

Miller-Abbott Tube Drainage (Non-obstructed bowel)
> 80-130 m.Eq. per litre.

Ileostomy

Diarrhœal Stools
> 150-350 m.Eq. per day.

Formed Fœces
> Less than 10 m.Eq. per day.
> > (Moore and Ball.)

There is good experimental and clinical evidence that chloride and potassium deficiencies in the plasma may well play an important part in the production of paralytic ileus (Marriott, 1947; Streeten, 1950; Streeten and McQuaid, 1952) and these ions should be replaced as far as possible in the prevention and treatment of paralytic ileus. Since it has been shown that sodium is retained in the immediate post-operative period, the infusion of large quantities of sodium chloride intravenously may actually be deleterious, leading to hypernatræmia, hyperchloræmia, œdema and hypoproteinæmia and an increasing potassium loss via the kidney. Indeed it may be impossible to correct chloride deficiency unless any deficiency of potassium is made good at the same time. Potassium is most easily and safely replaced by mouth in the form of potassium citrate mixture, but unfortunately this is not feasible in a patient with paralytic ileus. It should also be remembered that since potassium is normally excreted by the kidney, it should never be administered where there is oliguria or anuria without strict bio chemical control. On account of the complexities of these electrolytic balances, some simple rule of thumb methods are necessary for prescribing intravenous therapy in the average case of general peritonitis. The principles in giving such fluids are three: to make up past deficits, to maintain the patient, and to replace abnormal losses. For the average adult, depending on his size, age and cardiac condition, a basic daily intake of four to five pints of intravenous fluid should be given. This should consist of one pint of Ringer's solution or normal saline to cover approximately such salt losses as occur into the urine and the bowel, the remaining volume being made up of 5 per cent. glucose solution. In addition to this, every pint of vomit or gastric secretion aspirated should be made good daily by an equivalent volume of Ringer's solution or normal saline. If, at the end of three days, the patient is obviously doing well, the gastric aspirations are minimal and bowel sounds are heard, the patient will have begun to absorb the fluid taken by mouth and the remaining deficiencies of electrolytes will shortly be made good without recourse to any special measures. If, however, at the end of three days, the progress of the patient is not satisfactory and if large gastric aspirations indicate a paralytic ileus, it is essential to continue with the intravenous therapy as before, and in addition to replace the potassium, the depletion of which at this period, will be approximately equivalent to some 3-12 grammes. The potassium may be administered as Darrow's solution (NaCl 6 grammes and KCl $2 \cdot 7$ grammes per litre) two or more pints daily or 40 m.Eq. (approximately 3 grammes) of potassium chloride should be added to a litre of saline or glucose twice a day. The solutions should be administered slowly. Ringer's solution alone contains too little potassium to be effective with this degree of potassium deficiency. The progress of the patient should be controlled by biochemical estimation until such time as the intravenous therapy is discontinued and the patient can take fluids by mouth. An alternative and simple method of dealing with potassium and salt losses has been devised by Cooke and Crowley (1952) who have prepared two solutions to match the electrolyte composition of fluids aspirated or lost from the stomach or intestine. Which solution is used is determined by the surgeon on the basis of the position of the drainage tube and type of drainage. They are given in amounts equivalent to the aspirate so that severe depletion is prevented from the start, the solutions being in addition to those used for maintenance therapy. Rob (1946) has drawn attention to the loss of protein which occurs in general peritonitis, and he recommends that every case whose peritonitis is so bad that an intravenous infusion is necessary, should be given plasma as a prophylactic against peripheral circulatory failure. Though it is difficult to raise the plasma protein level by intravenous plasma especially in the immediate post-operative days, there is no question that it is an exceedingly useful measure and that many moribund patients who would not otherwise survive may be saved by this means. Although theoretically the starvation phase of seriously ill patients should not extend beyond five days without providing an adequate calorie intake, about 2,500 daily, in practice this is by no means easy for the patient who depends entirely on the intravenous route for nutrition. Rice and his associates (1952) have, however, prepared a solution for intravenous use containing 1,000 calories per litre which has given excellent results in 109 patients without undesirable reaction, and it is hoped that this may be useful in long and complicated illnesses.

General Management

As may be surmised from the previous paragraphs, modern treatment is apt to be formidable and indeed alarming to the bewildered patient waking from his anæsthetic surrounded by tubes and assailed by injections. Encouragement and explanation will do much to carry the patient through his ordeal for a great deal of the ancillary treatment is more distressing to him than the discomfort of his operation wound. The following points are worthy of consideration in treating the patient during the post-operative period.

Sedation. As soon as the patient is well round from the anæsthetic and able to cough effectively, an injection of morphine should be given. This may be repeated once, but it has been suggested from experimental work by Vaughan Williams and Streeten (1950, 1951) that repeated injections of morphine are likely to prevent the return of normal intestinal propulsion and may actually cause tonic contraction of the intestine. Amidone and pethidine have little effect on intestinal motility, and it is recommended that after the first twelve hours or so these drugs should be used as analgesics.

Position and Mobility. Although doubt has been cast by Spalding (1946) on the value of Fowler's position in protecting the patient from subphrenic abscess, the more important feature has emerged that the patient should be allowed to lie in whatever position is most comfortable, provided that frequent movement and change of position is ensured so that the lung bases are not immobile nor the veins of the calf stagnant. Regular breathing exercises under the supervision of a physiotherapist or nurse do much to reduce the incidence of pulmonary complications which were so commonly found with peritonitis.

Gastric Suction. It is customary for a large stomach tube to be used during the actual operation but as soon as possible afterwards, this should be replaced by an intranasal tube of smaller calibre—a Ryle's or duodenal tube being customary. It is debatable whether stomach suction is adequate or whether one of the longer intestinal tubes (Miller and Abbott, 1934; Harris, 1945; Cantor, 1946) is not more efficacious in relieving distension. The great majority of patients are afforded symptomatic relief from vomiting and distension by a Ryle's tube. The Miller-Abbott tubes should be reserved for those cases where great distension of small bowel is found at the time of the operation and for mechanical post-operative obstruction. This complication is by no means uncommon during the convalescent period. The adherent and distended loops tend to kink and where in addition the contractile power is poor, mechanical obstruction may easily occur. The aspiration from gastric or intestinal tubes may be intermittent or continuous. Continuous suction should be changed to intermittent as soon as the colour of the aspirate returns to normal and the usual hourly interval between aspirations should be prolonged to two and then four hours as soon as there is evidence that intestinal movements are returning. The patient is, of course, allowed small drinks during the period of gastric suction and these need not necessarily be of water. Bovril, weak tea or lime juice are more appetising.

Intravenous Therapy. Intravenous therapy has become so widely used that there is a tendency to regard its technical management too lightly. The very high incidence of thrombo-phlebitis with the rubber tubing at present available in this country (Handfield-Jones and Lewis, 1952) is stimulating research into alternatives of which polyvinyl chloride plastic tubing is probably one of the best. Nearly half the patients who receive intravenous infusions through the standard giving sets suffer this painful complication and frequently complain more of their arms than of their abdominal wounds. Needles and cannulæ should be introduced into veins away from joints and preferably in the arm than the leg. In the latter, immobility and phlebitis may result in a deep thrombosis with all its unpleasant sequelæ. The needling of a vein must be conducted as a sterile operation on a shaved limb. When the drip is running, precise instructions should be given with regard to rate and quantities, for all too often the prescribed daily quota is not actually delivered into the circulation unless a close and repeated watch is kept on the rate of drip. In those cases where all the superficial veins have been thrombosed or cannot be found, an intramuscular drip of saline or glucose with the addition of Hyalase is satisfactory and may be the only method whereby fluid can be given.

Nutrition and Vitamins. In the majority of patients who are making a normal recovery, a few days starvation is well tolerated and the lost ground is soon made up by ordinary diet. Where the onset of normal feeding is delayed by reason of complications such as residual abscesses, mechanical obstructions and secondary operations, the rapid weight loss and breakdown of endogenous protein is a very serious feature. If the patient can take by mouth, a diet of adequate calories and a high protein content must be given. If he cannot, the best use must be made of the intravenous route. Amino acid solutions are probably only of value as such if sufficient calories are administered concurrently to prevent their metabolism for basal requirements. These patients are often helped by post-operative transfusions, but the decision to transfuse rests purely on the degree of anæmia and its benefits derive solely from the infused red cells and plasma protein.

The transfusion of stored blood has no "stimulating effect" as such, and there is little evidence for the survival of the more delicate elements of blood in transfused fresh blood. Generally speaking a patient with a hæmoglobin of 70 per cent. ($1\cdot 0\cdot 4$G) will recover well on iron alone. Both Vitamin B and C should be given in the post-operative period parenterally at first and later by mouth, especially if antibiotics are being used. There is good evidence that antibiotics, whether given orally or parenterally, may produce deficiencies of the Vitamin B complex. One manifestation of this deficiency is stomatitis which is particularly distressing in patients recovering from general peritonitis as it restricts feeding by mouth. The relation of Vitamin C to wound healing is well known and ascorbic acid is, therefore, given in doses of 500 mgm. daily. During the period of gastric suction these preparations may either be given by injection or added to the intravenous fluid.

A. S. TILL

References:

CANTOR, M. O. (1946) *Amer. J. Surg.* **72,** 137.
COOK, R. E., and CROWLEY, L. G. (1952) *New Engl. J. Med.* **246,** 637.
CORRY, D. C., BREWER, A. C., and NICOL, C. (1939) *Brit. med. J.* **ii,** 561.
CRILE, G. (1946) *Surg. Gynec. Obstet.* **83,** 150.
DOMAGK, G. (1936) *Klin. Wschr.* **15,** 1585.
FANTUS, B. (1936) *J. Amer. med. Ass.* **107,** 14.
GARDINER, R. H. (1944) *Brit. J. Surg.* **32,** 49.
GILMOUR, I. E. W., and LOWDON, A. G. R. (1952) *Edinb. med. J.* **59,** 361.
HANDFIELD-JONES, R. P. C., and LEWIS, H. B. M. (1952) *Lancet* **i,** 585.
HARRIS, F. I. (1945) *Surg. Gynec. Obstet.* **81,** 671.

HUDSON, R. VAUGHAN, and SMITH, R. (1942) *Lancet* i, 437.
HUNTMAN, J. B. (1027) *Diit. med. J.* i, 808.
MARRIOTT, H. L. (1947) *Brit. med. J.* i, 285.
MILLER, T. G., and ABBOTT, W. O. (1934) *Ann. intern. Med.* 8, 85.
MOLONEY, G. E., RUSSELL, W. T., and WILSON, D. C. (1950) *Brit. J. Surg.* 38, 52.
MOORE, F. D., and BALL, M. R. (1951) "The Metabolic Response to Surgery."
   Springfield, Ill. Charles C. Thomas.
MURPHY, J. J., RAVDIN, R. G., and ZINTEL, M. A. (1946) *Surgery* 20, 445.
PULASKI, J., ARTZ, C. P., and REISS, E. (1952) *J. Amer. med. Ass.* 149, 35.
REID, M. R., POER, D. H., and MERRELL, P. (1936) *J. Amer. med. Ass.* 106, 665.
RICE, C. O., STRICKLER, J. H., and ERWIN, P. D. (1952) *Arch. Surg. Chicago* 40,
   20.
ROB, C. G. (1946) *Proc. R. Soc. Med.* 40, 126.
SPALDING, J. E. (1946) *Lancet* i, 643.
STREETEN, D. H. P. (1950) *Surg. Gynec. Obstet.* 91, 421.
STREETEN, D. H. P., and WARD-McQUAID, J. N. (1952) *Brit. med. J.* ii, 587.
TAYLOR, W. H. (1951) *Brit. med. J.* ii, 1125.
TURNER, G. GREY (1938) *Brit. med. J.* ii, 691.
VAUGHAN WILLIAMS, E. M., and STREETEN, D. H. P. (1950) *Brit. J. Pharmacol.* 5,
   584.
WHITBY, L. E. H. (1938) *Lancet* i, 1210.
WRIGHT, L. T., SCHREIBER, H., METZGER, W. I., and PARKER, J. W. (1951) *Surg.
   Gynec. Obstet.* 92, 661.
YEAGER, G. H., INGRAM, C. H., and HOLBROOK, W. A. (1949) *Ann. Surg.* 129,
   797.
YOUNG, M., and RUSSELL, W. T. (1939) "Appendicitis." Spec. Rep. Ser. med.
   Res. Coun., Lond., No. 233, H.M.S.O.

CHAPTER XIII

PORTAL HYPERTENSION

SUSTAINED increase of pressure within the portal venous system is the result of an obstruction to the free flow of blood through the portal vein or in its passage through the liver. These conditions are referred to as the extra-hepatic (or pre-hepatic) and the intra-hepatic types of portal obstruction respectively. Whipple, Blakemore and Lord (1945) drew attention to the possibilities of clinical cure by surgical means of patients suffering from both types, though removal of the cause or pathological cure is rarely possible. They demonstrated the successful clinical application of the Eck fistula, by constructing anastomoses between portal and systemic venous systems. (Interference with the return of blood from the liver to the heart, with a build-up of pressure proximal to the hepatic veins, will also be reflected in the portal vein, but this post-hepatic obstruction is rarely the concern of the surgeon.)

The majority of patients have certain definite *symptoms* conforming to the *syndrome* which carries the name of *Banti*—hæmorrhage from gastro-œsophageal varicosities associated with an enlarged and over-active spleen, as shown by persistent anæmia (apart from hæmorrhages), leukopenia and thrombocytopenia. To this may be added the symptoms of *advanced liver disease*, which may develop to the exclusion of part or all of the typical syndrome, depending on the severity of the cirrhosis. For example, a patient with rapidly advancing cirrhosis may have a raised portal venous pressure but may not develop œsophageal varices or an enlarged spleen. By contrast, the purest examples of Banti's syndrome occur in patients who have livers which are normal in fact or function; that is, those with extra-hepatic or mild static intra-hepatic obstruction. It is on this account that certain writers exclude from their definition of the symptom-complex patients with ascites or icterus or other evidence of gross hepatic derangement. From time to time cases occur in which not only is the liver cirrhotic, but also the portal vein itself becomes obliterated by clot. Yet again, only a tributary of the portal vein may be permanently obliterated, whether or not the liver is cirrhotic.

In considering portal hypertension, therefore, it is necessary to group the patients according to the causes and effects of the portal obstruction and to assess the results of treatment in relation to each group; bearing in mind that each patient is an individual problem within his particular group.

146

The normal *portal venous pressure* varies between 50 and 150 mm. of 3·8 per cent. sodium citrate solution when taken from an accessible radicle of the portal vein. It is dependent to some extent on the systemic arterial pressure and the pressure within the inferior vena cava. It can be estimated by means of a manometer to give a direct reading, or by rapid electrical recording of the pressure itself (Gray, 1951). In portal hypertension, the pressure varies from just above normal to 600 mm. of citrate (Hunt, 1952a).

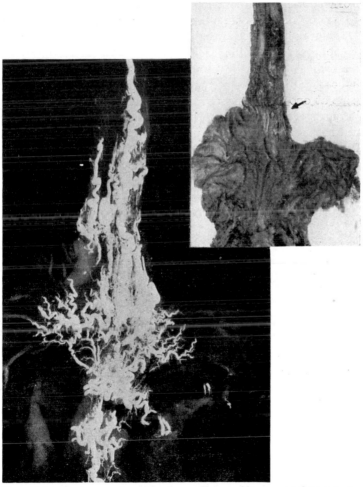

FIG. **13.1.** *Gastro-oesophageal varices.* X-ray of lower œsophagus and proximal stomach injected with a bismuth-gelatine suspension post-mortem to show the varices. The bleeding point (just proximal to the cardia) is arrowed on the photograph, which covers exactly the same portion of gut as the X-ray.

The most significant and vulnerable of the *anastomotic channels*, which connect the portal with the systemic venous systems (Figs. 1 and 2B), develop at the lower end of the œsophagus and the cardiac end of the stomach (Butler, 1951). Their extent may bear little relation to the height of the portal pressure. Large varices which have bled profusely have been encountered with a pressure of no more than 180 mm., whereas in other cases, with portal pressures extending up to 400 mm., no œsophageal varices have been found.

It is often possible at operation to demonstrate a rapid fall in pressure along collateral anastomotic channels, however large these may be or wherever they are situated. Such a circumstance may be encountered in the region of the umbilicus. The size of a caput medusæ, which is even more inconstant in development than œsophageal varices, may be no indication of the size of the other communicating channels. Thus large veins at one site often develop to the exclusion of others. However, all surgical approaches to deal with portal hypertension should be placed so as to conserve as many collaterals as possible with the exception of those around the cardiac end of the stomach, so that the natural compensatory channels, such as they are, are preserved.

Causes of Portal Hypertension

Extra-hepatic (17 out of the first 100 consecutive cases seen by the author (Fig. 1).

Congenital (11 cases). The obstruction to the portal vein in this condition is generally considered to be due to an extension of the process by which the ductus venosus and the umbilical vein are obliterated at birth (Thompson, 1940). Clinically it makes itself evident in childhood. The blood continues to reach the liver by way of thin-walled varicose channels of irregular size and number situated in the gastro-hepatic omentum, the so-called "cavernoma" (Fig. 2A), which is no more than an enlargement of the venous plexus associated with the biliary passages and their containing peritoneal folds. These channels sometimes are of considerable size but are usually useless for the construction of a porta-caval anastomosis. A shunt of sorts can occasionally be made with them, but it is very liable to thrombose. Further, in dissecting these veins, the bile ducts are in danger of injury.

Since the liver is normal, the immediate risks to life are simply those of hæmorrhage which can usually be controlled. These patients, therefore, tend to live for years in a reasonable state of health, though under the constant threat of a serious bleed (Reynell, 1951). In the past it was the common practice for splenectomy to be done, but it can now be categorically stated that the splenic vein is usually the most suitable

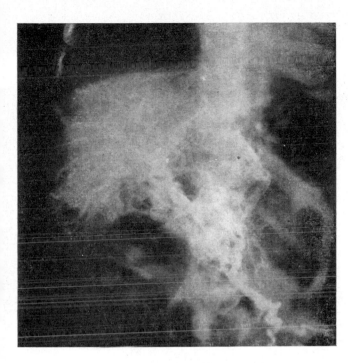

Fig. **13.**2A. A portal "cavernoma" demonstrated by venography at operation, in a boy aged 2½.

For comparison.

Fig. **13.**2B. Portal venogram in cirrhosis hepatis, to show a relatively normal portal vein, the left gastric leading to the gastro-œsophageal varicosities.

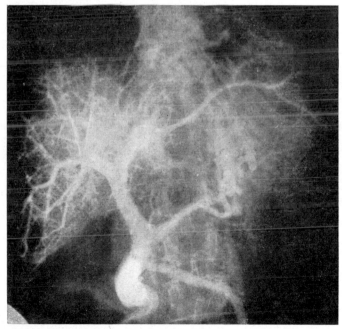

(The splenic vein shows in neither picture.)

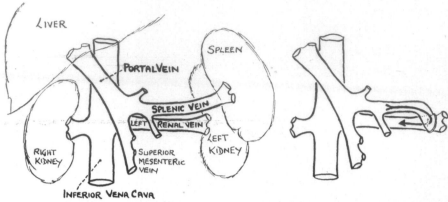

A. Diagram of the normal anatomy.   B. Spleno-renal anastomosis (end-to-side).

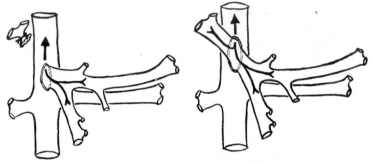

c. Porta-caval anastomosis (end-to-side).   D. Porta-caval anastomosis (in continuity).

FIG. 13.3.

and often the only available portal venous channel. It is, therefore, imperative that a spleno-renal shunt should be constructed (Fig. 3B). If this fails, some operation other than portal-to-systemic venous anastomosis is required. Portal venography (Dreyer and Budtz-Olsen, 1952; Hunt, 1952b) is of the greatest value in demonstrating the type and extent of the obstruction (Fig. 2).

Thrombotic (4 out of the 17 cases, one also occurring in association with congenital obliteration). Trauma may lead to thrombosis of one of the main portal venous channels, usually the splenic vein, or even the trunk of the portal vein itself. On occasions and given time, the clotted vein may recanalize, but the patient is liable to be left with part of the portal bed obliterated. In one of the author's patients the proximal half of the stomach alone remained in a hypertensive state after the portal vein had recanalized following splenorenal anastomosis. Proximal gastric resection removed the hypertensive area and has apparently effected a cure.

FIG. 13. 4.
CAUSES OF PORTAL HYPERTENSION
(100 consecutive cases)

I. EXTRA-HEPATIC (pre-hepatic).
Congenital portal vein obliteration 11
Thrombosis: Traumatic .. .. 1 ⎫
                Lymphosarcoma .. .. 1 ⎬ 3
                Myeloid leukæmia .. 1 ⎭
Compression by: Hypernephroma of right kidney .. 1 ⎫ .. 2
                   Displaced left kidney .. .. .. 1 ⎭
Splenic arterio-venous aneurysm 1

17

II. CIRRHOTIC (intra-hepatic).
Cause undisclosed 36
Following infective (viral) hepatitis of all types 19
Following cholangio-hepatitis 1
Following nutritional deficiency 4
Syphilitic 3
Toxic: Alcoholic .. .. .. 6 ⎫
         Arsenical (inorganic) .. .. 3 ⎬ 10
         Carbon Tetrachloride .. .. 1 ⎭
Biliary: Congenital atresia .. .. 3 ⎫ 7
           An acquired obstruction .. 4 ⎭
Cardiac 2
Following toxæmia of pregnancy 1

83

1. Some of the above causes of cirrhosis are considered as no more than probable. For instance, serum hepatitis, occurring during the treatment of syphilis and in the absence of cirrhosis, but succeeded later by the development of cirrhosis, must be regarded as the factor of greatest ætiological significance.

2. The patients suffering from nutritional deficiency had all been prisoners of war and suffered from a multiplicity of infections as well as starvation.

3. The significance of past contact with hepato toxic drugs was sometimes difficult to assess. The patient who had worked with industrial solvents (carbon tetrachloride) for many years, had also been in the habit of taking a tonic containing arsenic. Those labelled as arsenical all had pigmentation or hyperkeratosis or both.

4. The significance of a mild toxæmia of pregnancy is problematical. There was no other evident cause in this patient.

5. It must be recognized that such a list is of interest only so far as patients seen in Britain is concerned. Findings will be very different in other parts of the world. The above figures are not intended to represent percentages.

Thrombosis may also develop as a result of portal stasis in cirrhotic patients (it occurred demonstrably in 8 out of 83 cases), particularly following splenectomy when the platelet count is high. The comparatively common complication of mesenteric thrombosis is another aspect of this problem which must always be borne in mind when intestinal obstruction (usually sub-acute or insidious in its onset) develops in the presence of portal hypertension. Abdominal distension following operations for portal hypertension is also commonly encountered and it cannot yet be said to what extent this is due to interference with intestinal conductivity brought about by partial venous occlusion. The problem is complex and emphasizes the need for most careful and complete investigation and supervision at all stages of treatment of these patients.

Thrombosis of the portal vein is also encountered in conditions where the primary abnormality is a blood dyscrasia (one case).

Extra-hepatic portal obstruction caused by compression or displacement of the vein (two cases). The flow of blood in the portal vein may be obstructed by an adjacent swelling, e.g. tumour of the right kidney or of the pancreas. In one of the author's cases the left kidney had been pushed over to the right by an enlarged spleen, thereby compressing the portal vein at its origin.

If the effect on the portal vein is one of displacement and compression by a smooth structure, removal of that structure will probably effect a cure. Thrombosis usually only occurs in the presence of constriction, such as when a carcinoma or an inflammatory lesion embraces and, as it were, strangulates the portal channel. The treatment of this comparatively uncommon group of patients will depend very largely on the nature of the primary pathological process. The portal hypertension is often of no more than incidental importance. If the tumour can be removed, the portal hypertension will probably be relieved and the patient may be cured of both the original disease and its effects.

Portal hypertension due to arterio-venous communication, particularly of the splenic vessels (one case) (and Welch, 1950).

Intra-hepatic Obstruction. All types of cirrhosis may lead to portal hypertension, but its degree appears to bear little relationship to the extent of the liver disease or of the ascites (Hunt, 1952a). Eighty-three out of the first 100 of the author's patients were cirrhotics. An attempt was made to discover the cause of the cirrhosis in every case, and the findings are set out in the table (Fig. 4).

In cirrhosis, the prognosis following major operative procedures to relieve portal hypertension depends on the extent of the liver damage, irrespective of the cause of the cirrhosis. However, in comparable patients, the outlook appears to be better for those in whom the cause of the cirrhosis is reversible (as in toxic conditions) than for those who must be presumed to have a post-necrotic cirrhosis.

In some cases, 15 out of the 83, the hepatic fibrosis was mild and appeared to have reached a static phase (cf. Walker, 1952). Compensatory changes occur which enable the liver to function apparently normally. Clinically and as a result of biochemical investigation these patients are difficult to distinguish from those with extra-hepatic portal obstruction except that they are usually adult. From the point of view of surgical treatment, however, they are a more favourable group in that both the portal and the splenic veins are available. Only those with an associated portal thrombosis give rise to the mechanical difficulties which are encountered in patients with the congenital type of obliteration. The feel of the liver, liver biopsy by puncture (Terry, 1949), peritoneoscopy and pre-operative portal venography (Dreyer and Budtz-Olsen, 1952) may be of value in distinguishing between the two groups.

It is necessary that all patients with hepatitis shall receive sufficient medical treatment to enable the liver to recover as much as possible before elective major surgery is undertaken. Reversible parenchymatous changes should be given time to resolve under treatment with a diet containing a high proportion of animal protein and carbohydrate, with the additional support of lipotropic amino-acids (Himsworth, 1947) and preparations such as "Casinal". Anæmia should be treated with iron and transfusions of fresh blood. Deficiencies of blood prothrombin should, if possible, be made good. All vitamins, especially B, should be taken liberally. Gross ascites should be relieved by more rather than less frequent paracentesis so that the functions of the heart and lungs are not unduly impaired. Fluid and salt intake should be restricted and peripheral œdema reduced with the aid of mercurial diuretics If the liver disease is seen to be progressing so that deterioration occurs in spite of the treatment, some form of surgery may be undertaken in the hope that the process may be arrested or even reversed. In this respect it is important to emphasize that recurrent œsophageal hæmorrhages have a disastrous effect on a cirrhotic liver and must be prevented.

Biliary cirrhosis is a somewhat different problem in that it may be possible to remove the cause of the biliary obstruction and allow the liver to recover. In this type of cirrhosis relief of congestion within the biliary passages also appears to have a rapidly beneficial effect on the increased pressure within the portal vein and it may not be necessary to resort to surgery to relieve the associated portal hypertension.

It is through the portal tracts that blood is conducted to the liver lobules from the branches of the hepatic artery and the portal vein, in close association with the lymphatics and the bile passages. When these tracts become fibrotic, inelastic and distorted, as they do in cirrhosis (Kelty *et al.*, 1950), it is probably correct to deduce that relief of congestion in one of these channels will enable the blood or bile or lymph to flow more readily in the others. The converse of relief of portal hypertension following restoration of biliary flow can be observed in the amelioration of icterus that occurs following the successful construction of a portal-to-systemic venous anastomosis or common hepatic arterial ligature.

Congenital biliary atresia, in which no serviceable biliary passage can be discovered at operation, is a circumstance which has so far defied all efforts at successful treatment.

Patients with mild or moderate cirrhosis will tolerate a diversion of the portal blood from the liver very well indeed. After such a shunt operation, the liver may pass through a phase in which its function is temporarily impaired, but later to improve. Prolonged follow-up of such patients over the years will be necessary before it can be conclusively shown that such improvement is maintained.

Patients with more advanced cirrhosis, particularly those suffering from gross ascites, will not usually tolerate diversion of the portal blood stream. The liver fails within the first few days of operation. It is this group which requires the most careful medical treatment, for at least three months, before operative intervention is seriously contemplated. The type of operation to be done must be designed with the failing liver constantly in mind. The problem is in the nature of a dilemma, because the most effective way of preventing further œsophageal hæmorrhages—reduction of portal hypertension—is also, unfortunately, the very procedure most liable to precipitate acute hepatic failure.

Classification of these patients according to the intimate pathology of the cirrhotic process and according to the degree of liver damage will in the future undoubtedly enable those with good prospects to be separated from those for whom the operative risks are prohibitive. The results of operative treatment will inevitably be disappointing until accurate liver function tests are available. It is justifiable to take risks, however, because the patients live useless, miserable, invalid lives, with such time as remains to them usually limited to a matter of months.

Further, the dangers associated with the treatment of the advanced case must not be allowed to prejudice clinicians against the radical surgical treatment of Banti's syndrome in the mild or moderate cirrhotic, in whom the prognosis is excellent, provided that the portal pressure is reduced.

Investigation of Patients Suffering from Portal Hypertension

The investigation of patients who suffer from portal hypertension must of necessity be elaborate in order to decide whether or not the liver is diseased and how extensive this disease is; whether or not the effects on the spleen are sufficient to produce a material degree of secondary hypersplenism; what the intimate nature of the underlying disease process may be; whether or not the portal hypertension per se is of material significance; and perhaps to demonstrate an anatomical anomaly. Extensive and valuable co-operation with the ancillary departments, radiological, biochemical and hæmatological, must not lead to neglect of full and careful clinical assessment. For instance, where the liver apparently functions normally, a decision as to whether mild cirrhosis is present or not often rests on an accurate physical examination of the liver. An enlarged, adherent spleen may not extend below the costal margin, but may be detected by deep percussion of the left chest. That the liver is at fault must not blind the clinician to the fact that other vital organs may also be seriously deranged.

Liver function tests are of great value as indications of the degree of failure. Blakemore (1952) attaches most importance to the absolute level of albumen in the blood and the retention of bromsulphthalein. A blood albumen of 3·3 to 3·5 gm. per 100 ml. and a bromsulphthalein retention of less than 25 per cent. at the end of three-quarters of an hour (5 mgm. to the kilo body weight) are of good prognostic import. However, a comparatively satisfactory clinical state is sometimes encountered in the presence of a surprisingly low blood albumen. The prognosis following shunt operations appears to be good in this uncommon group. It is not proposed to set out in detail a complete list of investigations. Reference should be made to the third (1953) edition of 'Abdominal Operations' for a working guide and for details of operative technique.

Clinical assessment and pathological investigation are not only of value diagnostically, but also provide valuable information as to when the operation should be done. In this respect good risk patients do not present a problem. They should be operated upon as soon as their physical state has reached a point at which they may be judged capable of withstanding any major surgical procedure. It is the bad risk patients that require the most careful treatment and considered judgment. The general well-being of the patient, reduction of anæmia and improvement in secondary hypersplenism are satisfactory findings. An assessment of the rapidity of the formation of ascitic fluid related to repeated estimations of its protein content will provide valuable information as to the patient's progress or deterioration.

Indications for Operation

Hæmorrhage. Gastro-œsophageal varices bleed, sometimes with lethal effect (Fig. 1). The interval between hæmorrhages varies, but tends to become shorter and the hæmorrhages more profuse. The immediate risk to life is considerable. Work and activities are seriously interfered with. The patient and his relatives live in a state of constant anxiety and rightly feel that they must always remain within easy access of skilled hæmatological treatment. When the liver is cirrhotic, each hæmorrhage tends to produce a further deterioration of liver function. Ascites or irreversible liver failure is often precipitated by a hæmorrhage. For all these reasons, it is imperative to operate to prevent hæmorrhage.

Certain factors must be borne in mind concerning the causes of the bleeding, of which the presence of varicosities and the increased pressure within them are the most important. Thrombocytopenia and hypoprothrombinæmia should be considered as aggravating the bleeding. Erosions or ulcers of the œsophageal or gastric mucous membranes must necessarily be present before hæmorrhage can occur. It is often found that a common cold or an acute specific fever precipitates a bleed, particularly in children. Peptic ulcers appear to occur more frequently in association with portal hypertension than in the population at large.

The immediate treatment while the patient is bleeding is to stop the hæmorrhage with the help of opiates, transfusions and parenteral administration of fluids and nutriment. Compression of the lower end of the œsophagus with the balloon on a Miller-Abbott tube (Sengstaken and Blakemore) may be of assistance, but the bleeding often starts again when the balloon is removed. If these measures fail, it may be necessary to operate as a life-saving emergency. Nothing more is done than a direct or indirect ligation of the bleeding segment.

Hypersplenism. A much enlarged, over-active and congested spleen requires to be removed, usually as a preliminary to spleno-renal anastomosis. Lesser degrees of hypersplenism tend to resolve after porta-caval anastomosis.

Ascites. The causes of ascites are as yet incompletely understood. A raised portal pressure and a reduction in the blood albumen increase the hydrostatic filtration pressure and reduce the osmotic pressure of the plasma respectively. Fibrosis or congestion of the portal tracts obstructs hepatic lymph flow. Alteration of the metabolic processes within the liver produces or fails to remove substances responsible for the retention of fluid. Operations designed to reduce portal pressure should only be done in patients whose livers function well enough to enable them to tolerate diversion of their portal blood. Hepatic congestion can also be relieved, with less effect but perhaps with less immediate risk to the dropsical patient, by ligaturing the common hepatic artery. Neither of these operations, however, should be done until the liver has been given every opportunity to recover under medical treatment. It is during this phase of pre-operative therapy that hæmorrhages are of very serious import.

Sometimes ascites disappears under medical treatment and the patient is enabled to return to a fairly normal life. At present most workers would agree that such improved patients and certain cirrhotics, who have not had a hæmorrhage nor developed ascites and who are able to remain at work, should not be operated on, but should remain under close medical supervision. This opinion may require to be modified when knowledge of the pathology of liver diseases has advanced sufficiently for the early progressive cases to be segregated from the static.

Certain other pathological conditions which are related to portal hypertension require to be dealt with from time to time, e.g. the relief of obstructive jaundice; the removal of the pericardium in constrictive pericarditis. Yet other operations may need to be done on patients with portal hypertension such as the removal of an extrinsic cause, e.g. hypernephroma; or to relieve a complication such as a duodenal ulcer. The surgeon undertaking such operations should, if possible, be familiar with the special problems raised by the portal hypertension and its effects.

Methods of Surgical Treatment

It is, therefore, clear that no single operation is suitable for all cases of portal hypertension. The most effective procedure may prove to be impossible or may fail. Sufficient time has not yet elapsed for the value of the different operations to be fully assessed. The surgeon must, on occasions, be prepared to regard the patient as a problem which may require a number of different tactical approaches before the correct solution is found. This applies particularly to the patients with extra-hepatic portal obstruction. In general, however, it may be stated:

(i) That if the raised portal pressure *per se* is the cause of the symptoms, then reduction of this by an adequate portal-to-systemic venous anastomosis is undoubtedly a most successful method of restoring the patient to a normal state of health and preventing further hæmorrhages.

(ii) That if the elevated portal pressure is associated with a markedly enlarged and over-active spleen, splenectomy should be done as part of the planned treatment.

(iii) That if the function of the liver is severely deranged, the portal pressure can be reduced by the less drastic though much less satisfactory procedure of common hepatic arterial ligation.

(iv) That hæmorrhage can be stopped by interrupting the flow of blood from the portal bed to the bleeding segment. This operation is usually reserved for patients who have no portal channel of sufficient size for the construction of an efficient shunt, but may also be of value as an emergency measure to stop uncontrollable bleeding.

(v) That if only a segment of the portal bed is in a hypertensive state, as in splenic vein thrombosis, splenectomy alone or combined with proximal gastric resection may remove the hypertensive area and effect a clinical cure.

No attempt will be made here to give details of surgical techniques. However, certain considerations require to be borne in mind in comparing the different operative procedures.

Portal-to-systemic venous anastomoses.   (*a*)   *Porta-caval shunt* (Fig. 3c and D).   The portal vein and the inferior vena cava are both large veins which are easily handled. They are strong and hold stitches well. A large shunt can be unhurriedly constructed. The direction of flow in the portal vein is not reversed. The stoma is unlikely to thrombose (Blakemore, 1952). It is an operation which is suitable for most patients with hepatic cirrhosis of mild and intermediate degree. Moderately enlarged spleens shrink and become less active after successful porta-caval anastomosis. The spleen should be preserved when there is no thrombocytopenia, because of the increased risk of thrombosis after splenectomy in such cases.

It is usually best to make the shunt by end-to-side anastomosis (Fig. 3c) (Welch, 1947). Sometimes, however, the portal vein and inferior vena cava can be joined "in continuity" (Fig. 3D), thus allowing reflux of blood from the liver.

The results of porta-caval anastomosis are excellent in suitable cases.

(*b*) *Spleno-renal shunt* (Fig. 3B) (Linton *et al.*, 1947; Linton *et al.*, 1948) is indicated in the congenital type of extra-hepatic portal obstruction when it is likely that the splenic vein is the only portal venous channel which can be utilized. It should also be done for cirrhotic patients when the spleen is very large and over-active and has led to such a degree of hypersplenism that it is necessary to regard splenectomy as the first step in any major operation. Platelets return in fair numbers to the circulation very soon after the spleen has been removed. An alternative approach to this group is to remove the spleen and later do a porta-caval anastomosis (Rousselot, 1949; Stock, 1952).

(*c*) *Other portal-to-systemic venous anastomoses* may be necessary when neither the portal nor the splenic vein is available. Blakemore and Fitzpatrick (1951) describe the union of splenic vein stump to renal vein or inferior vena cava by way of a vein graft, with regional heparinization. Anastomosis of superior or inferior mesenteric vein to inferior vena cava has also been practised, but there have been few successes attendant on these indirect or small shunt operations.

Common hepatic arterial ligation (Rienhoff, 1951) is an operation of recent development which appears to be effective in relieving ascites in a proportion of patients. The proved long-term success of the venous shunt operations morally obliges surgeons to restrict hepatic arterial ligation to patients suffering from advanced cirrhosis. The results are worth while, bearing this in mind, that it is an operation practised on patients who are considered too ill to tolerate a shunt. About one-half of the patients survive and some of these are relieved of their ascites. Aureomycin (or other suitable antibiotic) must be administered for the first post-operative week (Markowitz *et al.*, 1949).

Porta-azygos interruption. The alternative to diversion of portal blood from the bleeding segment is division of the portal vessels below the dangerous area, at and above the cardia. This latter type of operation can take many forms, e.g. gastro-oesophageal resection (Phemister and Humphreys, 1947); transthoracic peri-oesophageal venous ligation (Allison, Personal Communications); sub-diaphragmatic gastric transection (Tanner, 1950); and transthoracic gastric transection. The purpose of these operations is to prevent high pressure portal blood from reaching the lower end of the oesophagus. Theoretically the most logical of such operations is that in which all vascular communications to the proximal half of the stomach and distal few inches of oesophagus are severed, sparing only safe venous communications to the abdominal parietes. The diaphragm must be incised and detached entirely from the alimentary canal, because the veins of the proximal stomach, spleen, diaphragm and oesophagus communicate freely. The stomach is then divided just below the cardia to complete the interruption between portal and azygos veins and re-anastomosed after careful ligature of the submucous gastric veins. The vagus nerves should be severed in the hope that this may reduce the risks of peptic erosions and ulcerations. The diaphragm is repaired. It is not yet known how long these operations remain effective in preventing hæmorrhage. The portal congestion persists unaffected, with its attendant troubles such as ascites, jaundice and the risk of thrombosis.

The interruption operation is clearly indicated:

(i) when there is no available portal venous channel for a shunt;

(ii) when it is imperative that bleeding should be stopped in a child whose veins are too small for the construction of a spleno-renal anastomosis that will carry him through life;

(iii) as an emergency operation to stop uncontrollable hæmorrhage in the case of cirrhotic patients who are undergoing pre-operative medical treatment. Some less extensive modification of the interruption operation may be sufficient in this last group of patients. Linton and Blakemore both advocate distal œsophagotomy with multiple ligature of the œsophageal varices under direct vision; and Tanner an abbreviated form of the transthoracic proximal gastric transection operation (personal communications).

(iv) in the rare case when hæmorrhage occurs from large œsophageal varices in the presence of a low portal venous pressure.

Splenectomy was until recently regarded as the standard operation for Banti's syndrome. It is now recognized that removal of the spleen should be reserved for the relief of hypersplenism, as a preliminary to a portal-to-systemic venous anastomosis, or when a venogram demonstrates clearly that splenic vein thrombosis is the only abnormality of the portal venous tree.

Splenic arterial ligation by itself produces a most uneven effect on the spleen, dependent upon the anatomy of the splenic artery and its branches. Collaterals from the pancreatic vessels may enable the spleen to continue functioning fully. On the other hand, ligature of the artery sometimes leads to a degree of ischæmia tantamount to massive infarction with sloughing of part or most of the spleen. This is an undesirable effect which may have serious consequences.

Injection of œsophageal varices with sclerosing solutions (Crafoord and Frenckner, 1939) is a method which approaches the problem, as it were, from the wrong end. It is occasionally attended by some degree of success.

Many other operations require to be mentioned but cannot be recommended. They were all intended to relieve ascites, but the little benefit that may on occasions be derived from them is transient. Repeated paracentesis abdominis is preferable to any one of them. The list includes the Talma Morison omentopexy, the peritoneal button operation, peritoneum-to-saphenous-vein anastomosis and peritoneum-to-renal-pelvis anastomosis. Lastly, the intravenous infusion of ascitic fluid is not practicable.

Anæsthesia

It is only with the aid of expert anæsthesia that major operations are successfully done on cases of portal hypertension. The agents should be selected so that adequate relaxation is maintained with the very minimum of hepato-toxic drugs. The patient must be kept fully oxygenated throughout the operation and during the phase of recovery.

Post-operative Care

The principles of post-operative treatment are:

(i) To prevent infection.

(ii) To retain full nutrition, by intravenous therapy in the first place and then by mouth.

(iii) To observe closely for complications such as paralytic ileus and mesenteric thrombosis and to treat them with all available means as early as possible. Hepatic coma is best treated with plasma and glucose infusions, supplemented with vitamins after the method of Latner (1950). Aureomycin and heparin should be added in the belief that the protection of the liver against infection is of vital importance in maintaining an adequate degree of function and that the coma is in part due to intra-hepatic thrombosis. Systemic heparin should not be given in the absence of coma unless active thrombosis has been demonstrated. It is unwise to start such treatment until forty-eight hours after operation.

Results of Surgical Treatment

Selection of cases by different workers according to different standards renders any detailed assessment of results at the present time valueless statistically. Significant, accurate, long-term follow-up is not yet available.

(1) *Congenital extra-hepatic portal obstruction* carries a good prognosis provided a large enough shunt can be well constructed. Circumstances are unfavourable in a number of these cases, the mechanical difficulties forestalling all but the most painstaking or ingenious of operations. On the whole the results are disappointing though the patients may survive for many years (Reynell, 1951).

(2) The outlook in cases of *cirrhosis of mild and moderate extent* is very favourable. A good shunt (using the portal or the splenic vein) can almost always be constructed. The operative mortality should not exceed 5 per cent. The great majority of these patients do not bleed again and are enabled to return to normal, vigorous lives.

(3) *Advanced cirrhosis* still presents a comparatively gloomy picture. Some patients deteriorate so rapidly that the opportunity for surgical intervention never occurs. In numbers these are about balanced by those that improve under medical treatment so that operation becomes, for the time being, unnecessary. Of the remainder, the majority are grossly ascitic and some also suffer from repeated hæmorrhages. The return of nearly one-third of this group of bed-ridden patients to active, useful lives is fair compensation for an immediate operative mortality

of about 30 per cent., with a smaller proportion of late deaths. Their only hope of reasonable life, rather than restricted and limited survival, lies in operative treatment, so that risks are justified. Surgery is used in an attempt to break the vicious circle of decline. Continued functional recovery of the liver depends on the persistence of medical treatment.

ALAN H. HUNT

References:

BLAKEMORE, A. H. (1952) *Surg. Gynec. Obstet.* **94,** 443.
BLAKEMORE, A. H., and FITZPATRICK, H. F. (1951) *Ann. Surg.,* **134,** 420.
BLAKEMORE, A. H., and LORD, J. W. (jun.) (1945) *Ann. Surg.* **122,** 476.
BUTLER, H. (1951) *Thorax* **6,** 276.
CRAFOORD, C., and FRENCKNER, P. (1939) *Acta oto-laryng. Stockh.* **27,** 422.
DREYER, B., and BUDTZ-OLSEN, O. E. (1952) *Lancet* i, 530.
GRAY, H. K. (1951) *Ann. R. Coll. Surg. Engl.* **8,** 354.
HIMSWORTH, H. P. (1947) "The Liver and its Diseases," Oxford, Blackwell Scientific Publications.
HUNT, A. H. (1952a) *Brit. med. J.* ii, 4.
          (1952b) *Proc. R. Soc. Med.* **45,** 722.
          (1953) "Portal Hypertension" in "Abdominal Operations" (3rd edition), edited by Rodney Maingot. New York, Appleton-Century-Crofts, Inc.
KELTY, R. H., BAGGENSTOSS, A. H., and BUTT, H. R. (1950) *Proc. Mayo Clin.* **25,** 17.
LATNER, A. L. (1950) *Brit. med. J.* ii, 748.
LINTON, R. R., HARDY, I. B. (jun.) and VOLWILER, W. (1948) *Surg. Gynec. Obstet.* **87,** 129.
LINTON, R. R., JONES, C. M., and VOLWILER, W. (1947) *Surg. Clin. N. Amer.* **27,** 1162.
MARKOWITZ, J., RAPPAPORT, A., and SCOTT, A. C. (1949) *Amer. J. digest. Dis.* **16,** 344.
PHEMISTER, D. B., and HUMPHREYS, E. M. (1947) *Ann. Surg.* **126,** 397.
REYNELL, P. C. (1951) *Lancet* ii, 383.
RIENHOFF, W. J. (jun.) (1951) *Bull. Johns Hopk. Hosp.* **88,** 368.
ROUSSELOT, L. M. (1949) *J. Amer. med. Ass.* **140,** 282.
SENGSTAKEN, R. W., and BLAKEMORE, A. H. (1950) *Ann. Surg.* **131,** 781
STOCK, F. E. (1952) *Ann. R. Coll. Surg. Engl.* **10,** 187.
TANNER, (1950) *Proc. R. Soc. Med.* **43,** 150.
TERRY, R. (1949) *Brit. med. J.* i, 657.
THOMPSON, W. P. (1940) *Ann. intern. Med.* **14,** 255.
WALKER, R. M. (1952) *Lancet,* i, 729.
WELCH, C. S. (1947) *Surg. Gynec. Obstet.* **85,** 492.
          (1950) *New Engl. J. Med.* **243,** 598.
WHIPPLE, A. O. (1945) *Ann. Surg.* **122,** 449.

CHAPTER XIV

PROGRESS IN PANCREATIC SURGERY

THE situation and anatomical relations of the pancreas must be regarded as singularly discouraging to the surgeon hoping to adopt the same principles of treatment as in dealing with other more accessible organs. Nevertheless, surgery in this field has shared in the general progress made possible by the very important developments in such ancillaries as anæsthetic technique and measures to counter surgical shock, and the last ten or fifteen years have seen a most remarkable expansion in the scope and variety of pancreatic surgery.

In this chapter, progress in the knowledge and treatment of the following lesions will be considered:

Acute and chronic pancreatitis.
Cysts of the pancreas.
Carcinoma of the pancreas.
Islet cell tumours and hyperinsulinism.

Acute Pancreatitis

The term acute pancreatitis is probably an inaccurate one, for although in many cases infection plays some part, the condition is not essentially an inflammatory one but a necrosis and autodigestion of the gland caused by activation within its substance of trypsinogen. It has been suggested that reflux of infected bile up the main pancreatic duct is the precipitating factor and it seems likely that in many cases this is true, though the mechanism producing this reflux is probably more often spasm of the sphincter of Oddi than impaction of a minute gall-stone at the very exit of the ampulla.

Pathology

The severity of the local changes varies greatly from case to case. The gland becomes swollen, hard and œdematous. Digestion of the walls of blood vessels may lead to extravasation of blood, in the gland and in the retro-peritoneal tissues. Local sloughing and liquefaction may occur and be followed by the development of a local abscess or a widespread retro-peritoneal cellulitis. The peritoneal cavity contains a turbid and sometimes blood-stained fluid and areas of fat necrosis appear in the great omentum, mesenteries and retro-peritoneal fat. Coincident biliary disease, often with stones, is common.

163

Symptoms, Signs and Diagnosis

Like the pathology, the severity of the clinical manifestations varies considerably. Typically, the attack starts soon after a heavy meal, the patient being seized with upper abdominal pain and collapse. The suddenness of the onset and the degree of circulatory failure may be so dramatic that a diagnosis of coronary thrombosis is made. More commonly a perforated peptic ulcer is suspected, though the build of the patient, usually overweight, lack of previous symptoms suggestive of an ulcer and perhaps the presence of symptoms referable to the biliary tract, rigidity less marked and much more obvious in the upper abdomen and absence of air under the diaphragm are all factors which may help to make a correct diagnosis, even though no one of them alone can rule out the possibility of a perforation. Occasionally the extravasation of blood may lead to discoloration in the flanks or around the umbilicus.

If the onset is less dramatic and an abscess develops, with fever and leucocytosis in addition to upper abdominal pain and tenderness and signs of peritoneal irritation, acute cholecystitis is often suspected, and indeed infection of the biliary tract may well be present in addition.

After the first week a fixed, tender epigastric mass may slowly develop.

Investigations

Valuable confirmatory evidence is obtained by the demonstration of diastase in abnormal amounts in the blood or the urine.

Treatment

Laparotomy must be undertaken in all cases of doubt, when not to operate may mean to miss some other intra-abdominal catastrophe. If the diagnosis can be made with relative certainty, it is probably better to rely upon antibiotics, oxygen and blood transfusion, morphine being given in full doses to control the pain, for there is no evidence that surgical intervention increases the chances of survival. If the diagnosis is made at operation, little is to be gained by draining the region of the pancreas itself, though sloughing detached portions of the gland should be removed and a drain inserted if a local abscess is entered.

Routine interference with a normal biliary tract is to be deprecated, but stones in the common bile duct should be removed and the duct drained with a T-tube. Cholecystectomy should not be performed, for in the possible event of recurrent bouts of pancreatitis leading to fibrosis of the head of the gland and obstructive jaundice, It may be necessary to use the gall-bladder for a biliary short-circuit.

Chronic Pancreatitis

This is becoming rather a fashionable diagnosis, liable to be attached to any patient with dypsepsia and upper abdominal pain with negative results from a barium meal and cholecystogram. The temptation to use chronic pancreatitis as a diagnostic waste-paper basket must be resisted. Two main types are seen:

(a) Recurrent Non-obstructive Pancreatitis

Recurrent bouts of low-grade pancreatitis similar to but less severe than the attacks described above may lead to scarring, thickening and hardening of the gland, and even to calcification. The condition appears to be a good deal more common in the United States than in this country, where cases are infrequent. Treatment should be directed to eradication of coincident biliary infection and if symptoms persist and particularly if pain is very severe, excisional surgery may have to be contemplated, a drastic remedy for a non-malignant condition. Recently, denervation has been practised with success for pancreatic pain

(b) Chronic Obstructive Fibroid Pancreatitis

Blockage of the main pancreatic duct leads to dilatation of the main ducts and a low-grade inflammatory process throughout the gland, which becomes larger and harder than normal, microscopically containing much fibrous tissue, less acinar tissue and a normal amount of islet tissue, which is therefore relatively increased. The condition may be non-malignant in origin, associated with intraductal epithelial hypertrophy or multiple papillomata, but in a high proportion of cases this variety of pancreatitis is caused by an ampullary carcinoma. Most surgeons will have seen patients with "chronic pancreatitis", even confirmed by biopsy, who have been treated by biliary short-circuit for obstructive jaundice, and who have a few months later developed metastases from a small carcinoma missed at operation.

The treatment of this variety of pancreatitis is the treatment of the causative lesion. If a carcinoma is present, it is treated by excision or a palliative operation, according to its extent and the age and condition of the patient. If obstructive jaundice is present and if no carcinoma can be demonstrated after a careful search has been made, including opening the duodenum to inspect and palpate the papilla of Vater from within the lumen, the biliary obstruction should be short-circuited by cholecyst-jejunostomy.

Pancreatic Cysts

Cysts of the pancreas can be divided into true and false, of which the latter are the more common.

False Cyst

This is, strictly speaking, nearly always a cyst of the lesser sac caused, it is thought, by previous injury or inflammation. A swelling grows slowly in the upper abdomen and may attain a considerable size, bulging forward above or below the stomach, usually pushing the latter upwards and the transverse colon downwards to present through the gastro-colic omentum. Symptoms are often rather vague and not in the main severe. Epigastric discomfort, indigestion, vomiting and loss of weight are not uncommon, whilst the cystic nature and retro-peritoneal situation of the mass should allow a diagnosis to be made. If help is needed, a barium meal and enema will demonstrate the relation of the mass to the stomach and colon.

Treatment.   Early attempts to treat the cyst in the same way as a true cyst, by enucleation, usually ended in discomfiture of the surgeon and occasionally in disaster, for the cyst has no true lining membrane and is surrounded by no plane of cleavage, its wall consisting of compressed fibrous tissue densely adherent to the boundaries of the lesser sac with its many blood vessels, so easily torn if removal is attempted.

Less dangerous and more rational is to treat the cyst by marsupialization, the cavity being opened, usually through the gastro-colic omentum, and packed with gauze after evacuation of its contents, with the edges of the incision into the cyst sewn to the edges of the wound. Three days later the gauze is removed and a smaller pack inserted. Finally a drainage tube is substituted and when this is removed fluid drains away for a variable time but nearly always ceases eventually. The trouble with this treatment is that in some cases a pancreatic fistula remains indefinitely unless further surgery is undertaken and in other cases the wound eventually heals but the cyst recurs.

If a pancreatic fistula does persist, it can be cured by implanting the fistulous track into the stomach or small bowel, establishing internal drainage, and this leads to a third method of treating a false cyst, primary internal drainage. Anastomosis of the cyst to the stomach is often a very simple process, for its fibrous envelope is already densely

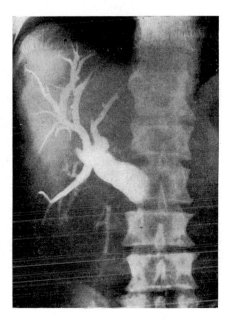

FIG. **14**.1.   Choledochogram obtained by injecting 35 per cent. diodrast directly into the dilated intrahepatic ducts. This shows a greatly dilated obstructed common bile duct. Diagnosis : Carcinoma of the pancreas.

FIG. **14**.2. Choledochogram followed up by an immediate barium meal showing the site of the obstructed common bile duct in relation to the duodenum.

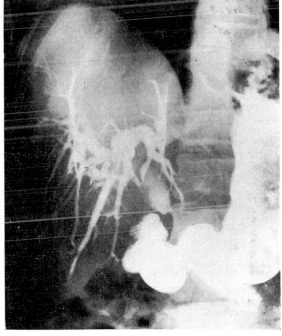

adherent to the back of the stomach and there is no need to suture the two together. The lumen of the stomach is entered through the anterior wall and an opening is made into the cyst by excising a disc or an oval segment of the whole thickness of the posterior gastric wall. A few interrupted sutures are necessary to control bleeding, but none for the purpose of anastomosis. The anterior gastric incision and the abdomen are closed and the operation is over.

A theoretical objection to this operation is the possibility that gastric contents might escape through the stoma into the lesser sac and introduce infection, but in practice this does not seem to happen and, indeed, post-operative studies with a barium meal have seldom shown any escape of barium through the stoma.

True Cysts

True cysts of the pancreas are uncommon, but retention cysts and cystic neoplasms do occur. Cystadenoma and cystadenocarcinoma are tumours resembling similar lesions in the ovary and may grow to a considerable size (Figs. 1 and 2). A pre-operative diagnosis is seldom possible, for symptoms are usually without characteristic features. The existence of a mass in the pancreas may be demonstrable radiologically and if the mass is large enough its site may be obvious clinically, even though the exact nature remains obscure.

Treatment. The possibility of malignancy makes exploration advisable and local excision, enucleation if a plane of cleavage exists, or partial or subtotal pancreatectomy should be carried out.

Carcinoma of the Pancreas

Great progress has been made in the last two decades in the treatment of carcinoma of the pancreas, but there is room for doubt whether the long term results always justify the performance of some of the major resections whose technical difficulties appear to have been largely overcome.

Carcinoma of the Head of the Pancreas, including Ampullary Carcinomas

Carcinoma of the head of the pancreas should be considered separately from carcinomas arising in the body or tail of the gland. The clinical manifestations are well known, the onset in a patient of mature years of obstructive jaundice without evidence suggesting gallstones or a gastro-intestinal carcinoma which might have led to secondary malignant glands in the portal fissure, accompanied by a palpable enlargement of the gall bladder.

Various points in diagnosis are worthy of comment;

(1) The term "painless jaundice" used in this connection is a bad one, for it is most unusual for a patient with a carcinoma of the head of the pancreas to be free from pain, which is often severe and often the first symptom, preceding the jaundice in onset. Pain is less prominent in the so-called ampullary carcinoma but is a complaint in about 50 per cent. of cases.

(2) The palpable gall-bladder in a case of obstructive jaundice is, of course, strongly suggestive of malignant obstruction, but occasionally palpable enlargement of the gall bladder is present with obstruction by a gall-stone, while absence of a palpable gall-bladder by no means excludes a pancreatic carcinoma. The gall-bladder may, for instance, be rigid from past inflammation and incapable of dilatation or it may be cut off from the main biliary tract by malignant involvement of a low junction of common bile duct and cystic duct.

(3) Various biochemical tests are commonly employed to confirm the obstructive origin of the jaundice and to exclude a hepatitis. Estimation of serum alkaline phosphatase is an empirical test of value, while tests based upon the alteration in albumin: globulin ratio caused by liver damage, such as the thymol turbidity test, are also useful.

Moderate elevation of the serum alkaline phosphatase and a thymol turbidity test beyond the normal range suggest a hepatogenous jaundice, while in obstructive jaundice marked elevation of serum alkaline phosphatase and a normal thymol turbidity are usual. The writer relies in the main upon these two tests alone to support clinical evidence.

(4) Absence of pancreatic ferments from the digestive

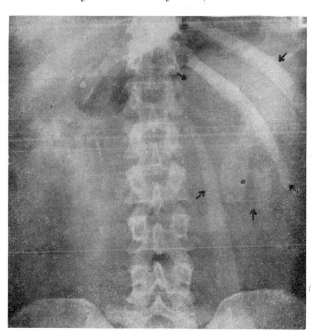

Fig. **14.3A.** Large soft tissue shadow. Cystadenocarcinoma of the pancreas.

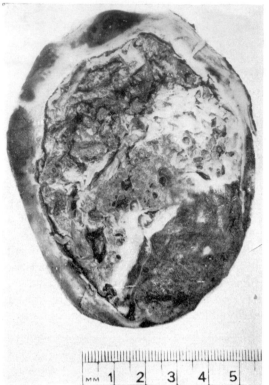

FIG. **14.3**B.   Cystadenocarcinoma of the pancreas.
The excised specimen.

tract is seldom demonstrated by finding unsplit fat or undigested meat fibres in the stools or by examination of fluid aspirated directly from the duodenum.

(5) Occult blood in the stools is present in more than 50 per cent. of cases of ampullary carcinoma and less than 50 per cent. of cases of gall-stone obstruction.

(6) Positive radiological evidence, by means of a barium meal, is obtained by an expert in this field in nearly 50 per cent. of cases.

(7) Per-hepatic choledochography may be of help in diagnosis (Fig. 3).

Treatment.   Patients believed to have a carcinoma of the ampulla or the head of the pancreas should undergo laparotomy, unless this is contra-indicated by grave intercurrent disease or manifest widespread metastases.   Even if the tumour proves irremovable, a palliative operation may well be possible and an even more cogent reason is that the diagnosis may prove incorrect and biliary obstruction by a gall-stone be found.

Preparation for operation should, of course, include the administration of vitamin K and this should continue after operation, whether a resection or a biliary short-circuit is performed, for about one week.

On opening the abdomen, the dilated gall-bladder and common bile duct will be noted.   In examining the head of the pancreas, the posterior peritoneum should be incised to the right of the duodenum, which is mobilized forward and to the left so that the gland can be palpated between finger and thumb.   It may be clear that a hard irregular growth surrounds the lower end of the common bile duct. Alternatively, the pancreas may appear to be normal.   A third possibility is that the gland may be the site of a generalized fibrosis and almost stony hard from head to tail. As has been stated, chronic pancreatitis is only too often caused by a small carcinoma obstructing the main pancreatic duct. If biliary obstruction is obvious but no carcinoma clearly present, the matter must not rest here, but further evidence must be sought, and this is best done by opening the common bile duct and passing a probe down it to the site of the obstruction and opening the duodenum so that the region of the papilla of Vater can be directly inspected and palpated. A small ampullary tumour will nearly always be demonstrable in this way, but if doubt still exists *trans-duodenal biopsy* should be performed, employing the technique described in detail elsewhere (Rodney Smith, 1953), followed by cholecyst-jejunostomy, which relieves the jaundice and can serve as the first stage of a two-stage resection if the biopsy reveals a carcinoma and the condition of the patient warrants radical excision.

If exploration reveals an undoubted carcinoma, the following procedures may be considered:

(1) External biliary drainage, cholecystostomy.
(2) Biliary short-circuit, anastomosis of the gall-bladder or common bile duct to stomach, duodenum or jejunum.
(3) Conservative resection.
(4) Radical pancreato-duodenectomy, including total pancreat-ectomy.

Cholecystostomy. This operation is mentioned only because it has been claimed that it is simpler and carries a lower risk to life than biliary short-circuit and that it should therefore be preferred as a palliative operation. In fact, an operation which leaves the patient with a fistula through which pours his entire biliary output is hardly described accurately as palliative, a word implying that the patient is made more comfortable.

Biliary Short-Circuit. If the growth is not to be excised, the jaundice should be relieved by biliary-intestinal anastomosis. The gall-bladder is employed for this junction unless grossly diseased, cut off from the common bile duct by extension of the growth or already removed, in which case the common bile duct is used. The best operation is probably a long-loop cholecyst-jejunostomy en-Y, though a loop in continuity with entero-anastomosis is little inferior. The loop receiving the bile should be some eight inches long. In this way the chances of reflux of gastro-intestinal contents into the bile passages and ascending cholangeitis are much reduced.

Conservative Resection. A small ampullary tumour may sometimes be resected locally by the trans-duodenal or retro-duodenal route or by

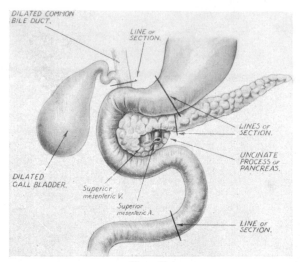

FIG. 14.4A.

cylindrical resection of the duodenum. Of these three operations, only trans-duodenal resection is at all satisfactory but, as was shown years ago by Gordon-Taylor, that pioneer in so many fields, this limited excision through the duodenal lumen is quite capable of giving good results in selected cases and is particularly applicable to the older patient in whom one hesitates to perform radical pancreato-duodenectomy.

Radical Pancreato-Duodenectomy. Time will not be spent upon a detailed discussion of surgical technique, but a few essential points must be mentioned. The modern radical operation consists of the block excision of the head of the pancreas with, around it, the pylorus, duodenum and lower end of the common bile duct and the associated cellular tissue and lymph nodes. The writer prefers to remove the whole of the duodenum, for the inferior pancreatico-duodenal artery often has a common origin from the superior mesenteric artery with the highest jejunal branch and, in securing it, the duodenal-jejunal flexure may be devascularized.

Local inoperability, when present, is usually the result of fixity to the portal vein or the superior mesenteric vessels and the technique adopted for the mobilization of the duodenum and pancreas should be so planned that no irrevocable step is taken until it is established that these vessels

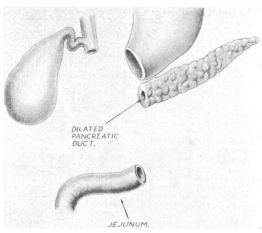

FIG. 14.4B.

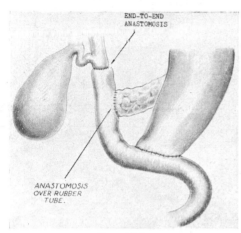

Fig. 14.4c.
One-stage radical pancreato-duodenectomy.

can be dissected free

Reconstruction after the excision of this block of tissue includes implantation of the common bile duct into the small bowel and end-to-side gastro-jejunostomy. The divided pancreas and pancreatic duct may be implanted into the jejunum or stomach or the duct may be tied off and the stump oversewn (Fig. 4).

To-day, the operation is usually performed in one stage but, if it is preferred, a procedure similar to the original two-stage Whipple operation can be selected, the first stage consisting of biliary short-circuit by a long-loop cholecyst-jejunostomy (Fig. 5).

Do the Results Justify Radical Pancreato-Duodenectomy? Although many of the technical problems of the radical operation have been solved, the results on the whole have proved disappointing. In the writer's view, radical pancreato duodenectomy should be performed for the ampullary growth without local fixity or metastasis and for the carcinoma of the head of the pancreas if mobilization opens up peripancreatic planes free of infiltration or œdema. In the presence of evidence suggesting direct or lymphatic spread of the tumour beyond the strict confines of the gland, the operative risk is high and the chances of escaping early recurrence of malignancy very remote. Many surgeons therefore feel that some tumours even though still technically just operable should be

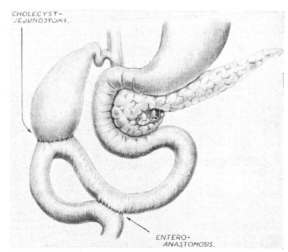

Fig. 14.5. Cholecyst-jejunostomy and entero-anastomosis as a first-stage in a two-stage radical pancreato-duodenectomy. (Figs. 4 and 5 published by permission of the Editor of the *Medical Press*.)

treated by cholecyst-jejunostomy rather than radical resection.

The older patient, considered unfit for radical resection, should be treated by short-circuit of a pancreatic carcinoma or possibly by trans-duodenal resection of a small ampullary tumour.

Total pancreatectomy should be reserved for cases in which very extensive carcinomatous infiltration is yet accompanied by freedom from peri-pancreatic involvement, an unusual finding. If total pancreatectomy is survived, the patient does, of course, become diabetic, but the amount of insulin necessary to control the diabetes is nearly always relatively small. Similarly, it is sometimes, but not always, necessary to give pancreatic extracts in order to control or prevent disorders of fat metabolism and fatty infiltration of the liver.

Carcinoma of the Body and Tail

Although the body and tail of the pancreas together constitute some three-fourths to four-fifths of the gland, carcinoma is less common here than in the head. From the purely anatomical point of view, resection is less complicated, for excision of the distal pancreas as far to the right as the superior mesenteric vessels, usually with the spleen, does not involve any reconstruction of the gastro-intestinal or biliary tract. Unfortunately, this advantage is more than offset in most cases by the lateness of the diagnosis and few cases reach the operating table with the growth still removable.

The reason for this is that either the clinical picture is so obscure and inconclusive that the complaint is not taken seriously until too late, or that a characteristic story is not correctly interpreted by the doctor consulted because, being unfamiliar with the condition, he is unaware that it is characteristic.

The history that should arouse suspicions is one of persistent, often constant pain, usually epigastric but sometimes substernal, sub-mammary, of a girdle distribution or felt in the back, frequently severe and made worse by lying down and little, if at all, affected by food. With this there is loss of appetite and loss of weight. Infrequently, and in the later stages, an abdominal mass is felt but, if so, the tumour is likely to be locally inoperable. Elevation of the erythrocyte sedimentation rate and a mild secondary anæmia may be detected.

Far too often, a patient giving this story but with no abnormal physical signs has a barium meal with negative results, a cholecysto-gram with negative results and nothing further is then done for several months when the appearance of metastases discloses simultaneously the tumour and its inoperability. This can only be avoided by earlier recourse to exploratory laparotomy in suspicious cases with negative results to investigations.

If at operation the tumour is still mobile, partial or subtotal pancreatectomy should be performed, the distal part of the gland being elevated by mobilizing the spleen and using it as a "handle". The stump is oversewn and there is no tendency for a pancreatic fistula to develop provided that there is no coincident obstruction of the outlet of the main pancreatic duct.

Islet Cell Tumours

These tumours are of interest to surgeon, physician and physiologist alike. Their existence was known as early as 1902 though naturally their physiological activity was not realized until insulin had been isolated and its properties demonstrated in the 1920's.

The islet cell tumour is usually single, though two or more are present in a small percentage of cases. It is nearly always small, often no more than 5 mm. across, and usually projects slightly from the surface of the gland, being rather darker in colour and bearing a network of tiny vessels. Very occasionally it grows to a large size.

Microscopically, it consists of clumps or strands of cells, less frequently exhibiting an alveolar pattern. The individual cells usually give the staining reactions of beta cells. It has been suggested that all physiologically active tumours are composed of beta cells and all functionally inactive tumours of alpha cells, but the correlation of histology and physiology may not be as clear-cut as this.

Most tumours are adenomas and benign. A tumour of undoubted malignancy is rare, but not infrequently some of the microscopic characteristics of malignancy, such as absence of a proper capsule and apparent invasion of blood vessels or lymphatics, are present in tumours which by their behaviour are clearly innocent, a very limited local enucleation resulting in complete cure with no subsequent recurrence or metastasis. The only real proof of malignancy is, in fact, metastasis.

Clinical Manifestations

Very rarely a large tumour causes pressure symptoms or a malignant tumour symptoms from local infiltration or metastasis. Much more commonly an innocent tumour of small size is diagnosed solely on account of the excessive production of insulin.

If this is the case, characteristic attacks of spontaneous hypoglycæmia occur, induced particularly by fasting or exercise and relieved by sugar. Many patients volunteer that attacks are most common before breakfast and that it has been noticed that they can be cut short by taking food or a sweet drink. The attacks vary in severity from patient to patient and from time to time in the same patient. As the higher cerebral functions are most sensitive to hypoglycæmia, the attacks are concerned first with judgment and behaviour and are characterized by silly, irrational, argumentative or quarrelsome episodes, followed if the attack increases in severity by inco-ordination in speech and gait, dizziness, faintness and sweating, finally drowsiness deepening into unconsciousness with convulsions, frothing at the mouth and incontinence.

An attack may be trivial enough to be regarded merely as eccentric behaviour or severe enough to cause death. Moderately severe episodes often lead to an early incorrect diagnosis of epilepsy or psychosis, but once the real cause of the trouble is suspected, a simple clinical test can be carried out which is likely to provide conclusive evidence.

A sample of blood for estimation of sugar is taken one morning from the fasting patient, who is then gently exercised until symptoms occur. A second sample of blood is taken and the attack cut short by giving sugar, by mouth or vein, after which a final sample of blood is taken. The classic findings are a low fasting blood sugar, often somewhere between 50 and 90 mgm. per 100 ml., a very low blood sugar at the onset of symptoms, 30 mgm. per 100 ml. or even lower having been described, and return to the previous level as the attack is stopped by giving sugar. Electro-encephalographic tracings are of interest and some value during this test, for although no particular pattern can be considered diagnostic, the findings usually provide strong evidence against a diagnosis of idiopathic epilepsy. Certain abnormalities in the glucose tolerance curve may also be detected, but do not provide the clear-cut information of the test described.

The three essentials on which diagnosis rests, often referred to as Whipple's Essential Triad, are:

(1) Attacks of spontaneous hypoglycæmia induced by fasting or exercise;

(2) A blood sugar during attacks below 50 mgm. per 100 ml.

(3) Prompt relief of an attack by giving sugar.

In completing the investigations, the possibility of pathology in other ductless glands should not be forgotten, but in general patients satisfying Whipple's essential triad should be explored for an islet cell tumour.

Surgical Treatment

At operation, the whole gland may have to be mobilized before the tumour is found and in any case even with one tumour found the surgeon must make sure that it is single. Removal is effected by enucleation or wedge resection. Post-operatively, the blood sugar often soars, but even if it reaches 400 to 500 mgm. per 100 ml. no alarm need be felt and, in the absence of ketosis, no insulin need be given. The level returns to normal within a day or two and it may well be that in the presence of a tumour producing insulin in excess of the body's normal requirements the islets become functionally dormant and do not immediately become active when the tumour is removed and that the stimulus necessary to restore activity is hyperglycæmia. The results of excision of the tumour are excellent.

If careful search reveals no tumour, it is customary to perform subtotal pancreatectomy, leaving the head of the gland protecting the common bile duct and the portal vein and its tributaries. If the excised pancreas is found on examination to contain a tumour missed at operation, a cure is very likely. If not, the result is much less easy to forecast. Hyperplasia of the islets has been described as an alternative cause of hyperinsulinism to an actual tumour and cases have been reported in which this hyperplasia was said to be present, without a tumour, in a specimen of subtotal pancreatectomy, operation having been followed by a clinical cure. Nevertheless, statistically if subtotal pancreatectomy is performed and no tumour is found, the chances of a cure are about equal in cases exhibiting histologically hyperplasia of the islets and in cases with normal islets.

RODNEY SMITH

Reference

SMITH, RODNEY (1953) "The Surgery of Pancreatic Neoplasms." Edinburgh, E. and S. Livingstone Ltd.

CHAPTER XV

MEDICAL INDICATIONS FOR SPLENECTOMY

THERE are only four clear medical indications for splenectomy—familial hæmolytic anæmia, acquired hæmolytic icterus, idiopathic thrombocytopenic purpura, and hypersplenism. The operation is justifiable as a last resort in cases of long-standing and intractable anæmia with a hypoplastic marrow, in which it rarely does harm and sometimes effects a dramatic cure (Whitby, 1952). Finally, a greatly enlarged spleen may become so intolerable a burden that the hazard of its removal is justifiable. Even in these cases splenectomy is usually considered unwise when, as in myelosclerosis, the organ has assumed a considerable hæmatopoietic function, although Edwards (1951) performed the operation with very good results in two cases of myelosclerosis.

Familial Hæmolytic Anæmia
(*Acholuric Jaundice*)

Splenectomy always cures familial hæmolytic anæmia, yet the spleen itself is not at fault. Normal red cells transfused into a patient with the disease survive for a normal time (Dacie and Mollison, 1943), but when the patient's spherocytic red cells are transfused into a normal individual they are quickly destroyed by his spleen (Loutit and Mollison, 1946). That the spleen alone is responsible for the rapid destruction of spherocytes is shown by the curative effect of splenectomy, after which spherocytes have a normal life-span in the patient, although they are still quickly eliminated by a normal recipient with an intact spleen. If, however, the "normal" recipient has had a splenectomy for some other reason, the spherocytes of familial hæmolytic anæmia survive as long in his circulation as normal red cells (Schrumpf, 1951).

The crises of familial hæmolytic anæmia are not due to intensified hæmolytic activity, but rather to a temporary arrest of red cell production. Owren (1948) believes that the marrow becomes aplastic, whereas Dameshek and Bloom (1948) ascribe the crises to hypersplenism (q.v.) with a consequent maturation arrest of red cell precursors. The characteristic neutropenia of crises is taken as further evidence of hypersplenism. Transfused red cells usually survive normally during a crisis, but occasionally their rapid destruction indicates excessive phagocytic activity of the spleen. Abnormal antibodies,

178

sensitizing the red cells as in acquired hæmolytic icterus, have occasionally been found during crises.

Splenectomy always cures familial hæmolytic anæmia (unless splenunculi have been left behind). The operation should be performed whenever the disease is diagnosed, except in early childhood, for even if symptoms are not severe the continued hæmolysis places a grave strain on the bone marrow, and gall-stones are more likely than not to form in time. Severe crises may necessitate an early operation in childhood, but in their absence splenectomy is best postponed until the age of ten. At all ages the operation should be performed in a phase of relative remission, although occasionally a severe and sustained crisis will demand an emergency splenectomy.

Acquired Hæmolytic Icterus

(*Acquired Acholuric Jaundice*)

The primary defect in acquired hæmolytic icterus is that the patient forms antibody to his own and most, if not all, other human red cells. The antibody may be demonstrable in the patient's serum, but often all has combined with his red cells. Red cells thus coated with antibody are said to be *sensitized*. The antibody is termed *incomplete* because it has no effect on red cells suspended in saline, although it does agglutinate red cells suspended in protein media such as 20 per cent. bovine albumin. (It is not always realized that the suspending medium influences the physical consequences of an antigen-antibody union. An anti-bacterial serum, for example, agglutinates bacteria if they are suspended in saline, but not in distilled water.)

Sensitization of red cells is detected by *Coombs' test*. The serum used, prepared by immunizing animals, contains precipitins to human globulin in saline suspension. The antibodies coating sensitized red cells are, like all antibodies, globulins. Thus if sensitized red cells are treated with the anti-globulin serum, the coating antibody molecules come together in precipitates that bind the attached red cells together in large clumps.

Sensitized red cells do not hæmolyse *in vitro*, but they are unduly susceptible to phagocytosis and so have a short life-span in the body. The patient's antibody quickly sensitizes transfused red cells, which are then as readily destroyed as his own. Often all the transfused red cells are eliminated in a week, and an exceptionally severe case may destroy 90 per cent. in a day (Loutit and Mollison, 1946). When the patient's red cells are transfused into a normal recipient, about half are eliminated in three or four days, but the remainder have a normal life-span (Selwyn and Hackett, 1949). At first the donated red cells are heavily sensitized and quickly destroyed, but they progressively share their antibody with the recipient's cells until eventually the antibody coat is too thin to provoke phagocytosis.

Acquired hæmolytic icterus is usually idiopathic, but some cases are secondary to other causes of splenomegaly such as chronic leukæmia, Hodgkin's disease and reticulo-sarcoma. About half the idiopathic cases, and a rather smaller proportion of secondary ones, are clinically cured or greatly benefited by splenectomy. (There is no means of foretelling which cases will do well and which will not.) The operation should not be too hurriedly undertaken, for not uncommonly a spontaneous remission follows a few blood transfusions. The patient's red cells usually remain sensitized after splenectomy even when clinical cure seems complete; probably the degree of sensitization is diminished until it no longer suffices to provoke phagocytosis.

Adequate doses of cortisone or ACTH produce a dramatic remission in most cases of acquired hæmolytic icterus, whether idiopathic or secondary. With continued hormone therapy the remission may be sustained for long periods, especially in idiopathic cases (Rosenthal *et al.*, 1952). A prolonged trial of hormone therapy is preferable to splenectomy when the hæmolytic anæmia is secondary to some other disease, such as leukæmia, that must in itself soon be fatal. When the anæmia is idiopathic, the risks of prolonged therapy with ACTH or cortisone must be weighed against the fact that splenectomy will cure half the patients and will not harm the remainder.

The preoperative preparation of cases for splenectomy has been greatly eased by the use of ACTH or cortisone, which will usually restore the blood count to normal and obviate the need for transfusions. When hormone therapy fails it may be very difficult to raise the hæmoglobin to a safe pre-operative level, for in severe cases transfused red cells are eliminated in a very few days. Sometimes it is possible to find donor red cells which are not sensitized by the patient's serum and which survive more normally in his circulation (Whitby, 1952).

Thrombocytopenic Purpura

Thrombocytopenic purpura may be idiopathic, or secondary either to other blood diseases such as acute leukæmia and aplastic anæmia. or else to sensitization by drugs. The distinction between the two (largely by blood and bone marrow examinations) is of great importance, for whereas splenectomy usually cures idiopathic cases, the operation is never beneficial and often harmful in secondary thrombocytopenic purpura.

The ætiology of idiopathic thrombocytopenic purpura is unknown, although the spleen clearly plays a major part. The disease has been regarded as a type of hypersplenism, both by those who believe in splenic inhibition of the marrow and by those who stress splenic phagocytosis (*vide infra*). Certainly the diagnosis should not be made unless the number of megakaryocytes in the sternal marrow is at least normal. Some (e.g. Dameshek and Miller, 1946) have claimed to recognize specific morphological abnormalities of the megakaryocytes indicative of a maturation defect, but others have found these cells to be normal. Other workers regard the disease as analogous to acquired hæmolytic icterus and claim to have demonstrated anti-platelet agglutinins in patients' sera (Evans *et al.*, 1951). It is perhaps significant that both diseases, unlike hypersplenism, are favourably influenced by ACTH or cortisone therapy.

The diagnosis of frank idiopathic thrombocytopenic purpura is not difficult, although it must be remembered that the spleen is usually not palpable. The most difficult cases are those in which the only manifestation of the disease is bleeding from a single surface, e.g. menorrhagia, and the platelet count rises to normal levels between hæmorrhagic episodes.

The indications for splenectomy are comparatively clear. The operation should not, except in desperation, be performed during the acute phase of a fulminating case, for the operative mortality is very high. A transfusion of fresh blood will usually check bleeding for two or three days, and most acute cases pass into a relative remission after repeated transfusions.

Spontaneous remissions of long duration, and even complete cure, are common in children, in whom the disease is most often seen. They should not, therefore, be submitted to splenectomy unless a remission fails to follow repeated transfusions, or unless a relapse follows remission. Adults are in considerable danger of fatal cerebral hæmorrhage as long as there is bleeding from the mucosæ. Splenectomy should, therefore, be performed on them at the first favourable opportunity.

The results of splenectomy are usually dramatic. Obvious bleeding may stop as soon as the splenic vessels are ligated, the platelet count rises rapidly and may pass the normal level in 24 hours, and purpura disappears. The platelet count may fall again in convalescence to subnormal values, but clinical cure is usually complete. Some 60 per cent. of cases of idiopathic thrombocytopenic purpura are cured by splenectomy and a further 20 per cent. are greatly improved (Welch and Dameshek, 1950). The remaining fifth pass with difficulty through a convalescence complicated by repeated hæmorrhages and delayed wound healing, and are left no better for the operation. There is, unfortunately, no way of telling in which cases splenectomy will fail.

ACTH and cortisone therapy produce remissions in about half the cases of idiopathic thrombocytopenic purpura, and in rare instances have even been effective after splenectomy has failed (Davidson *et al.*, 1952). The remission is occasionally sustained, but the patient usually relapses after therapy is stopped.

Hypersplenism

Hypersplenism may be defined as a condition in which certain blood cells (either red cells, neutrophils, platelets, or all three) are consistently depressed in number, the marrow contains a normal or increased number of their precursors, and splenectomy is curative. The disease may be idiopathic, or it may be secondary to splenic enlargement from other conditions such as leukæmia, Hodgkin's disease, reticulo-sarcoma and Banti's syndrome.

The role of the spleen in hypersplenism is undecided. Doan (1945) believes it to be purely phagocytic, the marrow hyperplasia being compensatory to increased blood destruction. "Sequestration" of blood cells in the splenic pulp is a prelude to, if not the cause of, the excessive phagocytosis. Dameshek, on the other hand, believes that the spleen normally secretes a hormone that hinders the release of blood cells from the bone marrow or inhibits maturation of their precursors. He regards hypersplenism as excessive splenic inhibition of the marrow, with over-active phagocytosis playing only an occasional and minor part. The histology of the spleen in hypersplenism has been claimed to support either theory. Usually sections show only lymphoid and reticulo-endothelial hyperplasia, perhaps with fibrosis, but Doan claims that excessive phagocytosis can always be demonstrated by supravital staining if not by routine histological techniques.

Hypersplenism is subdivided into *splenic pancytopenia* with depression of red cells, neutrophils and platelets, and *splenic neutropenia* with a normal red cell count and an inconstant and minor thrombocytopenia. Idiopathic thrombocytopenic purpura may be regarded as a third variety of the syndrome.

Splenic Pancytopenia. The association of anæmia, neutropenia and thrombocytopenia with a palpable spleen and a normal or hyperplastic marrow is presumptive evidence of splenic pancytopenia. The anæmia is in some degree hæmolytic in about half the cases. Sometimes the hæmolysis is associated with the presence of antibodies of the type seen in acquired hæmolytic icterus. In other cases it can be demonstrated only by observing the abnormally rapid elimination of transfused red cells.

There are two major diagnostic problems. First, to show that an apparently idiopathic pancytopenia is not in reality secondary to some more lethal condition such as aleukæmic leukæmia. Second, to show whether secondary hypersplenism exists in some established disease such as chronic leukæmia. The first problem need not detain us—it is largely a matter of thorough investigation and elimination. The importance of the second problem has not long been recognized. For example, the course of chronic leukæmia, especially the lymphatic variety, may be suddenly changed by the development of severe anæmia that outpaces any feasible programme of transfusion. If hypersplenism is the cause of the anæmia, it will be cured by splenectomy and the leukæmia proper can be controlled by other means for a further year or two (Hagen and Watson, 1951). If the patient's red cells are sensitized the case may be regarded as secondary hæmolytic icterus and treated accordingly (p. 180). If not, the diagnosis is best made by observing the shortened life of transfused red cells (Berlin, 1951). It is not always necessary to label the transfused red cells by minor blood group differences, for in a severe case the hæmoglobin after transfusion falls far more than 6 per cent. a week—the maximum with a completely non-productive marrow and normal red cell destruction.

The *adrenalin test* of Doan and Wright (1946) for hypersplenism is now somewhat discredited. A positive result—a sharp increase in the formed elements of the blood during the hour after a subcutaneous injection of 0·5-1·0 ml. of 1:1,000 adrenalin —seems not to be as firmly diagnostic of splenic sequestration as the originators believed.

Splenectomy relieves some 80 per cent. of cases of idiopathic splenic pancytopenia and some 70 per cent. of secondary cases. The symptoms may be greatly improved even when the blood picture does not return completely to normal.

Splenic Neutropenia is three or four times less common than splenic pancytopenia. The peripheral neutrophil count is greatly depressed, often with such symptoms of agranulocytosis as mouth ulcers and inter current infections. There is little or no anæmia but some degree of thrombocytopenia, insufficient to cause symptoms, is usual. The normal or increased cellularity of the sternal marrow, usually with a well-marked maturation defect of myelocytes, distinguishes splenic neutropenia from the types due to drugs and toxins. Splenectomy is as successful as in splenic pancytopenia. Even if the neutrophil count falls again after its post-operative rise, the patient usually remains free from symptoms of agranulocytosis.

Felty's syndrome of rheumatoid arthritis, splenomegaly and neutropenia may be regarded as a type of secondary splenic neutropenia. Splenectomy has usually cured the neutropenia and has greatly improved the general health of the patient (Hutt *et al.*, 1951).

Banti's Syndrome

Banti's syndrome of splenomegaly with gastro-œsophageal varices is now regarded as the consequence of portal hypertension. In older patients cirrhosis of the liver is the usual cause of the portal obstruction, whereas extra-hepatic obstruction is more common in children and young adults. Extra-hepatic obstruction may be secondary or, more commonly, due to a primary obliteration of the portal vein—probably an extension of the neo-natal obliteration of the umbilical vein and ductus venosus. Hypersplenism may complicate either type of portal obstruction.

The portal hypertension of Banti's syndrome (leading so often to fatal hæmatemesis) can rarely be relieved by any means short of a spleno-renal or porta-caval venous shunt (Blakemore, 1947). Simple splenectomy is justified only when, rarely, the portal obstruction consists solely of splenic vein obliteration—a point that can only be proved by portal venography at operation (Hunt, 1952). In other cases splenectomy alone cannot ameliorate the major symptoms and may well make a future venous shunt impossible.

Hypersplenism, evinced mainly by neutropenia and platelet deficiency, is common in Banti's syndrome. When it is present the portal anastomosis should be combined with splenectomy.

MARTIN HYNES

References:

BERLIN, R. O. M. (1951) "Proceedings of the 3rd International Congress of the International Society of Hematology." Grune and Stratton, New York, p. 99.

BLAKEMORE, A. H. (1947) *Surg. Gynec. Obstet.* **84,** 645.

DACIE, J. V., and MOLLISON, P. L. (1943) *Lancet* **i,** 550.

DAMESHEK, W., and BLOOM, M. L. (1948) *Blood* **3,** 1381.

DAMESHEK, W., and MILLER, E. B. (1946) *Blood* **1,** 27.

DAVIDSON, L. S. P., GIRDWOOD, R. H., and SWAN, H. T. (1952) *Brit. med. J.* **ii,** 1059.

DOAN, C. A. (1945) *J. lab. clin. Med.* **30,** 385.

DOAN, C. A., and WRIGHT, C. S. (1946) *Blood* **1,** 10.

EDWARDS, H. C. (1951) *Lancet* **ii,** 601.

EVANS, R. S., TAKAHASHI, K., DUANE, R. T., PAYNE, R., and LIU, C. K. (1951) *Arch. intern. Med.* **87,** 48.

HAGEN, P. S., and WATSON, C. J. (1951) "Proceedings of the 3rd International Congress of the International Society of Hematology," p. 95. New York, Grune and Stratton.

HUNT, A. H. (1952) *Brit. med. J.* **ii, 4.**

HUTT, M. S. R., RICHARDSON, J. S., and STAFFURTH, J. S. (1951) *Quart J. Med.* **20,** 57.

LOUTIT, J. F., and MOLLISON, P. L. (1946) *J. Path. Bact.* **58,** 711.

MAINGOT, R. (1952) *Lancet* **i,** 625.

OWREN, P. A. (1948) *Blood* **3,** 231.

ROSENTHAL, M. C., SPAET, T. H., GOLDENBERG, H., and DAMESHEK, W. (1952) *Lancet* **i,** 1135.

SCHRUMPF, C. A. A. (1951) "Proceedings of the 3rd International Congress of the International Society of Hematology," p. 94. New York, Grune and Stratton.

SELWYN, J. G., and HACKETT, W. E. R. (1949) *J. clin. Path.* **2,** 114.

WELCH, C. S., and DAMESHEK, W. (1950) *New Engl. J. Med.* **242,** 601.

WHITBY, L. E. H. (1952) *Lancet* **i,** 623.

CHAPTER XVI

SURGICAL INDICATIONS FOR SPLENECTOMY AND TECHNIQUE OF THE OPERATION

VARIOUS indications for splenectomy may be recognized which can be loosely grouped together as surgical:

A. *Mechanical.*   (i) Rupture.
                    (ii) Penetrating wounds.
                    (iii) Torsion of the splenic pedicle.
B. *Neoplasia.*   (i) Malignant; Lymphosarcoma.
                    (ii) Rare benign neoplasms.
C. *Cysts.*   (i) Parasitic; Hydatids.
                    (ii) True cysts lined by epithelium or endothelium.
                    (iii) False cysts; Neoplasm with degeneration; Hæmangioma and lymphangioma.
D. *Inflammation.*   Splenic abscess.
E. Aneurysm of the splenic artery.
F. With gastrectomy or œsophago-gastrectomy for carcinoma of the stomach.
G. In the so-called *Banti's Syndrome*, with or without some form of portal-systemic shunt. (See Chapter XIII).

Rupture or Penetrating Wound

Spontaneous rupture of the spleen occasionally occurs if the organ is already the site of some gross pathological change. It is thus rare in this country, though an occasional case has been described in association with glandular fever.

Damage to the spleen from a penetrating wound is obviously rare in civil practice, but most large series of battle casualties contain examples, usually in association with a left abdomino-thoracic wound. Splenectomy is carried out in the course of an operation which will very probably bring to light injuries of a more serious character to stomach, diaphragm, colon, left lung, pancreas, left kidney or great vessels.

Direct violence to the left lower chest may cause rupture of the spleen in accidents on the road or playing field or sometimes from a fall which at first seems trivial. Diagnosis is made by finding:

(*a*) Evidence of trauma applied to the region of the spleen.
(*b*) Evidence of internal hæmorrhage.
(*c*) Evidence of blood in the peritoneal cavity.

The classic features, based upon these three elements, are too well known to require setting out in full, but certain aspects are worth stressing:

(*a*) The degree of violence is not infrequently less than that which might reasonably be considered necessary to cause a splenic rupture.

(*b*) In the early stages, signs of blood loss may be absent and signs of peri-splenic leakage of blood minimal. Subcapsular tearing may precede splitting of the capsule and sudden severe hæmorrhage.

(*c*) Associated injuries of a more obvious nature may direct the attention of both patient and doctor away from the abdomen, for instance a painful fracture or dislocation in a limb.

Taken together, these three factors combine to lay a trap for the unwary and are a not infrequent cause of discomfiture of the newly qualified Casualty Officer, who reduces the Colles fracture of a man knocked off his bicycle and complaining only of the pain in his wrist, and sends him home, where he goes to bed and dies in the night of a ruptured spleen, the Sunday papers usually commenting "Doctor sends home dying patient".

(*d*) Evidence of leakage of blood from the spleen can usually be obtained by altering the posture of the patient during examination. Tipping him head-down will often cause irritation of the diaphragm with blood and the sudden onset of a sharp pain referred to the left shoulder-tip. This most valuable sign is not sufficiently stressed in standard textbooks.

(*e*) Blood in the peritoneal cavity can cause inhibition of peristalsis, but normal peristaltic sounds heard with a stethoscope do not prove the absence of intraperitoneal blood.

(*f*) Rectal examination must not be omitted, blood clot in the pouch of Douglas giving a characteristic feel.

(*g*) A plain X-ray film of the abdomen may demonstrate an effusion of blood between the splenic flexure and the diaphragm.

Treatment is splenectomy, combined with blood transfusion as may be required. In an emergency, if cross-matched whole blood is not readily available, auto-transfusion of unclotted blood from the peritoneal cavity may be indicated.

Torsion of the Splenic Pedicle

Torsion of the splenic pedicle is usually recurrent and leads to bouts of splenic congestion, perisplenitis and sometimes infarction. The condition is uncommon and when diagnosed should be treated by splenectomy. The ligaments are necessarily long and lax and the operation technically easy.

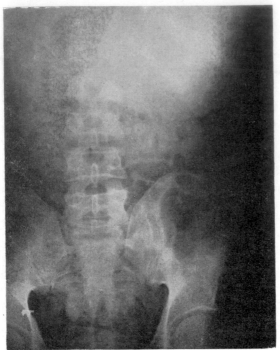

FIG. 16.1A. Soft tissue radiograph showing outline of large upper abdominal tumour which proved to be a hæmangioma of the spleen.
(Reproduced by permission of the Editor of the *British Journal of Surgery.*

Neoplasm

Splenic neoplasms may necessitate splenectomy but are very rare. Lymphosarcoma is almost invariably accompanied by manifest evidence of widespread dissemination, contraindicating operation.

Cysts

Cysts, too, are uncommon, but examples are encountered from time to time and may grow to a considerable size. Fig. 1 shows a very large cystic hæmangioma of the spleen, weighing 8 lb. 12 oz., removed by the writer.

Aneurysm of the Splenic Artery

This may occasionally be diagnosed when large as a pulsatile swelling with a bruit and sometimes exhibiting calcification visible in an X-ray film. Treatment should aim at excision of the spleen and the aneurysmal vessel.

Carcinoma of the Stomach

Splenectomy is now a routine part of gastric resection for carcinoma of the upper part of the stomach. It allows a more thorough ablation of lymph nodes and is combined in the operation advocated by Allison with partial pancreatectomy and excision of the posterior peritoneum of the lesser sac and the cellular tissue around the branches of the cœliac axis.

The Technique of Splenectomy

Except as described in Chapter XV, it is not usual for any complicated pre-operative treatment to be necessary, but emptying and keeping empty the stomach by suction is valuable, for a distended stomach may add to technical difficulties.

General anæsthesia, rather than spinal or local, is usually preferred, good muscular relaxation being important and obtained by an intravenous relaxant. A left paramedian incision is perfectly adequate in most cases, though some surgeons prefer a transverse or subcostal incision, either of which does, in fact, give particularly good access to the spleen.

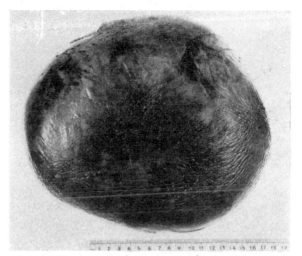

FIG. 18.1M. Hæmangioma of the spleen. The excised specimen.
(Reproduced by permission of the Editor of the *British Journal of Surgery*.

Before the spleen can be drawn into the wound, the lieno-renal ligament must be divided, and the first step in the operation is therefore to pass the left hand over the convexity of the spleen, which is depressed and retracted to the right so that this avascular peritoneal fold is put on the stretch and can very simply be cut through with curved scissors under direct vision.

A very large or very adherent spleen is said occasionally to call for a left abdomino-thoracic incision for its adequate exposure and removal, but the necessity for this has not arisen in any of the writer's cases. Gross adhesion of the spleen to the parietal peritoneum is rare but, if present, and if an attempt is made to draw the organ into the wound by force, tearing of the splenic pulp may easily occur with severe hæmorrhage, often incorrectly attributed to bleeding from "vascular adhesions". The difficulty can be overcome by incising the parietal peritoneum anterior to the area of adhesion and carrying out an extraperitoneal mobilization of the spleen.

The vascular attachments should be dealt with by individual ligation of the vessels, both in the pedicle and the gastro-splenic ligament, mass ligatures being avoided. In order to conserve blood, the splenic artery is secured before the vein and some surgeons inject 0·5 ml. of 0·001 per cent. adrenaline in order to make the spleen contract and empty into the circulation its reservoir of blood. Ligatures in the hilum should carefully avoid damage to the tail of the pancreas.

If the operation is performed for some disorder of function, it should end with a search for accessory spleens, which may be present in the hilum of the spleen, the transverse mesocolon or greater omentum, or retroperitoneally.

Given a dry field at the end of the operation, the abdomen should be closed without drainage, but if there is any risk of vascular oozing or leakage of pancreatic juice from a damaged pancreatic tail, a corrugated rubber drain through a stab incision for a day or two is a safety measure.

Post-operative Treatment

Convalescence is not often complicated, but post-operative acute dilatation of the stomach and reflex paralytic ileus do seem rather more common after splenectomy than some other upper abdominal operations and an indwelling gastric tube for 24 hours is a good investment.

RODNEY SMITH

CHAPTER XVII

MODERN DEVELOPMENTS IN THE SURGERY OF THE SKULL AND ITS CONTENTS

Introduction

In the past five years progress in the field of neurosurgery has been on three main fronts: improvements in the technique of angiography and its extension to the vertebral arterial system; the surgery of intracranial vascular abnormalities which has been made possible by the use of arteriography; and the modifications of leucotomy in the treatment of mental illness and intractable pain. It is mainly with these advances, which are in effect extension and elaborations of existing techniques, that this chapter will be concerned, as the surgery of brain tumours and the management of head injuries has seen little change in the past five years. There is only one completely new development of note, which is the use of radioactive isotopes in the localization of cerebral tumours.

Neurosurgical Investigation

For the localization of brain tumour delineation of the ventricles and subarachnoid space by air or oxygen still remains the most accurate method and this method has not been supplanted by arteriography, although a great deal of additional information may often be obtained by the latter procedure.

Air Study

For the performance of an air study the gas is introduced either directly into the ventricle (ventriculography) through burrholes in the posterior parietal areas, or indirectly via the subarachnoid space by lumbar or cisternal puncture (encephalography). In the latter method the air collects in the cisterna magna below the vermis of the cerebellum and because of local anatomical relations tends to be directed through the Foramen of Majendie into the ventricular system. Providing the air is introduced sufficiently slowly and the head is carefully positioned the ventricles can be filled in more than 90 per cent. of cases, and then with movement of the head air can also be directed into the subarachnoid space round the brain. Encephalography will thus give information not only about the ventricular system, but also about the subarachnoid space and cisternæ, but the procedure will not be used if the intracranial pressure is raised.

The indications for ventriculography and encephalography can be summarized in this manner:

Ventriculography for the investigation of:
  (1) Tumours with raised intracranial tension,
  (2) Ventricular obstruction with hydrocephalus, and
  (3) When encephalography has failed.

Encephalography for the investigation of:
  (1) Tumours without raised pressure,
  (2) Atrophic lesions of the cortex (such as occur in the organic dementias),
  (3) Sequelæ of cranio-cerebral injuries,
  (4) Epilepsy.

Arteriography

The method of arteriographic visualization of the carotid or vertebral vascular systems is being increasingly used both for its essential value in demonstrating malformations of the blood vessels, such as aneurysm and angioma, and also for the investigation of brain tumours.

Its important feature in tumour investigation is that it does not alter the intracranial pressure as does ventriculography, and so is less likely to precipitate the need for urgent operation. Although remarkably safe it does carry the occasional danger of embolism or thrombosis of the intracranial vessels, particularly in old people. Sensitivity to Diodone is fortunately very rare.

Carotid Arteriography (Fig. 1).   The details of the technique of injection of the common or internal carotid artery are now well known and in experienced hands successful films are obtained in over 90 per cent. of cases. It is the usual practice to take three exposures in the lateral projection, showing roughly the arterial, capillary and venous phases, and two exposures in the antero-posterior plane. Recently machines have been devised which take a large number of films automatically from which more precise information about the circulation can be obtained.

In the investigation of brain tumours the site of the neoplasm will be revealed by a displacement of the main arterial, and to a lesser extent venous, trunks, or by a demonstration of the small vessels actually within the tumour, or both. If the neoplastic vessels happen to fill with contrast material, as is more likely with the highly vascular tumours such as meningiomata (Fig. 2) or the more malignant groups of gliomas, not only will the situation of the tumour be disclosed with great accuracy but also its pathological nature.   More commonly,

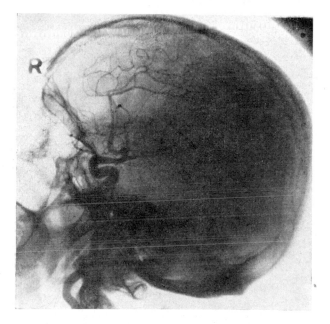

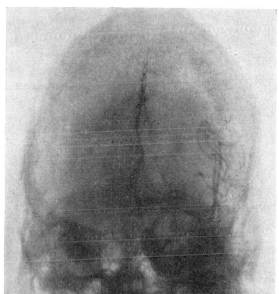

FIG. **17.1.** The normal carotid arteriogram. Lateral and antero-posterior views. In this case the posterior cerebral artery has filled in addition to the middle and anterior cerebral arteries. This occurs in approximately 25 per cent. of patients.

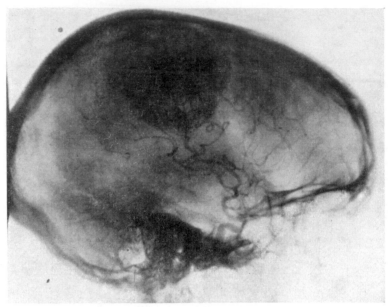

Fig. 17.2. Carotid arteriogram showing a meningioma in the parietal region. The precise situation and size of the tumour is revealed as well as its pathological nature.

however, the location has to be deduced from the shift of the main vessels and except in the cases of temporal lobe and subfrontal neoplasms the method generally is not as precise as ventriculography (Fig. 3).

With tumours situated in the parasagittal area, in the occipital lobes and in the midline producing hydrocephalus, the method is often of very limited value.

Vertebral Arteriography (Fig. 4). This procedure can usually be performed under local analgesia (Sutton and Hoare, 1951). The vessel is punctured through an intervertebral foramen, between the 3rd/4th, 4th/5th or 5th/6th cervical vertebræ. This procedure is successful in about 70 per cent. of cases when performed by skilled operators, but as there is this 30 per cent. failure rate alternative methods for injecting the artery are available; such as percutaneous puncture of the artery as it winds round the lateral mass of the atlas, exposure of the vessel by operation at the root of the neck just after it leaves the subclavian artery, or by the insertion of a fine catheter via the right radial artery up to the subclavian trunk under radiographic control, where it has a tendency to pass directly into the vertebral artery (Radner, 1951).

Vertebral arteriography has its greatest value in investigation of

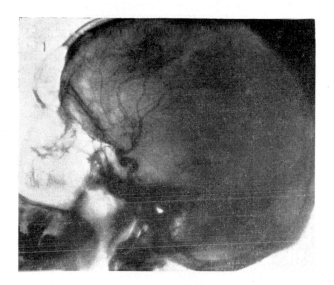

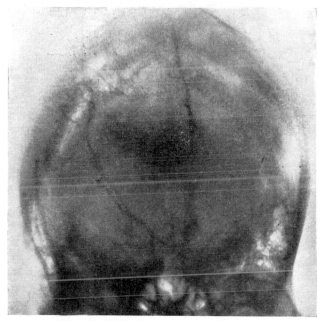

FIG. **17.3.** Carotid arteriogram demonstrating a temporal lobe tumour. Considerable displacement of the middle cerebral artery can be seen, forwards and upwards in the lateral view and medially in the antero-posterior projection.

The anterior cerebral artery is bowed across the midline.

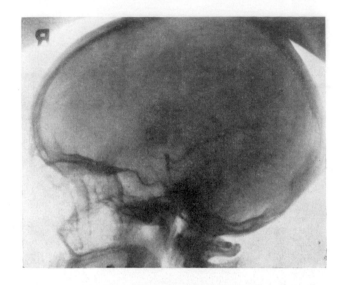

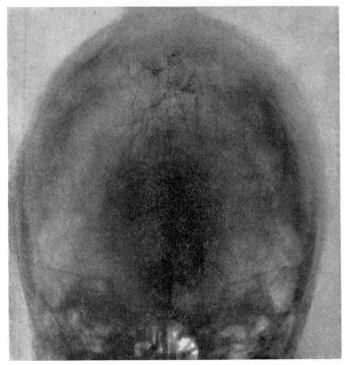

FIG. **17**.4. Normal vertebral arteriogram. Injection of one vertebral artery will fill both posterior cerebral arteries unless there is an anomaly of the Circle of Willis.

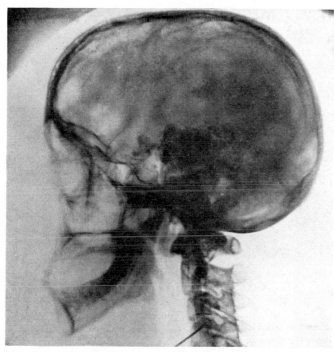

FIG. **17.5.** Vertebral arteriogram demonstrating a large angioma of the brain stem and cerebellum. The dilated left vertebral artery has been punctured through the intervertebral foramen between the 3rd and 4th cervical vertebrae.

angiomata of the occipital lobe, cerebellum and brain stem (Fig. 5) and aneurysms of vertebral, basilar and posterior cerebral arteries. Its use in diagnosis and localization of posterior fossa tumours is more limited partly owing to the fact that the density of the petrous and mastoid temporal bones tend to obscure the details of the small-calibre blood vessels in this situation. Meningiomata are commonly outlined, occasionally a nodule in a hæmangioblastoma may show up, and it may be helpful in tumours in the region of the pineal body. A shift of the basilar artery may be demonstrated with acoustic neuromata but without reliable frequency, and it is of little value in the presence of the medulloblastomata, cystic astrocytomata or cerebellar abscess.

Radio-active Isotopes. The need for a method of recognition and accurate localization of brain tumours without disturbing the intracranial pressure and with less discomfort and risk to the patient than ventriculography or arteriography has long been recognized, and the advent of radioactive isotopes gives some promise in this field (Ashkenazy *et al.*, 1951).

The principle determining their use is that intracranial tumours tend to concentrate certain isotopes more than the surrounding normal brain, the proportion varying with the type of isotope and the nature of the tumour, but it is roughly 6 to 8 times to 1, with an extreme range of about 100 to 1. With a Geiger-Müller counter applied to various areas of the head it should be possible to map out the site of greatest activity. There are, however, many technical difficulties of which an important one is that other structures such as the liver, the thyroid gland, muscles, etc., may take up the isotope in much greater concentration than the brain, and the emanation from them may swamp that from the head and give rise to inaccurate readings.

Radioactive Iodine (I^{131}) has been commonly used for this method in the form of Di-iodo fluorescin or more recently as iodonated human serum albumen. Peyton *et al.* (1952) using both of these substances found that accurate localization was possible in 94 per cent. of cases when the information obtained was interpreted in conjunction with clinical data, but the method was unfortunately not specific for brain tumours, as demyelinating conditions and lesions affecting the blood-brain barrier could also give positive results. On the other hand it was found that cystic and necrotic tumours would not concentrate the isotope.

Another application of the method is for localization and demarcation of subcortical tumours during the course of operation, utilizing a specially designed probe-counter of about the same diameter and length as an ordinary brain needle. The isotopes used with this method have been Radioactive Phosphorus (P^{32}) and Potassium (K^{42}). Radioactive Phosphorus emits only beta rays of short penetrating powers (5 to 7 mm. in brain tissue) so that a fairly accurate demarcation of the margin of the tumour is possible. Selverstone and White (1951) report that with its use they have located 150 tumours and demarcated 74 of them with less than 5 per cent. of error.

A further use for this probe-counter is for precise localization of a tumour through a small burrhole in the skull as a guide for the insertion of the biopsy needle when confirming the pathological nature of a tumour prior to operation.

Spontaneous Intracranial Hæmorrhage

The frequent occurrence and high mortality of spontaneous intracranial hæmorrhage coupled with the advances made by arteriography in the investigation of vascular lesions has stimulated a great deal of interest in, and expansion of, this field of neurosurgery in recent years.

The important three causes are rupture of (1) a "congenital" aneurysm, (2) an angioma, or (3) an atheromatous vessel in hypertensive vascular disease.

Congenital Aneurysms

These arise from a congenital weakness of the media of the arterial wall either at the branching of main arteries or at the original site of attachment of an embryonic vessel.

The common situations for aneurysms which can give rise to intracranial hæmorrhage are: (1) on the supraclinoid portion of the internal carotid artery, (2) on the anterior cerebral artery at or about its junction with the anterior communicating vessel, and (3) on the middle cerebral artery near the first bifurcation. These three sites give origin to over 80 per cent. of intracranial aneurysms.

An aneurysm in its unruptured state may cause (*a*) an isolated cranial nerve palsy, (*b*) attacks of migraine-like headache, and rarely (*c*) compression of the brain by great enlargement of its sac; but it is when it bursts and blood at high arterial pressure enters the subarachnoid space that it produces its most devastating symptoms. The high mortality resulting from aneurysmal rupture has been brought to light in recent years, and it appears that about 50 per cent. of patients who are admitted to hospital and treated conservatively die from the initial or from early recurrent hæmorrhage.

Subarachnoid hæmorrhage is the commonest manifestation of rupture, but bleeding may also occur into (1) the brain substance, to produce an intracerebral hæmatoma, from aneurysms set deeply in the interlobar fissures, or (2) into the ventricles (with a rapidly fatal outcome), or (3) into the subdural space.

Surgical treatment. The present trend in the management of cases of subarachnoid hæmorrhage from aneurysm is to carry out bilateral carotid arteriography as soon after the initial hæmorrhage as the patient's co-operation will permit, but if the bleeding is severe and the patient appears likely to die, angiography will be required as an emergency during the course of the hæmorrhage. If no aneurysm is disclosed on the carotid system vertebral angiography is performed a few days later. Once the aneurysm has been demonstrated and its position, size, and presence or absence of a "neck" defined, there are two main lines of surgical treatment available, that of ligation of a carotid artery (Internal or Common) in the neck, or that of a direct attack on the aneurysmal sac through a craniotomy flap.

It must be emphasized that at the present time the principle of surgical treatment is concerned more with the prevention of recurrent hæmorrhages, of which the peak incidence occurs during the second and third weeks after the first bleed, than with the immediate arrest of hæmorrhage during the initial rupture of the aneurysm.

It is, however, the uncertainty in the individual case regarding the chances of recurrent hæmorrhage that make the surgical management so difficult.

As the mortality and morbidity of surgical treatment (as will be shown later) are not inconsiderable, the present trend is to advise operative treatment for the more severe hæmorrhages, and to treat the minor bleedings more conservatively with rest in bed for four to six weeks, and to operate on these cases only if a further hæmorrhage occurs.

On the other hand there is the minority view that all aneurysms should be treated surgically once they have ruptured, but it is unlikely that this attitude will be generally adopted until the mortality rate from surgery is reduced to a much lower figure than it is at present.

Carotid Ligation.   This method will reduce the blood pressure in an arterial trunk and aneurysm, and so minimize the chance of a further leak and also will permit the aneurysm to shrink in size. Undoubtedly in some cases actual thrombosis occurs within the sac.   After common carotid ligation the mean arterial pressure in the internal carotid is reduced about 50 per cent. (Sweet and Bennett, 1948). The method will be most effective for aneurysms arising directly from the carotid artery, less effective for those on the circle of Willis, and least for those on the peripheral branches.   Its main hazard lies in the fact that if the anastomosis across the circle of Willis is inadequate ischæmia of the cerebral hemisphere results with the disastrous neurological symptoms of hemiplegia, aphasia, etc.   Manual compression of the carotid artery in the neck for 10 minutes will disclose the more severe grades of collateral inadequacy and is practised as a routine prior to ligation, but a hemiplegia may still develop despite a normal test.

The results that may be expected from carotid ligation in the treatment of intracranial aneurysms have recently been demonstrated by Jefferson (1952) in a series of 142 cases.

There were twelve deaths within six weeks of the procedure of which six were due to recurrent hæmorrhage from the same aneurysm. There were only two late deaths (after six weeks) from recurrent bleeding, at two and six years respectively after ligation.   Eleven patients developed hemiplegias of which four recovered and seven remained permanently.   It would seem that this method is remarkably effective as a prophylactic against a further early bleed, but is not an absolute bar to its occurrence, and the risks of a late recurrent hæmorrhage are remote. The chance of the development of a permanent hemiplegia is about 5 per cent.

Open Operation. This consists in turning a craniotomy flap, removing the intracerebral clot if one is present, exposing the aneurysm and then if feasible placing a clip or ligature round its neck at its junction with the parent vessel and so excluding it from the circulation (Fig. 6). It is, however, sometimes difficult to define a neck whatever the angiographic appearances may have suggested, and the ligature may have to be placed on the sac distal to its point of origin thus leaving a little pouch which may possibly lead to the redevelopment of the aneurysm. In a number of cases the aneurysm is truly sessile or is obscured by a number of small but important branches, and the surgeon is reduced to wrapping the wall of the aneurysm round with muscle which may have some effect in strengthening it and preventing rupture.

The mortality from these open operations is in the region of 16 per cent. (Falconer, 1952) although some striking results have recently been achieved by Norlen (1952) who recorded 44 patients operated upon with only three deaths and three permanent hemiplegias. Whether these methods will prevent further enlargement and rupture of the sac, particularly in those cases where a pouch is left, is not known, for the follow-up is still too short and until this is known and until a lower mortality is obtained the indications for open operation must remain unsettled.

It may be generally stated that at the present time the trend is to reserve the direct attack for those aneurysms which are situated more peripherally on the arterial tree and to employ carotid ligation for aneurysms arising from the internal carotid trunk. For those on the circle of Willis there is no general rule, if a narrow well-defined neck is seen on arteriography exploration is justified, but for others ligation in the neck still remains the best method.

Angiomata

These are congenital lesions but tend to enlarge and to give rise to symptoms in adult life, and rarely manifest themselves in childhood. They usually lie on the surface of the brain but may be deeply situated in close relation to the basal ganglia or ventricles and some occur on the brain stem or in the cerebellum. In size they vary from almost microscopical dimensions (but still capable of producing fatal hæmorrhage) to a very large size sometimes covering half a hemisphere.

The usual presenting symptom is that of epilepsy, either focal or generalized, which may exist for many years without demonstrable physical signs, but eventually a progressive neurological deficit or

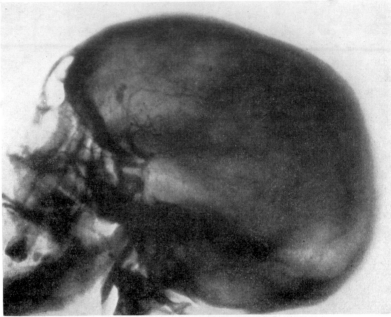

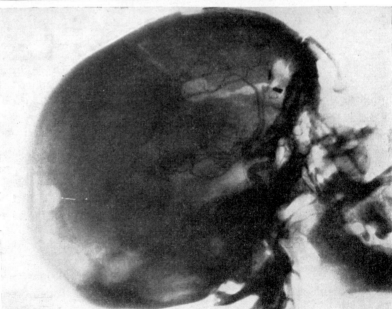

FIG. 17.6.   The pre-operative arteriogram on the left shows a bilocular aneurysm
arising from an anomalous calloso-marginal branch of the right anterior cerebral
artery. The neck of the aneurysm was ligated and the post-operative arteriogram shows the parent artery still to be patent but there is no filling of the sac.

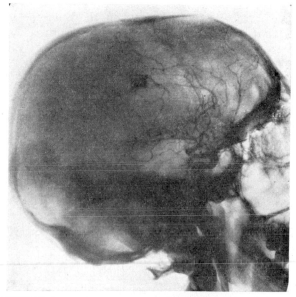

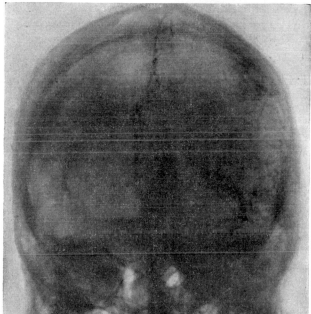

FIG. **17**.7.   Carotid arteriogram showing a small angioma in
the left parietal area which had ruptured into the brain substance to produce a large intracerebral hæmatoma as indicated
by the displacement of the anterior cerebral artery across the
midline. The angioma is supplied by two branches of the
middle cerebral artery and its single draining vein can be seen
emerging at its posterior border.

dementia appears. It is, however, when the angiomata give rise to hæmorrhage that attention is drawn more dramatically to their presence.

With the larger malformations the bleeding tends to occur into the subarachnoid space in a similar fashion to aneurysms, sometimes recurring at intervals of months or years. In other cases, and particularly with a small angioma deeply hidden in a sulcus, the blood erupts into the substance of the brain producing gross neurological symptoms (Fig. 7). As the effused blood tends to follow the projection fibres from the cortex towards the internal capsule the tracts are displaced and distorted rather than transected, and the amount of recovery that may take place from an initial severe neurological disability is often surprisingly great.

These lesions, despite the rapid circulation through them, can usually be well demonstrated by arteriography and their arteries of supply easily located. Whatever their symptomatology it is possible to remove them in about one-third of the cases (McKissock, 1950) and the use of hypotensive drugs to lower the blood pressure has made the surgery of them much more safe. The large arterial channels are first ligated and then the resultant shrunken tumour mass can be dissected off the brain surface with little or no damage to the latter and, if care is taken, without hazard to the normal blood supply of the hemisphere.

Hypertensive Vascular Disease

This is a much less rewarding field of surgical endeavour. The patients are usually older than in the previous two groups and even if surgery is successful the hypertension of course persists, and recurrent fatal hæmorrhage a few weeks or months later is a common sequel. Moreover, the hæmorrhage from the usual source of rupture, the striate vessels, tends to transect the fibres in the internal capsule so that the neurological disabilities which result are usually profound and the degree of recovery disappointingly small. Intellectual function is often severely and permanently reduced and personality changes are common.

Some 80 per cent. of patients with this type of hæmorrhage die within 2 to 24 hours, and of the remainder a small number cease bleeding spontaneously but remain with a large hæmatoma in the cerebral hemisphere, and it is this group which may come to surgery. The hæmatoma can then be aspirated by means of a brain needle introduced through a frontal or parietal burrhole. An occasional brilliant result is obtained with the patient making an almost complete recovery, but more often he is left severely crippled and survives for a few months only until the next hæmorrhage.

Abscess

A recent survey by Jooma *et al.* (1951) of 291 cases of brain abscess has confirmed the value of antibiotics in the treatment of these lesions, and has also brought to light some interesting facts concerning the late results of treatment.

There are three methods of treating brain abscess in general use: (1) Continuous drainage by tube or marsupialization, (2) aspiration (and sterilization with antibiotics), and (3) excision (usually following aspiration). A strict comparison of the mortality between these varied methods is not feasible, but it is evident that the mortality generally has been substantially reduced by the use of antibiotics, for in the series quoted above the death rate dropped from 58 per cent. to 27 per cent. with the use of penicillin.

The important late complications after successful treatment are those of recrudescence of the abscess, and epilepsy. In this series recurrent abscesses formed in 8 per cent. of cases treated by aspiration (and all died) whereas none formed following excision of the abscess.

Epilepsy occurred in about 47 per cent. of patients whatever the method of treatment and, surprisingly, irrespective of whether the abscess capsule was left in the brain or removed, with the sole exception of abscesses in the frontal lobe where excision of the capsule did result in a significant lowering of the risk of seizures.

The present trend in treatment of brain abscess, whether secondary to ear and sinus infection or metastatic from the lung, is to use aspiration in the first instance. This method will be a life saving procedure, it will control the size of the abscess while its capsule is forming and will permit sterilization of its contents by the introduction of antibiotics. The changes in size of the abscess can be followed by X-rays after the insertion of thorotrast which is "taken up" by the capsule within 7 to 14 days. In over one-third of the cases there is more than one loculus in the abscess, and the antibiotic may not penetrate into all of these so this condition should be borne in mind if the patient's symptoms and signs do not improve with shrinkage of the demonstrable abscess.

When it is judged that the capsule is well formed, usually between 3 to 6 weeks after the commencement of treatment, the abscess should be excised if readily accessible. If situated deeply within the hemisphere or in an evocative area of brain treatment by aspiration without excision will give the best functional result. Whatever treatment is adopted anti-convulsant drugs should be taken for several years.

Leucotomy

For certain types of psychiatric disorders pre-frontal leucotomy and allied procedures have achieved an established place in treatment, and providing there is careful selection of cases the effects of the operations are generally predictable and the results satisfactory.

The operation which up to the present time has been most commonly used has come to be known as the "standard" operation and as advocated originally by Freeman and Watts (1942) was a blind procedure, the white fibres being divided in the plane of the coronal suture by an instrument inserted through a burrhole placed 3 cm. behind the orbital margin and 5 cm. above the zygomatic arch. This operation has the greatest therapeutic effect but is also more liable to be associated with undesirable personality changes. As the extent of the incision in the frontal lobe tended to vary from patient to patient and often from surgeon to surgeon an "open" operation through a craniotomy flap was devised by Poppen (1948), and the division of the fibres was made under direct vision which made the extent of the section more precise and also permitted complete hæmostasis to be achieved.

The modern trend in psychosurgery, however, has been concerned with the search for certain areas in the frontal region, division of whose connections might produce the desired therapeutic result without any personality change. These operations were based on the hope that there was some selectivity of function in the frontal areas and that the effects of leucotomy were not decided solely by the amount of cortex detached, i.e. that there was a qualitative as well as a quantitative relationship.

The modified operations all have one feature in common, that of interruption of the cortico-thalamic connections at some part of their course, and they have been inspired and influenced mainly by the knowledge obtained from stimulation and ablation experiments in animals and the effect of these on autonomic reactions and behaviour.

These selective operations have been directed at four main sites in the brain:

(1) The supero-lateral convexity of the frontal lobe (Brodmann Areas 9 and 10 partly or completely).

(2) The orbital surface of the frontal lobe.

(3) The anterior cingulate gyrus (Brodmann area 24).

(4) The thalamus.

The precise type of operative interference has also varied; some surgeons have advocated actual excision of the cortex of the area concerned, "Gyrectomy" (Penfield, 1948) or "Topectomy" (Pool, 1949) by open exposure. Although a precise method in some ways it has the disadvantage of interfering with the blood supply of adjacent cortex, and more importantly, of leaving a raw area which may act as an epileptogenic focus— and in fact the operation has an incidence of epilepsy of 14 per cent.

Another method, also by open operation, is to make a small incision in the cortex and then divide the white fibres at their junction with the grey matter, a comparatively avascular plane— "Cortical undercutting" (Scoville, 1949). This has the advantage of avoiding a large scar, and should not interfere with the blood supply either of the cortex which has been undercut or that adjacent to it.

A third method is a closed or "blind" procedure, similar to the "standard" operation in which the white matter is divided on a deeper sub-cortical plane through a burrhole on the convexity of the skull, or in the case of areas 9 and 10 by an instrument inserted through the conjunctival sac and orbital roof—the controversial operation of transorbital leucotomy.

In general the open operations are more precise in the amount of tissue damaged and less liable post-operatively to be followed by intracerebral hæmorrhage, for any bleeding points can be seen and arrested, but it is a major procedure for the patient and can only be done in a fully equipped neuro-surgical department. The "blind" procedures are less precise and more uncertain in the degree of fibre interruption, and post-operative bleeding may occur from un-witting damage to vessels, but the nature of the operation is a more minor one.

A further method and one which is quite separate in its approach from those already mentioned, is that of destruction of the dorso medial nucleus of the thalamus by electro-coagulation, a needle electrode being inserted into the nucleus by means of a stereotaxic apparatus (Spiegel and Wycis, 1949). Orientation of the apparatus and needle is obtained by reference to a fixed part in the brain, the pineal body if it is calcified, or other anatomical features at the posterior end of the third ventricle which can be demonstrated by air encephalography.

Although a most ingenious method its results so far do not appear to be any better than the other procedures, the mortality is certainly no lower, and it is a method which can only be used in special centres by teams skilled in the procedure.

The various sites and procedures can now be summed up in this fashion:

(1) Standard operation of Pre-frontal Leucotomy:
    (a) "Blind".
    (b) "Open" method.

   (2) Superior Frontal Convexity (Areas 9 and 10 Brodmann):
       (*a*) Gyrectomy or topectomy.
       (*b*) Open undercutting.
       (*c*) Blind subcortical section
           (i) from above, or
           (ii) transorbital.
   (3) Orbital Surface:
       (*a*) Topectomy.
       (*b*) Open undercutting.
   (4) Cingulate area (Brodmann 24):
       (*a*) Gyrectomy.
       (*b*) Open undercutting.
   (5) Thalamotomy. Stereotaxis.

The results of these diverse operations have tended to confirm the fact that there is little selectivity of function in the frontal lobes and that as far as the frontal operations are concerned it is the amount of brain detached rather than its situation which is the important factor in the result.

In general the present tendency is to advise the "standard" operation for patients with severe symptoms, and to employ a lesser procedure in patients with milder symptoms who are not insane. The lesser operation commonly favoured at the present time is that directed at the superior frontal convexity (Brodmann areas 9 and 10) because of its easy accessibility, either by "open" or "blind" operation.

Complications

Severe personality changes have already been mentioned. The mortality rate is between 2 and 3 per cent., although higher and lower rates have been recorded from different clinics. Death is usually a result of hæmorrhage or sepsis, although it occasionally occurs later as a result of neurological damage (Meyer and McLardy, 1948). The incidence of epilepsy is probably in the neighbourhood of 8 to 10 per cent. but the fits tend to improve and are usually easily controlled with anti-convulsants.

Results

Since leucotomy is essentially the treatment of a symptom—that of emotional tension, the benefit obtained in any mental illness will depend largely on the emotional state associated with it.

The results in specific syndromes have recently been assessed by Curran and Partridge (1952) from their own extensive experience and their conclusions can be summarized as follows:

Schizophrenia. In general rather more than one-third of any series of well-selected schizophrenics who would otherwise be permanent hospital inmates, are benefited sufficiently to be able to leave hospital, although by no means necessarily cured. About one-third of the remainder are improved in that they would be able to lead a less restricted life and become less difficult nursing problems. Persons of good previous personality whose symptoms were of sudden onset and which pursued a fluctuating course have the best prognosis whereas those with the simple deteriorating type of illness, of insidious onset and with emotional flatness, show the least improvement. In paranoid patients where the personality is relatively well preserved the tension and distress associated with the delusions may lessen considerably although the delusions persist.

Affective disorders. In involutional melancholia about two-thirds of the patients may be restored to near normality, always providing that the pattern of the illness has not become fixed and that it has not persisted without fluctuation for more than two years.

In manic-depressive psychosis those cases with a previous history of only depressive phases (the larger group) tend to do better than those with manic attacks. In the latter type of illness the tendency for the attacks to recur after operation is greater, and difficult post-operative personalities are common.

Obsessional states. Some of the most striking results are seen in this group, and providing the symptoms have not become too entrenched the vast majority of these patients will show symptomatic improvement. The obsessional pattern remains but the distress which it causes the patient is much reduced. Those cases in whom the obsessions take the form of rumination, phobias and compulsive thinking, usually have a better prognosis than those presenting with ritualistic behaviour.

Leucotomy for Pain

This procedure is of great value in the treatment of intractable pain where operation on the peripheral nerves or spinal cord is either not feasible or has failed.

Leucotomy does not interfere with the perception of pain and certainly does not abolish the normal reaction to painful stimuli, but it does eliminate the distressing emotional over-reaction to continuous pain. For instance a patient after a successful leucotomy will not complain spontaneously of pain, but if pressed usually admits that his pain is still present and possibly as bad as it ever was, but will state that it no longer worries or distresses him, and he can put up with it.

The operation has its best use in the treatment of those patients with painful progressive malignant disease for whom life expectancy is comparatively short and who do not obtain adequate relief from analgesics, but it has also been successfully used for the crises of tabes dorsalis, the thalamic syndrome, causalgia and phantom-limb pain.

The extent of the leucotomy is important, for although modified procedures have been advocated for the successful control of pain it will often be found that their effect is shortlived, and although a more extensive operation can always be done as a second step for patients who have a longer life expectancy, the use of the "standard" operation in the first instance will usually be found to be the best. It must be realized, however, that with this type of patient, who is otherwise mentally normal, the degree of "flattening", apathy and lack of drive that results is considerably greater than in a patient suffering from a psychiatric disorder, and a successful cure of the pain is not often associated with a return to full work.

VALENTINE LOGUE

References

Neurosurgical investigations:
Arteriography:
SUTTON, D., and HOARE, R. D. (1951) *Brit. J. Radiol.* **24,** 589.
Radner, S. (1951) *Acta Radiol. Stockh.*, Suppl. **87.**
Radio-active isotopes:
ASHKENAZY, M., DAVIS, L., and MARTIN, J. (1951) *J. Neurosurg.* **8,** 300.
PEYTON, W. T., MOORE, G. E., FRENCH, L. A., and CHOU, S. N. (1952) *J. Neurosurg.* **9,** 432.
SELVERSTONE, B., and WHITE, J. C. (1951) *Ann. Surg.* **134,** 387.

Spontaneous intracranial hæmorrhage:
Aneurysm:
FALCONER, M. A. (1952) *Proc. R. Soc. Med.* **45,** 298.
JEFFERSON, G. (1952) *Proc. R. Soc. Med.* **45,** 300.
NORLEN, G. (1952) *Proc. R. Soc. Med.* **45,** 290.
SWEET, W. H., and BENNETT, H. S. (1948) *J. Neurosurg.* **5,** 178.
Angioma:
MCKISSOCK, W. (1950) *Ann. R. Coll. Surg. Engl.* **7,** 472.

Brain Abscess:
JOOMA, O. V., PENNYBACKER, J. B., and TUTTON, K. (1951) *J. Neurol. Neurosurg. Psychiat.* **19,** 308.

Leucotomy:
CURRAN, D., and PARTRIDGE, M. (1952) "Surgical Progress," p. 162.   London, Butterworth & Co. Ltd.
FREEMAN, W., and WATTS, J. W. (1942) "PsychoSurgery." Springfield, Ill. Charles C. Thomas.
MEYER, A., and McLARDY, T. (1948) *J. ment. Sci.* **89,** 194.
PENFIELD, W. (1948) "The Frontal Lobes." *Res. Publ. Ass. nerv. ment. Dis.* **27,** 519.
POOL, J. L. (1949) *Proc. R. Soc. Med.* Suppl. **42,** 1.
POPPEN, J. L. (1948) *Dig. Neurol. Psychiat.* **16,** 403.
SCOVILLE, W. B. (1949) *J. Neurosurg.* **6,** 65.
SPIEGEL, E. A., and WYCIS, H. T. (1949) *Proc. R. Soc. Med.* Suppl. **42,** 12.

CHAPTER XVIII

THE SURGICAL TREATMENT OF HYPERTENSION

DURING the last twenty years the surgical treatment of Hypertension has been attempted on a large scale, reaching a climax in the years 1948-51. Lumbo-dorsal sympathectomy, varying from the lower operation of Adson to the total sympathectomy of Grimson, has been performed in an attempt to reduce the blood pressure by opening up the "splanchnic pool", to improve the renal circulation and perhaps to denervate the adrenal glands. The author has had considerable experience of an operation involving removal of the sympathetic chain from the 4th dorsal ganglion to the 1st or 2nd lumbar involving complete removal of the splanchnic nerves.

Undoubtedly many patients have been greatly benefited by the operation, which is severe and involves two stages, one for each side; but also many patients have received little or no permanent reduction of blood pressure level and a few, 2·6 per cent., have died as the result of the operation.

The important stage of the treatment by sympathectomy is not the operation itself, of which many varieties have produced both good and bad results, but in the assessment and selection of patients for surgery. Many of the most startlingly beneficial results have been obtained in patients with "malignant" complications of papilloedema, retinitis and impaired renal function. In such patients the probable course of the untreated disease leading to blindness and an early death often justifies a major surgical procedure which may restore the failing sight and return the patient to a useful life which is prolonged, even at the risk of death or a long incapacity as the result of an unsuccessful operation.

The hardest patients to assess are those suffering from "essential hypertension". Certain factors are leading pointers in making the decision:

1. Symptoms may be entirely absent and the patient's general condition good. Such a case I am very reluctant to submit to operation.
2. Symptoms of headache, shortness of breath, dizziness and "palpitations" may be severe enough to cause invalidism. Such a patient will be considered.
3. Cardiac damage may be progressive as demonstrated by screening and by electrocardiography. In such cases a successful operation will delay the progress of the heart deterioration and

211

may frequently cause a definite improvement in the E.C.G. and the size of the heart.

4. Renal function must be good enough to stand two severe operations. I have usually set a standard as judged by the intravenous pyelogram—good enough concentration to see the anatomy, and the Urea Clearance Test—a minimum of 33 per cent. of normal, together with a blood urea of not above 90 mgm./100 ml.

These last figures, of course, represent a poor risk case, but if the other indications are positive, still allow operation.

Macroscopic hæmaturia I regard as an absolute contra-indication.

5. The age of the patient is not very material, but the younger the better the operation is taken as a rule and, within the limitations of physical damage to heart and kidneys, the better the result. As a general rule the arbitrary age of 50 is taken as limit to the major sympathectomy, after that age I recommend a more limited type of subdiaphragmatic procedure on the lines of Adson's operation. This is quite arbitrary and depends on the patient's general condition, remembering that women usually do better than men.

Some of the best results are obtained in women who have been found hypertensive during pregnancy, the condition persisting after delivery but not being accompanied by albuminuria. The best result so far is in a child of 12 who had a stroke at the age of 11 with a hemiplegia which had mostly cleared; he had hæmorrhage and exudate in the retina, but normal renal function. This boy was thought to have a phæochromocytoma, but gave no positive tests and, indeed, none was found on exploration; the sympathetic chains were therefore removed from T.4 to L.2 at an interval of two weeks. Now, four years later, he has a blood pressure of 120/80 (pre-operatively 200/150) and is a normal boy of his age except for a footdrop being the remains of his right hemiplegia.

6. Attacks of heart failure are not a contraindication and may be relieved by operation, but such a patient may be undergoing a grave risk of death during or shortly after the operation.

7. A stroke is not a contraindication provided that the patient has made sufficient recovery to be nearly or quite back to normal.

Summing up these points and trying to estimate the probable untreated life of the patient will require considerable investigation and observation. I will not operate upon such patients as have rapidly advancing renal disease, whom I expect to die within six months. On the other hand, if I think that the kidneys will last long enough for the patient to enjoy a possibly successful result of the operation, such as restoration of eyesight and cure of other disabling symptoms, then I will try, even if only a subdiaphragmatic operation is performed.

A girl aged 17 was found to be virtually blind due to œdema of the optic discs and hæmorrhage into the retina. Her blood pressure was high, 220/160, and her renal function poor. (Urea Clearance 40 per cent. Blood Urea 60 mgm./100 ml.)

We judged her to have glomerulonephritis, but thought operation justifiable. After operation her eyesight recovered to 6/6 and she was symptom free for one year, when she went into coma and died of renal failure. During that year she was at work for nine months and could pursue her hobby of embroidery. We watched her renal function deteriorating at three monthly tests.

The hardest factor to estimate is the patient's state of mind. An introspective, worrying patient is not a good subject for operation; symptoms are magnified and post-operative disabilities are likely to be out of all proportion. On the other hand, many patients are much better mentally if they know that something may be done for them. It is important to get to know the patient before passing final judgment.

From this account of the selection before operation it will be seen that the physician and surgeon both play their part and make a decision, a unanimous decision, to operate.

The various tests to estimate the likely outcome of sympathectomy are quite unreliable and routine performance of sedation and cold pressor tests are not now considered worth while. Similarly, the response or not to hexamethonium compounds gives little indication of the operation result. It is important that the patient should not be misled into expecting a cure; someone will always divulge the blood pressure in after years, but they must expect a relief of symptoms and lessening of the danger of early cerebral catastrophe or cardiac or renal failure.

Crediting operation results on these lines, they are good in a series of 150 patients. All had been carefully selected and were co-operative, none expected to be a complete clinical cure, and I believe such a thing is impossible even though the blood pressure may be normal several years after operation.

The operation of my choice is transthoracic, through the bed of the ninth rib, opening the pleura and removing the sympathetic chain from the junction with the topmost root of the great splanchnic nerve to the 2nd lumbar ganglion, pursuing the chain behind the diaphragm by splitting the crus. The great splanchnic is removed down to the cœliac ganglion and the kidneys and adrenals can be palpated and, if necessary, inspected and pieces removed for biopsy. The two sides are done at a minimum of two weeks' interval.

In the immediate post-operative period the blood pressure may be very low, but the pulse should remain good and the colour pink. I am very much against any "boosting" of blood pressure by drugs, it will return to a working level and meanwhile the head-down position and very occasionally leg bandaging is all that is required. Urinary output may be very restricted for a few days if there is much kidney damage, but the blood urea usually returns to pre-operative normal within a week.

Chest complications are few, but an effusion which needs aspiration appears occasionally and on two occasions a chylothorax has developed after damage to cœliac lymphatics; both settled down with aspiration.

Post-operative pain is the real bugbear of the operation. Some degree of deep pain follows all operations on the sympathetic nervous system, but is usually transient and not very severe. After a large-scale ganglionectomy for hypertension the pain may be very severe and prolonged. Great care is taken to avoid damage to intercostal nerves by carefully raising the ganglion and cutting the rami communicantes, and the ninth nerve is divided proximal to the site of rib section. The severe pain is usually centred on the epigastrium and round the ribs, is worse at night and during inactivity and usually reaches a peak of intensity about the 7th-10th day after operation. No peripheral nerve blocks make any difference, it is ameliorated by hot or cold packs to the chest wall posteriorly and movement. Occasionally such a pain persists for weeks, but in that case an intercostal nerve has often been damaged and can be blocked or divided proximally.

In the immediate post-operative period anorexia, abdominal distension and flatulence are often annoying, but this is usually over by the fifth post-operative day. A duodenal or gastric ulcer may flare up and must be watched carefully, because lesions of the upper intestinal tract no longer cause pain. In spite of these troubles most patients are up and about in from 2-5 days and ready for the second operation in 2-3 weeks.

Convalescence is prolonged, 3-5 months, and arrangements must be made beforehand for relief of all domestic and business burdens from the patient. Postural hypotension is often troublesome for some time and may require an abdominal binder or leg bandages. Patients should be instructed to rise slowly from the lying or sitting position.

Symptoms of headache, "palpitations" and fear are relieved in nearly all patients suitable for operation; if the sight has been affected by papillœdema or retinitis there is frequently a dramatic subjective improvement within 10 days, even though the ophthalmoscopic appearances are unaltered for several weeks.

Eventually in about six months most patients feel and look much better than before operation and are grateful for the treatment. The blood pressure, as we know, will usually rise again, but often to a "safe" level, and undoubtedly more stable to emotional stimulation.

A few elderly patients, often men, with malignant hypertension, bad kidneys and failing sight respond to a limited subdiaphragmatic removal of the sympathetic chain from D.12 to L.2, together with the terminal parts of the splanchnic nerves. Both sides may be done at one session and even though the renal or cardiac failure eventually supervene, sight may be restored. In these patients the fall of blood pressure is not marked, but again it becomes much steadier.

Partial removal of the adrenals may be performed with both types of operation, but the value of such a procedure is doubtful and the risks of operation may be increased.

Chronic pyelonephritis is a lesion causing hypertension and, if it should affect only one kidney, then removal of that kidney may cure the hypertension. If the high blood pressure is of long standing, then the other kidney may be secondarily damaged and nephrectomy is contraindicated.

A unilateral renal lesion causing hypertension must obstruct the afferent arterioles or the main renal artery. Hydronephrosis or tuberculous lesions do not cause hypertension, although it may be superimposed.

"A patient with malignant hypertension was found to have a functionless left kidney, which proved to be destroyed by a longstanding hydronephrosis. The other kidney function was not normal but adequate. Left nephrectomy caused no improvement in signs or symptoms. Bilateral lumbo-dorsal sympathectomy was performed eight months later and the patient responded well. Now three years after the last operation she is symptom free, eyes normal, blood pressure 170/100, and feels and looks very well. The urea clearance of the remaining kidney is 50 per cent. normal, having improved from 40 per cent."

"Another patient with malignant hypertension and a functionless right kidney containing a large calculus had normal function in the left kidney. Right nephrectomy has improved her to such a degree that all symptoms have gone and the blood pressure, two years later, is 140/95. The removed kidney was small and atrophic with microscopic evidence of chronic pyelonephritis."

Patients with hypertension which respond well to nephrectomy are very rare; although the blood pressure may be within normal limits six months after such an operation, so it may respond in certain patients to any major operation. Unless the remaining kidney is good and the removed kidney had obstructed arterial flow the final result will be bad.

Removal of the worst of two damaged, but functioning, kidneys is a very bad operation. If any shadow is seen on intravenous pyelogram on the supposed bad side and the other kidney function is not within normal limits then all treatment should be directed at salvage and not destruction. There is no doubt that a suitable sympathectomy and splanchnicetomy may improve kidney function after a period of time. Particularly must the surgeon beware of the hydronephrosis that shows no shadow on intravenous pyelography, but yet is secreting when examined by ureteric catheterization and intravenous dye. A hydronephrosis on the other side may not be so large and may show on pyelography and tempt the unwary to remove the poorer of two poor kidneys. Lumbo-dorsal sympathectomy in such a case will often cause a remarkable contraction of the renal pelvis and a greatly improved pyelogram besides the benefit to the patient's hyperpietic condition.

A suprarenal medullary tumour, phæochromocytoma, will cause hypertension, spasmodic and rapidly becoming malignant. Such hypertension will be cured by removal of the tumour and the cure will be complete unless a second tumour is present.

E. G. TUCKWELL

References:

ADSON, A. W., CRAIG, W. McK., and BROWN, G. E. (1936) *Surg. Gynec. Obstet.* **62,** 314.

BOURNE, G., PHILPS, A. S., and TUCKWELL, E. G. (1948) *Proc. R. Soc. Med.* **41,** 728.

PEET, M. M., WOODS, W. W., and BRADEN, S. (1940) *J. Amer. med. Ass.* **115,** 1875.

THOMPSON, J. E., and SMITHWICK, R. H. (1952) *Angiology* **3,** 493.

WHITELAW, G. P., and SMITHWICK, R. H. (1951) *Angiology* **2,** 157.

CHAPTER XIX

CARCINOMA OF THE BREAST

Early Diagnosis

The breast remains the most frequent site of cancer in women. Diagnosis at an early clinical stage offers the greatest hope of combating the disease until some new and as yet undiscovered diagnostic method becomes available. Even early diagnosis does not ensure that we are dealing with an "early carcinoma"—a misleading term—but at least it makes this possibility more likely than if the disease is clinically well established when we first encounter it. Two tendencies in recent years have contributed significantly to an improvement in the outlook for carcinoma of the breast because they tend to lead to earlier diagnosis. The first has come from the patients themselves, many more of whom are now reporting their disease at an earlier clinical stage. The second has come from the teaching schools where the emphasis has passed from the academic contemplation of the refinements of differential diagnosis to the importance of recognizing the urgency of establishing by exploration the nature of a doubtful lump. The fallibility of clinical diagnosis is at last accepted and it is now recognized that however experienced we are, we cannot differentiate with certainty on *clinical grounds alone* between the non-malignant and the early malignant swelling. Exploration can alone reveal its true nature. Similarly it is now agreed that a period of *observation* is no longer justifiable in the treatment of the doubtful breast lesion. Exploration is the only proper procedure if there is the slightest uncertainty and we have therefore come to regard the "biopsy" of a lump in the breast as an emergency operation. It is for this reason that the names of all such patients as well as those with established carcinoma should be placed upon a special waiting list so that arrangements can be made for their very early admission.

Reorientation of our ideas of the presenting clinical picture of carcinoma of the breast is also resulting in earlier action. It is now accepted that a swelling in the breast of a woman of any age is cancer until it is proved otherwise—that on inspection the configuration of the breast is normal in "early carcinoma"—that on palpation a hard lump in the breast, unattached to the skin is the earliest sign of carcinoma—that the "cardinal signs", adherence to the skin, a retracted nipple, and palpable axillary glands are the signs of long standing advanced carcinoma—that the inaccuracy of the clinical findings is greatest in the stout patient, in whom fat conceals from palpation both the tumour

217

and the glands—that "no case is as early as it seems" and that negative axillary findings and non-adherence to the skin are compatible with the presence of metastases in glands which cannot be palpated clinically, and finally that the urgency for investigation is greatest in those patients in whom the cardinal signs are absent and the diagnosis is uncertain, because it is with these patients that the chances of cure are highest.

Biopsy

The term biopsy may not be entirely satisfactory, but in this connection is familiarly used by most surgeons to mean the exploration of a lump in the breast. In all doubtful cases a biopsy must be advised and the patient's permission obtained to remove the breast if in their interests this course seems advisable. An incision should be made directly over the lump when it will immediately become apparent whether it is solid or cystic. If the swelling is revealed to be a cyst this should be excised. If solid it is recommended that the incision should be carried through the centre of the swelling when it will be apparent to an experienced surgeon in eight out of ten cases on naked eye inspection whether the lump is definitely malignant or definitely innocent. If necessary the swelling can be completely excised with the diathermy and examined away from the breast. In the small proportion of cases in which doubt remains after cutting into the lump, two courses are open to the surgeon. He may either hand it over for immediate frozen section or close the wound and send the specimen to the laboratory. The frozen section technique is a great convenience, and in the hands of the few is reliable but it is a matter of experience that it is in just those cases in which the surgeon is still uncertain after cutting into the tumour, that the pathologist also has most difficulty in making up his mind. For this reason unless the facilities available are exceptional it is wiser to allow the pathologist the extra time necessary to dehydrate the specimen thoroughly, with the advantages in staining and examination which such preparation makes possible. While a second anæsthetic may be necessary the delay occasioned by this more cautious method is not great. An unhurried examination can be carried out and a reliable report obtained within 24 hours of sending the specimen to the laboratory.

Treatment
Stages I, II

Treatment is a radio-surgical problem, and the parts to be played by X-rays and by surgery must be determined separately before embarking upon either. This can only be done effectively if surgeon and radiotherapist first see and discuss the case together.

Radical Mastectomy

Radical mastectomy combined with radiotherapy remains the best treatment available for Stage I and II cases. Our objectives in carrying out this operation are to eradicate the disease and to achieve this without mortality or morbidity. It is not the purpose of this survey to describe the operation. A detailed technical account has been given by Riddell (1948).

Mortality. In 11,014 radical mastectomies performed by 22 British surgeons and collected by Cade (1948) there were 182 deaths a mortality of 1·65 per cent.

Morbidity. Curiously enough the morbidity is more worrying than the mortality following the operation of radical mastectomy. Such complications as *necrosis of the skin edges* and a *poor functional result* are still seen with greater frequency than one would expect following an operation which has been abundantly practised by innumerable surgeons all over the world for over half a century. These particular sequelæ are essentially a reflection on the judgment or the executive skill of the operator and not upon the operation itself. Furthermore such indifferent results become known, and because they lose nothing in the telling may have a serious deterrent effect upon patients contemplating advice about a newly acquired lump in the breast. It is to be remembered that we are operating under almost ideal conditions— the patients are constitutionally well and often near the prime of life, the anatomy of the area is normal and not distorted as it might be, and there are none of the embarrassments associated with operations within a body cavity. A very high degree of technical excellence should therefore be our aim, both in regard to the thoroughness of the dissection which has as its objective the extirpation of the disease, and in regard to the care with which the flaps are first raised and later approximated which can so much determine the degree of ultimate functional disability.

The Prevention of Functional Disability. Functional disability usually takes the form of restricted movement at the shoulder and is doubly undesirable, since it not only seriously reduces the range of usefulness of the limb concerned, but aggravates by constant reminder the psychological trauma resulting from the operation.

Following mastectomy, free movements at the shoulder depend upon the normal *laxity* of the skin of the axilla remaining unimpaired. Functional disability is due to *shortage of skin* in the axillary area which has the effect of tightening the axillary fold and so restricting movement. This can come about in two different ways:

By loss of skin. Marginal *flap necrosis* resulting in skin loss occurs if the blood supply of a flap is damaged during its elevation. This accident most commonly occurs to the lateral flap as the dissection approaches the anterior border of latissimus dorsi which corresponds with the deepest part of the wound; it is usually due to hurrying this part of the reflection in a field obscured by hæmorrhage. The blood supply may also be cut off from the edges of both flaps by the use of *tension* sutures and with the same result. Both are *surgical* injuries. Both result in varying degrees of marginal skin loss, which if not promptly excised and replaced with fresh skin will result in some loss of function at the shoulder.

As soon therefore as it becomes clear that an area of skin has been deprived of its blood supply no time should be lost in excising the dead portion. To wait for the devitalized area to slough off of its own accord is to prolong convalescence by many weeks. The denuded area should be skin-grafted as soon as the local bacteriology offers a reasonable chance of a "take".

By displacement of skin—in the "skin short" case. Functional disability is particularly liable to occur in the skin short case unless special steps are taken to prevent its development. The "skin short" case is one in which it is judged that it will not be possible to close the wound completely following mastectomy. A shortage of skin is commonly encountered in all men and in women with small breasts or with large tumours involving the four quadrants.

The circumstances which may arise are as follows:

In closing the wound at the end of the radical operation a shortage of skin becomes apparent; this can temporarily be overcome by bringing the arm down to the side: this action has the effect of relieving tension at the time and so allowing the flaps to be brought together. It should never be done (Fig. 1). By this manœuvre skin is borrowed—by displacement—from the axilla and upper arm to close the upper part of the chest wound, thereby creating a shortage in the axillary area and leaving the patient with the foundation of a permanent functional disability.

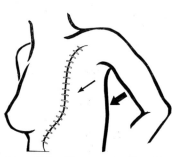

FIG. **19.**1. The arm to the side while closing the wound. This position predisposes to a stiff shoulder. The small arrow indicates the direction of displacement of the axillary skin.

The correct procedure to be adopted

before sewing up the flaps at the end of the operation is as follows: **Elevate** *the arm straight above the head;* in this position the upper limb makes its maximum demand upon the skin of the axilla: that is to say, this position gives the measure of the exact amount of skin required in the axilla to allow full and unrestricted movements at the shoulder post-operatively (Fig. 2). Start the approximation of the flaps by sliding the skin of the lateral flap well up into the axilla so that an adequate supply of skin

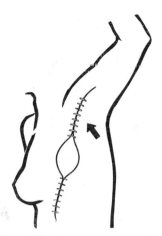

Fig. **19**.2. The arm raised. The drawing shows the correct position of the upper limb before closing the wound; the skin of the lateral flap should be pushed well up into the axilla (arrow) before suturing.

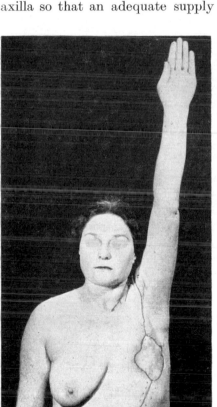

Fig. **19**.3. A "skin short" case. This patient was treated by pre-operative irradiation followed by radical mastectomy with an immediate skin graft. There is a full range of movement at the shoulder.

in this area is assured. This sliding manœuvre may result in a gap between the flaps lower down on the chest wall, but this is a small price to pay for ensuring full range of movement. The gap should be grafted there and then, unless the condition of the patient at the end of the operation is unsatisfactory. If this is the case, as it may be with an elderly patient, no harm is done by leaving a raw area and grafting early in convalescence, usually at the time of the first major dressing.

In concluding the review of this disability it should be emphasized that while it is not in our power to prevent physical disfigurement following mastectomy it is in our power to prevent physical *disablement*, and it is recommended that the following pre-

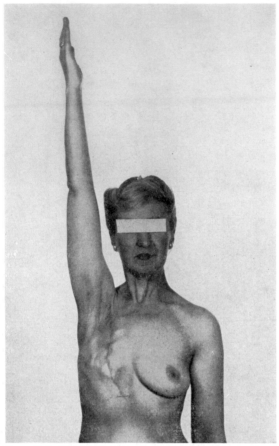

FIG. **19.**4. Full range of movement: The "arm raised" position is the most delicate test of function at the shoulder following mastectomy: six months should be allowed after the termination of all treatment for the skin to regain its suppleness before assessing function: inability to raise the arm vertically after such an interval must be regarded as an imperfect functional result.

cautions should be taken:

(1) Approximate the skin edges with the arm fully elevated and never down at the side.

(2) In the "skin short" case be prepared to insert a skin graft.

(3) In cases of "marginal necrosis" excise all dead skin as soon as it becomes obvious that it is devitalized and skin-graft the resulting raw area.

(4) Lastly, discourage all movements at the shoulder joint until the wound is healed, because too early movement may cause separation of the skin edges, and increases the liability to serum collection without any compensating advantages (Figs. 3 and 4).

The Extended Radical Operation

The observation by Handley and Thackray (1949) following a series of anterior mediastinal gland biopsies that 70 per cent. of cancers arising in the inner half of the breast in their series showed involvement of the internal mammary chain has stimulated some surgeons to extend the radical operation to an excision of the overlying part of the chest wall with subsequent dissection of the glands. While admitting the desirability of attacking the internal mammary chain it is questionable whether such a marathon surgical procedure is the right way of setting about it. Fortunately invaded anterior mediastinal glands do not always give rise to further trouble—witness the rarity of parasternal intercostal recurrence—a point to be borne in mind when trying to assess the significance of invasion of these glands. Similarly the operation has been extended to include clearance of the supraclavicular area with division of the clavicle, but again it is doubtful if the increased survival rate would balance the increased operative mortality and morbidity if the procedure became widely practised.

Simple Mastectomy

Simple mastectomy followed by post-operative irradiation to the chest wall and the undissected axilla is being practised by some surgeons in place of the radical operation.

In this method Stage I as well as Stage II cases are treated conservatively. The view is taken that if the disease has spread to the axilla surgery will serve only to disseminate it still further, and that if the disease is confined to the breast dissection of the axilla is unnecessary (McWhirter, 1948). The advantages claimed are a high survival rate, a lower operative mortality, a better functional result and a lower incidence of post-operative œdema of the arm.

The disadvantages are much the same as those with radium in particular the continued presence of living cancer cells in the axillary glands after the termination of treatment. The danger of these residual cells may be exaggerated and can be more potential than actual, but the possibility of their recovering their activity cannot be excluded. That they do persist at least for a time has been proved by carrying out a radical mastectomy after a full course of pre-operative irradiation and examining the axillary and breast material so obtained. Malignant cells were found to persist in the axillary glands of patients treated with X-rays alone in 92 per cent. of cases by Adair (1943) and in 65 per cent. by Richards (1948).

The question is, can X-rays in Stages I and II (the only stages in which radical mastectomy is done) restrain the local growth and spread of carcinoma in the axilla more effectively than operative clearance? The answer is not yet known. The advocates of X-rays believe that if the irradiated tissues are not disturbed by operation the cells will eventually either disappear or be rendered harmless by fibrous encapsulation. Those in favour of clearance of the axilla by operation contend that X-rays are only a "holding" technique, and that recurrences or dissemination must ultimately be expected. Until longer survival rates have been published it is not possible fairly to assess the final place conservative surgery combined with radiotherapy is likely to occupy in the treatment of early clinical cancer of the breast.

Indications. The foregoing remarks are not intended to imply that there is no place for conservative surgery in the treatment of Stage I and II cancers. This is far from the case. Simple mastectomy combined with irradiation of the undissected axilla should always be practised in all bad risk cases, and be considered whenever there is a combination of adverse factors present, such as age over 65, a history of rapid growth, wide attachment to the skin, diffuse involvement of the whole breast, or a peripherally situated tumour, more particularly if it is in the inner hemisphere.

X-Ray Treatment

Pre-operative X-ray Treatment

Pre-operative irradiation is given with the intention of sterilizing or restraining the activity of the tumour and the glands. It has been, and still is, used less than post-operative therapy and there are no hard and fast rules for its application. Theoretically, at least, it has the following advantages: (1) Pre-operative irradiation is more reliable in that there is no delay in starting the treatment, whereas post-operative irradiation may be long delayed by some complication of the operation, such as flap necrosis. (2) If X-ray treatment precedes operation any cells which may subsequently be disseminated may be either dead or so devitalized that they are not harmful. (3) It is probable that the skin will tolerate a heavier dose of X-rays if its blood supply has not been disturbed by previous operative trauma.

There are certain difficulties with pre-operative irradiation.

Positive diagnosis. A diagnosis of cancer is required before summitting a patient to a course of X-ray treatment. This information is automatically available with post-operative cases—not so with the pre-operative, unless the clinical signs of cancer are well established. If they are not a biopsy will be necessary to establish a positive diagnosis; to do this the tumour has to be disturbed; if it is found to be malignant most surgeons would deem it wiser to proceed to the radical operation rather than close the wound and give pre-operative X-rays.

Pre-operative delay. There is considerable—up to ten weeks—delay before the patient is able to undergo operation. This wait is very irksome to some patients.

Operation refused. If the lump disappears under X-ray treatment, some patients may refuse operation altogether.

Operating difficulties. It is stated by some that pre-operative irradiation makes subsequent operation more difficult because of increased bleeding. This has not been my experience. The tendency to ooze is a little greater and the tissues are slightly more friable, but on the whole the operation is quite straightforward.

Irradiation—operation interval. If mastectomy is carried out before the skin reaction has developed there is the risk that this may coincide with the healing of the skin flaps, in which case separation of the edges of the wound or sloughing may occur. The optimum irradiation—operation interval is not known. It must be long enough to allow the skin to regain its natural healing qualities but not long enough to allow regrowth of tumour cells. It would appear to be about six weeks.

Indications. Pre-operative X-ray treatment is indicated in the "skin short" case, for ulcerating carcinoma, and for the four quadrant tumour.

Skin short case. In this group, because of shortage of skin, removal of the breast, whether this is carried out before or after X ray treatment, leaves a gap between the skin edges which will require skin grafting. Unfortunately every skin graft does not take uniformly, so that a proportion of cases are left to heal—at least in part—by granulation, and this takes time; indeed, sometimes so much time that X-ray treatment may be delayed to a point where its usefulness is open to question. For this reason it is suggested that if by careful pre-operative clinical assessment we can anticipate and so forecast such a defect arising, we should consider giving the X-ray treatment before the operation. The use of pre-operative irradiation does not in any way absolve the operator subsequently from still adhering to the principle of excising a wide area clear of the growth. The argument is, that once the course of therapy has been given, delay in healing of the wound has not the same significance as it holds up nothing except the ordinary convalescence of the patient.

Ulcerating carcinoma. Primary radical mastectomy is absolutely contra-indicated in the presence of *moist* ulceration of the breast because of the risk of widespread infection of tissue planes opened up in the course of the dissection. By giving pre-operative X-ray treatment, the ulcerating surface is dried up and the subsequent mastectomy made easier and safer.

The four quadrant tumour. Many of the cases may not be judged suitable for the radical operation, but if it is contemplated the size of the tumour can be much reduced by X-rays and at the same time the skin and subcutaneous tissues will be at least partially sterilized of malignant cells.

All patients who have received a full course of pre-operative deep therapy should have chest and pelvis X-rayed before operation is decided upon.

Post-operative X-ray Treatment

Post-operative irradiation is given with the intention of destroying any islets of active cancer cells which may still remain in the field of operation after the primary tumour and the glands have been removed. The area irradiated includes the chest wall, the axilla and the supraclavicular region. Ideally the course should be started as soon as the wound is healed, which is likely to be any time after the tenth post-operative day.

Gland-free cases. Some surgeons exclude their gland-free cases from X-ray treatment on the grounds that the operation is sufficient in itself for these patients. In these circumstances they say they prefer to keep post-operative irradiation in reserve for the treatment of recurrences, should they appear. While such an opinion is controversial, it is also a considerable assumption, because it implies that all the axillary glands removed have been sectioned. This is possible, and it is certainly desirable, but it cannot always happen. In a busy department, it is the exception rather than the rule for the pathologist to have either the staff or the time to dissect, section and examine every gland in every mastectomy specimen, with the result that sooner or later a gland invaded case is going to be reported on as gland-free. If the presence or absence of nodal metastases is the criterion on which one decided whether to give post-operative irradiation or not, a number of patients who might have received the treatment with advantage are going to be denied it at the optimum time, unless the pathological services are exceptional. The only safe procedure is to arrange for all patients to have post-operative X-ray treatment unless there is some contra-indication. In the *frail*, in the *elderly* and in those who have had a *slow convalescence* following the operation it is better to withhold post-operative X-rays; the treatment can be exhausting and may defeat its own ends if we insist upon it regardless of the general condition of the patient.

Stages III, IV—Inoperable Cases

Radical surgery is absolutely contra-indicated in patients in these two groups. The common error in clinical diagnosis is to mistake a Stage III for a Stage II and so to submit a patient with advanced carcinoma to a major operative procedure which has no hope of eradicating a disease which has already spread beyond the boundaries of the operation area. It is of the greatest importance, therefore, to be aware of and so to search for those evidences of extension which convert the operable Stage II carcinoma into the inoperable Stage III. In addition the chest should always be X-rayed to include a silent pulmonary metastasis or a symptomless pleural effusion.

Stage III. This group comprises cases with a fixed mass of axillary nodes, enlarged supraclavicular nodes, enlarged axillary nodes on the opposite side or a lump in the opposite breast; deep fixation of the breast to the chest wall; secondary nodules in the skin, œdema of the arm and certain cases showing peau d'orange.

Stage IV. This group comprises cases with distant metastases in bones, viscera or lungs.

THE TREATMENT OF ADVANCED CARCINOMA OF THE BREAST

There are a number of palliative measures which may be used in the treatment of advanced carcinoma if the breast and they include: *local mastectomy, deep X-ray treatment, bilateral oöphorectomy* and *hormone therapy.*

Local Mastectomy. Local mastectomy should be practised in all ulcerating or fungating cancers which are not attached to the chest wall. The surrounding skin should be widely excised and a split skin graft dressing applied. Such treatment rids the patient at one sweep of a lesion which is not only painful and offensive but requires frequent change of dressings. A solitary recurrence either in the skin or of one gland should also be excised. If there are multiple skin nodules or several enlarged glands—axillary or supraclavicular—it is generally better that they should be treated by irradiation.

Deep X-ray Treatment. Deep X-ray treatment, judiciously applied, may be of great value in the treatment of the *ulcerating carcinoma* fixed to the chest wall, and for *multiple skin nodules, glandular masses* and *metastases in bone.* Although the ultimate prognosis is grave some of these patients survive for considerable periods with well-controlled X-ray treatment. The discharging ulcerating carcinoma is dried up so that the painful daily dressings can be stopped. The pain of brachial neuritis caused by a supraclavicular mass of glands is similarly relieved, and there may be complete relief of the pain caused by secondary deposits in bone, particularly when the metastatic process is confined to a solitary deposit—for example, a single vertebra.

There is, however, a limit to the scope of X-ray treatment to which attention should be drawn. Some hold that X-ray treatment can convert the case which has been judged clinically incurable by surgery into a surgically curable case. This is doubtful. The commonest example is the patient with a *fixed mass* of axillary glands. It is true that the effect of a full course of X-ray therapy can be quite remarkable, and that at the end of treatment in radiosensitive cases no lump may be palpable where previously there had been a fixed mass. It is tempting in these circumstances to proceed to radical mastectomy but this is wrong. Fixation of the glands implies penetration of their capsule by malignant cells. This in turn implies advanced malignancy, and it is reasonable to suppose that a subsequent attempt at clearance of the axilla will serve only to disseminate the disease. Pre-operative X-ray treatment may render these patients technically operable, but that is not the same thing as rendering them surgically curable.

Bilateral Oöphorectomy and Ovarian Irradiation. Bilateral oöphorectomy should be given serious consideration as a delaying measure in all pre-menopausal patients with advanced cancer of the breast. It is as old a procedure as radical mastectomy itself and was advocated by Beatson as long ago as 1896 and reported upon by Lett (1905) but later fell into disrepute as a result of its exploitation in unsuitable cases. The results are variable but occasionally dramatic. If removal of the ovaries by operation is not feasible sterilization by ovarian irradiation reinforced by androgen therapy is an alternative. Radiation sterilization can be achieved by a single exposure but the dosage required— 900 r.—can be very upsetting and is better split into three treatments when radiation effects are minimal. It is not as effective or lasting a method as surgical castration but is to be preferred when the hazards of anæsthesia are high as for example when pulmonary metastases are present.

Hormone Therapy—by Androgens and Œstrogens. *Indications.* Hormone therapy is so uncertain and unpredictable in its effects that it should only be considered in the treatment of the advanced case, that is to say for *inoperable, metastatic* and *recurrent carcinoma.* There is no convincing evidence that hormones have at present any useful part to play in prophylaxis so that the concurrent implantation or injection of hormones at the time of radical mastectomy cannot be recommended. This is not to say that hormones are not disturbing and powerful agents which may alter a patient physically, chemically, metabolically and emotionally. For these reasons they should be administered with a full sense of responsibility and knowledge of their various effects. At their best they are a palliative measure but one which during their period of influence—and in exceptional circumstances this may last for a year or more—may cause considerable regression of the primary tumour and the apparent disappearance of secondary deposits and relief of bone pain. Healing of ulceration may also occur, lymphatic deposits diminish in size, the general health improve and the weight of the patient may increase, no mean achievement in a patient in whom all other recognized methods of treatment are contra-indicated or have been abandoned. At their worst, and if injudiciously or carelessly administered, they accelerate the rate of growth of all carcinomatous tissue throughout the body.

Rationale. The incidence of carcinoma of the breast is greatest at the time of the menopause, and it has been suggested that the falling off of œstrogen production by the ovary at this time may play some part in the production of the carcinoma. It would seem rational, therefore, to replace this œstrogen therapeutically. On the other hand, some of the most rapidly growing carcinomas of the breast occur in young patients when ovarian activity is at its height. In short, their mode of action is not yet clearly understood for it is contrary and illogical that in a proportion of pre-menopausal patients the withdrawal of œstrogens either by castration or by inactivation by androgens produces regression of tumour and that in the post-menopausal the administration of œstrogens can produce the same effect. It is possible that œstrogens may exert their greatest effect through the anterior pituitary. Thus an increase of circulating œstrogen may inhibit pituitary gonadotropic activity leading to suppression of ovarian function—a form of medical castration— or withdrawal of œstrogens by oophorectomy or ovarian irradiation or their antagonization by testosterone therapy may stimulate the anterior pituitary to an increased output of gonadotropic hormone which stimulates extragenital sources of œstrin production such as the adrenals. The results of hormone therapy are so variable that it can only be regarded as established in the sense that it is a legitimate experimental method. It is not possible to say more than that it would seem probable that these substances exert their effect by temporarily upsetting the existing hormonal balance and general endocrine status of the host.

Androgens

Androgens, used as some form of *testosterone*, in contra-distinction to the œstrogens are effective regardless of age and so may produce beneficial effects in both *pre-menopausal* and *post-menopausal* patients. Androgens depress the function of the anterior lobe of the pituitary and antagonize the œstrogenic hormones. If given before the climacteric they induce an artificial menopause—so that the patient should be warned accordingly. In the post-menopausal patient androgens are to be preferred to the œstrogens in the younger patients, i.e. up to the age of 55. They can be administered by inunction, by mouth, by intramuscular injection or by implantation. In order to get an effect as quickly as possible it is usual to start with injections and later to give the androgens by mouth.

Injection. Testosterone *phenyl* propionate (T.P.P.) seems likely to become the androgen of choice in the treatment of advanced carcinoma of the breast if its claim to be four times as potent as its predecessor is maintained, as this will have the advantage of prolonging the intervals between injections. This new compound is also less viscous and so can with safety be injected subcutaneously. The dosage suggested is 100 mg. weekly but with growing experience this may need modification according to the reaction produced.

(Also by injection: Testosterone propionate: 150 mg. twice weekly. Methyl androstenediol: 50 mg. *daily*; said to have less virilizing effect.)

Oral. Methyl testosterone is given in the form of linguettes. These should not be swallowed but are placed under the tongue or in the buccal gingival sulcus and are absorbed through the mucous membrane. The dosage suggested is 30 mg. daily—in the form of two linguettes of 5 mg., each morning and evening. They take about half an hour to be absorbed. The results of using this method of administration are not entirely satisfactory and it is probably better to use it only as an adjunct to the other methods.

Implantation. Subcutaneous implantation of androgen pellets (100 mg.) have the advantage of a more prolonged effect and may be a more convenient form of therapy if it is difficult to arrange for regular intramuscular injections.

Side effects. Clinically virilism is manifested by hirsutism, voice changes, enlargement of the clitoris and increased libido. Any one of these changes can be very distressing to a sensitive patient. Increased libido can still occur in the elderly—I have had experience in a patient of 82—and they may find the experience almost more than they can bear. In such cases the drug should be stopped and œstrogens substituted.

Œstrogens

Œstrogens, used as Stilbœstrol or some variation of synthetic œstrogen, should only be given to the *post-menopausal* patient. Furthermore, experience suggests that its administration should be confined to the older post-menopausal subject with carcinoma, i.e. women over the age of 55.

Stilbœstrol has been the œstrogen preparation most frequently used up to the present time. It can be administered intramuscularly twice weekly, or by mouth, which is more convenient. Dosage varies in different hands but 5 mg. twice daily by mouth or 5 mg. by injection may be taken as an average. If intolerance is shown to this preparation a change to dinœstrol or stilbœstrol dipropionate in the same dosage may be more satisfactory.

Side effects. The side effects with œstrogen therapy are less distressing than those associated with the androgens. For this reason in those cases in which there is a choice of hormone therapy as between œstrogens and androgens, and this applies to the more elderly post-menopausal patients, the œstrogens are to be preferred for initial trial as their side effects are less unpleasant and may indeed be absent altogether. When present they may include gastro-intestinal disturbance in the form of indigestion, vomiting particularly in the morning, and vaginal bleeding. This latter is particularly prone to occur on withdrawal of the drug: elderly patients who have long since stopped menstruation should therefore be warned of this possibility or they may be alarmed unnecessarily. Locally the breasts may become engorged, the nipples tender and the areolæ pigmented.

Hormone Therapy—General Observations. *Response: duration of treatment: hypercalcæmia.* Objectively true progress can only be assessed in the primary tumour by observing an actual regression in its size or with visceral metastases, by their reduction in size or actual disappearance, or in the case of skeletal metastases by radiological evidence of recalcification and increased density. A subjective improvement may be noticeable at an early stage in hormone therapy with either androgens or œstrogens and shows itself in a sense of well being, relief of anorexia and insomnia and sometimes by a dramatic relief of bone pain, but helpful and encouraging as these results are, they must not be attributed to, or mistaken for, an anti-carcinogenic effect.

Improvement with hormone therapy, if it is going to occur, is usually manifest in two to four weeks after starting treatment; in cases showing such a favourable reaction treatment on full dosage should be continued until it appears that the maximum response has been obtained; thereafter the patient should continue indefinitely on a reduced maintenance dose. If no response is obtained within three months, the hormone under trial should be abandoned and the opposite variety substituted. Similarly if there is intolerance to one hormone it is worth trying the effect of switching to another preparation of the same hormone, or in post-menopausal patients, of giving androgen instead of œstrogen or vice versa. (In pre-menopausal patients it would clearly be unwise to substitute œstrogen for androgen.)

Both androgens and œstrogens tend to cause retention of sodium, potassium, and chloride so that œdema and even heart failure may develop during hormone therapy. It has been said by some that the increase in weight which may occur during this treatment is due to a temporary waterlogging of the patient as a result of salt retention. Care, therefore, must be exercised during their administration and particular watch kept on an existing pleural effusion which may be increased to the point of dyspnœa. If this should happen the treatment need not necessarily be stopped but the dosage of hormone should be much reduced, the fluid intake limited and diuretics given. Both hormones may also produce hypercalcæmia if bone metastases are present—with the syndrome of nausea, vomiting, dehydration, atony, drowsiness and coma. Treatment is by the intravenous injection of $2\frac{1}{2}$ per cent. sodium citrate.

Metastases. Androgens have developed a reputation for having a greater effect on osseous than soft tissue metastases. This selective behaviour is certainly not uniform and soft tissue metastases may also respond to androgen therapy. Œstrogens have similarly been credited with exerting their maximum effect upon the primary growth if this is present and on soft tissue metastases, but it is also true to say that an osseous metastasis which does not respond to androgen may show recalcification on œstrogen therapy (Douglas, 1952).

Summary. To summarize, it can be said that at the present time hormone therapy has no place in the early prophylactic treatment of cancer of the breast, and that it should be reserved for advanced cases only. There is no recorded case of a "cure" of a proven carcinoma of the breast that can be attributed to hormone therapy but there is good evidence that palliation can be produced in approximately one-third of patients with inoperable carcinoma of the breast even if this is short lived. The use of Testosterone implant at the time of operation in operable cases has been advised and employed but there is no evidence that it does any good, and the double indignity of radical mastectomy and masculinization is asking too much for the patient to bear psychologically.

So far as a constantly changing position can be judged, it would seem that œstrogens are contra-indicated in pre-menopausal patients but are to be preferred for the treatment of post-menopausal patients over the age of 55. Androgens should be used before the menopause and are first choice in post-menopausal women up to the age of 55 and in women over this age if œstrogens fail or are not tolerated. In addition bilateral oöphorectomy or radiation sterilization of the ovaries should be considered in all pre-menopausal patients (and up to five years after the menopause) who have advanced cancer of the breast.

Finally it must be firmly understood that hormone therapy does not in any way replace adequate surgical and radiotherapeutic treatment of carcinoma of the breast in Stages I and II.

Experimental Methods

Pituitary Irradiation. The effects of pituitary irradiation have been investigated. It has been given with the object of suppressing all gonadotropic hormones and so bringing about a cessation of œstrogenic activity. The results have been disappointing and the method of treatment is the least well tolerated of all irradiation methods because of the constitutional reaction produced (Douglas, 1952).

Adrenalectomy. Bilateral adrenalectomy has been carried out for advanced mammary cancer with metastases (Huggins and Bergenstal, 1952). In pre-menopausal patients the ovaries should first be removed. Regression of tumour and relief of pain have been observed but the remedy is a desperate one in a very sick patient and the results are unpredictable. The post-operative recovery phase requires highly skilled nursing and first class biochemical facilities. The mechanism whereby regression of some tumours occurs after adrenalectomy is not clearly established, largely because of uncertainty about normal adrenal function. The adrenalectomized patient has to be maintained for the duration of her life on cortisone so that the procedure cannot be envisaged unless hormonal substitution therapy is available.

Bilateral Carcinoma of the Breast

Simultaneous primary malignant neoplasia in the two breasts is exceedingly rare but the appearance of a second primary in the remaining breast some time after the first is not such a rarity. The sequence of events is as follows: a primary carcinoma appears on one side and is treated by mastectomy; some years later a carcinoma appears in the opposite breast. The question arises as to whether the second carcinoma is a new primary tumour or a secondary extension from the original primary. The interpretation is of practical importance as it affects the treatment. If the second cancer is regarded as a tumour arising *de novo* its removal by radical mastectomy is likely to be the proper treatment but if it is regarded as part of a metastatic process its treatment will be conservative. Recently Reese (1953) has examined the pathological material obtained from 20 cases of bilateral cancer of the breast and concluded that in 15 of these there was clinical and histological evidence that both were distinct primary tumours. Supporting evidence in favour of a diagnosis of a second primary would be: if the cancer appears in the second breast some years after the first had been removed: if both breasts contain cancer but no metastases can be found elsewhere: if the histological pattern of the two cancers differs: if the second cancer is seen to be arising as an intraduct carcinoma.

Carcinoma of the Male Breast

Carcinoma of the male breast is uncommon, only one case being seen for approximately every 100 in the female. Apart from its comparative rarity the disease behaves in essentially the same way as its female counterpart. The literature has been reviewed by Somerville (1952) who draws attention to four cases in his series in which the presenting symptom was a lump in the axilla. It is well known, owing to the scarcity of connective tissue in the area, that superficial and deep fixation occur early as well as early spread to the axilla. For these reasons the prognosis is not good. Treatment is by radical mastectomy. Carcinoma of the male breast comes into the "skin short" category so that a skin graft is almost certain to be required and should therefore be anticipated.

Fulminating Cancers

The rapidly growing types of cancer of the breast include the carcinoma occurring during pregnancy, lactation carcinoma and inflammatory carcinoma. Clinically the interest in these cases lies in the difficulty of diagnosing them from cases of acute mastitis and breast abscess, with which they may be confused and as such treated. The following points should be considered, when diagnosis is in doubt. Acute mastitis usually occurs in the early months of lactation, is associated with local tenderness and a general systemic reaction with fever and malaise. Carcinomatous lesions on the other hand are characteristically not tender and are unassociated with fever, leucocytosis or systemic reaction and are not responsive to the antibiotics.

Unfortunately this picture is much modified and the inflammatory nature of the lesion masked if antibiotics have already been given before the patient is first seen. If the nature of the swelling remains in doubt for more than a week it should be explored.

Treatment is difficult. In pre-menopausal patients, that is all cases of carcinoma in pregnancy or during lactation, and a proportion of the inflammatory carcinomas, a possible line of treatment is bilateral oöphorectomy, pre-operative irradiation to the breast followed by simple mastectomy and androgen therapy. A woman, well advanced in pregnancy, having her first baby, and anxious to keep it might be allowed to go to term, but each case must be assessed individually. Only a small proportion of the carcinomas arising in pregnancy or lactation are inflammatory in type. A full description of inflammatory carcinoma of the breast, which more commonly occurs in women over the age of 40, has been given by Chris (1950).

VICTOR RIDDELL

BIBLIOGRAPHY

ADAIR, F. E. (1949) *Proc. R. Soc. Med.* **42**, 468.
BEATSON, G. T. (1902) *Brit. med. J.* **ii**, 1300.
CADE, S. (1948) *Proc. R. Soc. Med.* **41**, 129
CHRIS, S. M. (1950) *Brit. J. Surg.* **38**, 163.
DARGENT, M. (1949) *Brit. med. J.* **ii**, 54.
DOUGLAS, M. (1952) *Brit. J. Cancer* **6**, 32.
HANDLEY, R. S., and THACKRAY, A. C. (1949) *Lancet* **ii**, 276.
HORSLEY, G. W. (1947) *Ann. Surg.* **125**, 703.
HORSLEY, J. S. (1944) *Surgery* **15**, 590.
HUGGINS, C., and BERGENSTAL, D. M. (1952) *Cancer Res.* **12**, 134.
KASDON, S. C., FISHMAN, W. H., DART, R. M., BONNER, C. D., and HOMBURGER, F. (1952) *J. Amer. med. Assoc.* **148**, 1212.
LETT, H. (1905) *Lancet* **i**, 227.
LOESER, A. A. (1941) *Lancet* **ii**, 698.
NATHANSON, I. T. (1952) *Cancer* **5**, 754.
NATHANSON, I. T. (1951) *Radiology* **56**, 535.
REESE, A. J. M. (1953) *Brit. J. Surg.* **40**, 428.
RICHARDS, G. E. (1948) *Brit. J. Radiol.* **21**, 109, 249.
RIDDELL, V. H. (1948) *Brit. J. Surg.* **36**, 113.
RIDDELL, V. H. (1950) *Brit. J. Cancer* **4**, 289.
SMITHERS, D. W., RIGBY JONES, P., GALTON, D. A. G., and PAYNE, P. M. (1950) *Brit. J. Radiol.*, Suppl 4.
SOMERVILLE, P. (1952) *Brit. J. Surg.* **39**, 296.
TAYLOR, C. W., and MELZER, A. (1938) *Amer. J. Cancer* **33**, 33.
WANGENSTEEN, O. H. (1949) *Ann. Surg.* **130**, 315.

CHAPTER XX

RENAL TUBERCULOSIS

IT is a reasonable assumption that tuberculous disease exists in a kidney which secretes urine containing tubercle bacilli. Tuberculous "Bacilluria" is thought to be the result of small embolic cortical lesions which give no pyelographic signs. This is the first stage of the disease, and such lesions may heal without serious damage to the kidney or may progress to its complete destruction. The rate of progress is always slow and the first stage may last for many years. The next stage is marked by changes in one or more calyces which ulcerate or communicate with cortical abscesses. Such lesions rarely heal and normally, in the end, spread to destroy the organ, and to involve the pelvis, ureter and bladder and also the prostate, seminal vesicles, epididymis and testis. This sequence of infection is normal but steps in it are often omitted; epididymitis for instance frequently results from a cortical lesion, the calyces, pelvis, ureter and bladder remaining unaffected. Contrary to earlier belief it is now thought that renal infection is commonly bilateral in its early stages. Both sides may heal; one may heal while the other progresses; or the progress of the disease in one side may lag far behind. The last phenomenon may be responsible for the all too frequent occurrence of disease in the remaining kidney after nephrectomy.

Spread to the ureter and bladder is at first confined to the epithelium and may heal without causing serious damage. When it spreads more deeply fibrosis eventually leads to permanent deformities.

Diagnosis

Bacteriological. Urinary tuberculosis may be symptomless or may show itself in such a variety of ways that it has no characteristic syndrome. It should always be suspected when there is persistent dysuria or unexplained hæmaturia and should always be excluded by the bacteriologist in routine urinary examinations, particularly when sterile pyuria is present. Patients suffering from tuberculous disease of other systems, particularly the hæmatogenous type such as bone and joint disease, should have frequent urological examinations at regular intervals.

Tubercle Bacilli appear sparsely and intermittently in the urine in the early stages and no reliance should be placed on single negative examinations. Deposits from the urine should be examined, cultured, and inoculated into a guinea pig. To get adequate samples it is best to "pool" the deposits from a series of early morning specimens. Twenty-four hour specimens are difficult to collect aseptically and unsuitable for modern bacteriological methods.

Radiological. Intravenous pyelography may show varying degrees of fluffiness and ulceration of the calyces, and sometimes cavitation of the renal cortex. In older lesions there may be irregular calcification here and there. With very advanced lesions, particularly "closed" ones, renal function may be absent. If, as often happens, excretion pyelograms are not clear, retrograde pyelograms should be done as it is essential to have an accurate picture—particularly when, with nephrectomy in view, the "sound" side is being investigated. There is very little evidence that harm has come from this if done with skill and care. It is important to avoid over-distension of the pelvis. This may do harm and may also give a misleading picture.

Cystoscopy. The bladder may appear normal in severe renal disease, and conversely may show typical tuberculous cystitis when only minor cortical lesions are present. Any part of the bladder may be affected with small tubercles, ulcers or areas of uncharacteristic cystitis. Ureters may be inflamed and œdematous, or retracted and dilated. With long established cystitis the bladder contracts and cystoscopy is difficult or impossible. The value of cystoscopy is chiefly as an aid in the management of the disease and as an estimate of the progress and efficiency of treatment both in the bladder and, by ureteric catheterization, in the kidneys individually.

Prognosis

Before setting a value on methods of treatment it is essential to know what is likely to happen without treatment. This is a difficult matter in tuberculosis, but in the urinary system some common patterns of behaviour may be expected:

(1) Tuberculosis confined to the cortex of the kidney often heals without treatment.

(2) Ulcerative disease involving calyces seldom does so.

(3) Renal tuberculosis is usually a very chronic disease, slowly progressive.

(4) Death from purely renal causes is long delayed unless complicated by back pressure from a contracted bladder.

(5) Urogenital tuberculosis frequently complicates serious disease elsewhere in the body in patients with low resistance. In such cases prognosis is very poor.

(6) Tuberculosis of the bladder epithelium will usually heal if the renal focus is removed.

(7) When the deeper layers of the bladder are involved healing is accompanied by fibrosis which, if severe, leads to progressive contraction of the organ.

Treatment

With these facts in mind treatment should obviously strive to combine the maximum chance of eradication of the disease with the minimum risk of shortening life by removal of renal tissue. When there are active lesions outside the genito-urinary tract their treatment is usually of greater urgency and importance, and the urinary lesion should be managed conservatively.

General. Urinary tuberculosis is a manifestation of a constitutional disease and all patients should have prolonged rest, fresh air and ample diet.

Nephrectomy. Radical surgery is never urgent as uncomplicated renal tuberculosis is never an urgent threat to life. It is important, however, to prevent spread to the bladder because severe tuberculous cystitis is the most troublesome and perhaps the most dangerous complication of the disease. Early nephrectomy may achieve this but unfortunately does not always do so. Nephrectomy is still the only certain means of eradicating established tuberculosis of a kidney, but the indication for it must be considered carefully.

The decision to remove renal tissue of good function is not to be taken lightly, and in early cases convincing evidence of health of the opposite kidney must be obtained. There must be a clear pyelographic picture which is completely normal and an absence of pus cells from an adequate ureteric sample; the latter preferably on more than one occasion. Even so disease may eventually be manifest in a remaining kidney.

Nephrectomy is never indicated unless there is pyelographic change. On the other hand a seriously diseased kidney, especially one with a poor renal function, should always be removed even when the other side is affected to a slight degree. Otherwise bilateral disease must be treated conservatively.

The most difficult problem is that of apparently unilateral disease showing pyelographic changes of a minor degree, and surgeons differ about the management of this type. Classically it has hitherto been treated by nephrectomy.

Another point of controversy has been the treatment of a kidney totally destroyed by disease and functionless. Such a condition may exist without obvious symptoms and the term "autonephrectomy" has been applied to the process. This implies that the disease is inactive—a dangerous assumption—for activity is often to be found histologically even when extensive calcification is present. Unless there are strong reasons to the contrary, functionless tuberculous kidneys should be removed.

The technique does not differ from that used for other inflammatory renal lesions except in dealing with the ureter. Here, again, opinions differ. It is reasonable to remove the whole ureter when it is found to be diseased, but probably unnecessary to do so when it is apparently healthy. Its complete removal involves a change of position on the table and a separate incision, oblique or paramedian, or a second operation at a later date. The ureter can and always should be removed as far down as the pelvic brim through the nephrectomy incision.

Partial nephrectomy, the removal of the obviously diseased part of a kidney, is often condemned. It is said that it does not necessarily eradicate the disease which may be present, though not obvious, in other parts of the organ. There is, however, much to be said for the preservation of renal tissue in a disease so apt to be bilateral.

If the disease is apparently limited to one part of the kidney, it seems worth while to remove this part without sacrificing the whole kidney, and this has been done successfully. When one kidney has been removed, partial nephrectomy has been used to remove an area of localized disease in the kidney remaining. There is a danger of hæmorrhage, but this can usually be controlled. The theoretical risk of acute hæmatogenous spread can be avoided by chemotherapy.

Chemotherapy. The assessment of the value of streptomycin and other chemotherapeutic agents is made difficult by the fact that urinary tuberculosis is a chronic and persistent disease which may improve without treatment and may recur or relapse after treatment. Many years must elapse before the value of these drugs is finally known. Meanwhile the results of clinical experiments (Jacobs and Borthwick, 1950; Ross *et al.*, 1951; Lattimer, 1952) have shown that the earlier claims that chemotherapy could replace surgery were exaggerated but that the results in some cases were encouraging.

The drug which has been most widely and successfully used is streptomycin, best given in conjunction with paramino-salicylic acid (P.A.S.). Newer compounds such as iso-nicotinic hydrazide are being tried but it is too early to assess effectiveness. There is evidence that resistance to streptomycin is readily acquired by tubercle bacilli in the kidney, especially in an acid medium, and that the concomitant administration of P.A.S. delays or prevents the onset of this resistance.

It is customary to treat all cases with these drugs whether or no operative surgery is undertaken.

In tuberculous bacilluria, without pyelographic changes, healing may take place spontaneously. It is therefore misleading to draw conclusions from the results of chemotherapy. Some encouraging results have been seen from the treatment of early or minor calyceal lesions. With more advanced disease, however, results have on the whole been disappointing, chemotherapy having apparently little effect on serious ulceration or abscess formation. On the other hand in bilateral cases where nephrectomy is contra-indicated, a prolonged course may help to slow the progress of the disease and to ameliorate symptoms, Tuberculosis of the ureters and bladder is much more susceptible and usually improves rapidly, but as healing takes place fibrosis increases and stricture of the ureter or contraction of the bladder may cause complications and distressing symptoms. Since the use of streptomycin "cover" pre- and post-operatively, non-healing or sinus formation in the wound is prevented or readily cured.

Dosage. This varies greatly in different clinics. An average total dose appears to be about 100 gm.—although sometimes much more is given, with 12 gm. of P.A.S. daily. The streptomycin may be given daily or may be spread out, 1 gm. being given every third day. There is some evidence that the more prolonged the course the better the result.

Treatment of Complications

Those calling for special surgical treatment are genital tuberculosis, stricture of the ureter and fibrous contraction of the bladder.

Tuberculous epididymitis should, when possible, be treated by epididymectomy. Only in very advanced stages is orchidectomy essential. It is often wise to cut a section out of the opposite vas deferens to avoid spread to a healthy testis.

Stricture of the ureter usually happens at the lower end and is frequently associated with fibrous contraction of the bladder wall. The condition often develops after nephrectomy and is of particular importance when it affects a single and comparatively healthy kidney. There are two indications for treatment:

(1) Back-pressure on the kidney will eventually cause renal failure and this will be greatly accelerated by secondary infection.

(2) Intolerable pain and frequency wears out the patient whose bladder may only be able to hold an ounce or two.

Although attempts have been made to enlarge the bladder by anastomosis of some isolated part of intestine to it, these have not generally been successful, and the standard treatment for both conditions is to divert the ureteric flow from the bladder. This may be done by cutaneous ureterostomy or by uretero-colic anastomosis. The latter is more comfortable for most patients but carries a serious risk of ascending infection especially when applied to a single kidney and ureter already damaged by disease.

M. F. NICHOLLS

References

JACOBS, A., and BORTHWICK, W. M. (1950) *Proc. R. Soc. Med.* **43,** 453.
LATTIMER, J. K., HERTZBERG, A., HARPER, J., BERMAN, M., BRADLEY, D., and VEENEIMA, R. (1952) *J. Urol.* **67,** 750.
Ross, J. C., GOW, J. G., and HILL, C. A. ST. (1951) *Lancet* **i,** 1033.

CHAPTER XXI

THE SURGERY OF PROSTATIC OBSTRUCTION

THE management of bladder neck obstruction due to affection of the prostate gland has changed greatly in the last decade both in technique and in results. These changes are due in the main to the effective use of chemotherapy which has made technical advances possible. Improved methods of anæsthesia have helped to lower the risks of radical operations on poor subjects.

At the present time the operation known as "prostatectomy" is unique in surgery for the variety of techniques practised with success by surgeons in this and other countries. Surgical procedures on most of the other systems and parts of the body have been standardized within fairly narrow limits, but in dealing with the abnormal prostate gland five main methods, apart from minor variations, are still widely used. These may be summarized as:

(1) Transvesical prostatectomy in one or two stages with open bladder drainage.
(2) Transvesical prostatectomy with bladder closure.
(3) Retropubic prostatectomy.
(4) Perineal prostatectomy.
(5) Endourethral prostatectomy.

Some surgeons employ one method for all types; others, in this country the majority, commonly use several—choosing in each case the one most suitable for the particular patient. This seems to be a logical standpoint and will be assumed in this chapter.

Assessment

The indications for prostatectomy cannot be set out categorically. They may vary with different surgeons and should vary with different patients. Operation is certainly advisable when more than an ounce or two of residual urine is persistent; when there have been incidents of acute retention, or, in the absence of any retention, when frequency is severe, especially at night. A most careful assessment of the patient's general and local condition is necessary before treatment is undertaken. The general investigation must include the cardio-vascular and respiratory systems, and the renal function. The last is perhaps the most important for, if renal function is adequate, few patients with urgent prostatic symptoms need nowadays be denied the chance of operative cure.

The most practical way to assess renal function in prostatic cases is by estimation of the blood urea. It is quickly done and is adequate. An intravenous pyelogram will show renal function, but when the blood urea is above 100 mg. per cent, the picture is usually so ill-defined as to be valueless. A clean sample of urine should be sent to the laboratory at the earliest opportunity for bacteriological examination and tests of the sensitivities of the organisms to various chemo-therapeutic drugs.

It is in cases of chronic retention and particularly of retention with overflow that the renal function is most likely to be impaired. If retention is absolute it is therefore of some importance to discover whether it is recent and acute, or whether chronic retention has culminated in complete stoppage. This may be learnt from the history and from comparison of the size of the distended bladder with the pain and discomfort it causes.

Next an attempt should be made by rectal examination to determine the type of prostatic lesion. When the lateral lobes are very large, when they are abnormally small and hard, or when obviously carcinomatous, this may be easy; but there are often difficulties which may lead to mistakes. The commonest is to overestimate the size of a gland which is congested and made prominent by a grossly distended bladder. Enlargement of the middle lobe when the lateral lobes are of relatively normal size can only be felt bi-manually, and then not in fat men. If encroachment within the bladder is large it may be shown as a filling defect in an intravenous cystogram. There remain many cases, however, in which the true state of affairs can only be seen by endoscopy. This should always be done, not only for the information it gives about the prostate but also to exclude urethral stricture and, most important, concomitant or over-riding vesical lesions such as new growths or diverticula. The risks of infection of the bladder with cystoscopy are not so serious as those of misdiagnosis and consequent maltreatment without it. It is important to know the size and the amount of encroach-ment on the urethral lumen of the lateral lobes and whether an intra-vesical lobe or prostatic collar or bar is present. If malignancy is suspected on physical examination more detailed investigations are necessary and are described later.

Treatment

Treatment of Complete Retention

Patients suffering from complete retention should be admitted to hospital as an emergency. Should this prove impossible, by tradition and in practice retention is relieved by the general practitioner with a catheter. There is no doubt that a single catheterization has often been successful, sometimes for an indefinite period. This seldom happens, however, when there has been any considerable chronic obstruction, and its success must be ascribed to the relief of a congestive and spasmodic incident. The danger of infection is greatly increased each time catheterization has to be repeated under such conditions, particularly when there is bleeding. Indwelling catheters should only be used under hospital conditions. Suprapubic aspiration through a fine-bored needle is much less likely to cause infection, but should not be repeated often for fear of extravesical leakage. The patient should be admitted to hospital as soon as possible and ideally before treatment.

Once admitted to hospital the patient's condition can be assessed rapidly and the first important decision made. The choice lies between immediate or "emergency" prostatectomy, or a preliminary period of bladder drainage. The practice of "emergency" prostatectomy originated in the realization (by Wilson Hey) that the most serious complications—especially fatal uræmia—arise from infection introduced from without, and particularly from urethral catheterization. Hey's technique is, in effect, a transvesical prostatectomy with wide resection of the trigone to avoid post-operative bladder neck obstruction and to facilitate hæmostasis—achieved by diathermy—in the prostatic bed. This is followed by the insertion through the urethra of a wide-bore tube or catheter from within the bladder, and then by complete bladder closure. The indwelling catheter is retained for a few days only. Even this cautious drainage leaves a loophole for infection from without and chemotherapy is freely used. The results of emergency operations by any standard method are good, but it is probable that with modern drugs similar safety can be achieved by methods which leave time for investigation and, particularly important in the "bad risk" case, for recuperation.

Each case must be judged on its merits, but a rough guide is that prostatectomy should be postponed if the blood urea is over 100 mg. per cent. Suprapubic drainage, except possibly with the "Riches" catheter, is usually reserved for patients whose bladders are already heavily infected or bleeding seriously, or for those for whom, for some reason, prostatectomy has to be postponed for an appreciable period.

The simplest and most convenient method of drainage is by an indwelling urethral catheter, and if this method is used with care, sepsis may be avoided. Slow decompression of the bladder is rarely necessary and never when the retention is acute. With the grosser degrees of distension found with retention and overflow it may be advisable, as hæmorrhage into the bladder when it is emptied is common and may cause blockage of the catheter. There seems little doubt that the uræmic fatalities ascribed to sudden changes of pressure were in fact due to rapid and fatal ascending infection through incompetent ureters of kidneys already at the point of failure. The aim should be to empty the bladder in 24 hours. A self-retaining catheter of the "Foley" type is the most convenient, but if this cannot be passed a Tieman's or bicoudé type may be used, and fixed by some external method. To avoid urethritis the catheter must not fit the urethra tightly and the "tying in" must not constrict the penis round it. Penicillin should be given as a routine and an aseptic closed drainage should be set up. Irrigation should be avoided if possible. Within seven days function is usually sufficiently improved to allow prostatectomy. This period may be used for thorough assessment of the condition. Cysto-scopy is best left as the first step in the radical operation.

Methods of Prostatectomy

The Two Stage Method. This is still used by many surgeons who claim it to be the safest. At the first stage the suprapubic tube should be placed as high as possible. At this stage it is convenient to cut and tie the vasa deferentia, a precaution against epididymitis advisable in all but endourethral methods of prostatectomy. The second stage is best done two or three weeks later before scarring becomes severe, but may be postponed for months or even years. It is advisable to excise the primary wound and track and to mobilize the parts as much as possible. A wedge of the posterior lip of the bladder neck should be excised but it is usually impossible to get an exposure of the prostatic bed good enough to stop all bleeding. Open drainage through a large tube is necessary, packing rarely so. Continuous suction may be used in after-treatment, or a suprapubic box may be fitted. The patient should pass water naturally and the wound should heal in about fourteen to twenty-one days. Persistence of suprapubic leakage is usually due to sepsis or bladder neck obstruction.

One Stage Operations with Bladder Closure. *Retropubic prostat-ectomy.* First described by Millin in 1945, this method is now widely used. It is not without difficulties and dangers, especially when unsuit-able patients, such as those with small fibrous prostates better treated endoscopically, are dealt with in this way. There is then little room retropubically for manipulation and the capsule is ill-defined, thin and difficult to sew.

The skin incision may be transverse or vertical, followed by a vertical incision between the recti. The main steps of the operation are:

The ligation of the veins (dorsal vein of penis) in the prevesical fatty areolar tissue, followed by clearing of the anterior and lateral sides of the prostate by gauze dissection. Then the prostatic capsule is incised transversely or vertically after securing the main capsular veins. The adenomatous prostatic lobes are freed by blunt dissection and the urethra is cut by scissors close to the apex of the prostate to avoid damage to the membranous urethra. Bleeding in the prostatic bed, which may be minimal or severe, is stopped by diathermy or ligation. A wedge of the posterior lip of the bladder neck must be excised and the prostatic capsule then closed by water-tight suture over an indwelling catheter. The retropubic space should be drained for a few days.

Hæmorrhage during the operation is sometimes brisk, particularly from unsecured vessels in the prostatic capsule. It is best in such cases to complete the removal of the enlarged lobes as rapidly as possible. The hæmorrhage often then becomes less and its origin is anyway more easily seen and secured.

Post-operatively the main complication is clot retention. This can usually be avoided by the installation of sterile 5 per cent. sod. citrate at the time of the operation. Gentle lavage at intervals with the same solution may be necessary post-operatively, but should be used only when absolutely necessary as infection is difficult to avoid. Should clot cause serious blockage it may have to be broken up and washed out through a catheter by a Bigelow's evacuator. The catheter should be removed as early as possible depending on the amount of hæmorrhage —but certainly within seven days. The patient should be up for short intervals within a few days. Suprapubic leakage occasionally happens but seldom persists. Slight incontinence is common at first but control is soon regained. Post-operative stricture is not common provided the bladder neck has been resected as described above. Osteitis pubis—the ætiology of which remains obscure—is a rare complication of this as of other methods of prostatectomy.

Transvesical Methods. These are associated with the names of Freyer, Thompson Walker and Harris, the pioneer of primary bladder closure. There are many individual modifications of each method; all have in common wide exposure with trimming of the bladder neck and hæmostasis of the prostatic bed by sutures or diathermy. In the Harris type an attempt is made to obliterate the prostatic cavity with deeply placed sutures. Transvesical methods have the advantage that concomitant lesions of the bladder such as neoplasm or diverticulum can be treated and are preferred by some surgeons when an enlargement is mainly of the intravesical type. Access to the lateral lobes is less good than by the retropubic route, even with a finger in the rectum to push the prostate forward; the hæmorrhage from the prostatic bed is less easy to control. Some surgeons use a catheter with a hydrostatic bag to give temporary pressure to the bed, and some use one of the hæmostatic fibrin compounds. Prolonged efforts to stop hæmorrhage in the prostatic bed during the operation may be deceptive, success being due to a fall in blood pressure. This may mean that subsequent resuscitation is followed by reactionary hæmorrhage and clot retention. If hæmorrhage is persistent it may be advisable to place a small suprapubic tube in the bladder at the end of the operation. If possible the bladder should be sewn up in two layers, the more superficial being a continuous suture of the "Lembert" type.

Perineal Prostatectomy. Although an established method, perineal prostatectomy is practised very little in this country. Its main advantage is that it is the least disturbing of all methods, including endourethral methods, of prostatectomy. Both hæmorrhage and shock are minimal and, there being no abdominal wound, post-operatively respiration is not embarrassed. The operation is most suitably done under low spinal anæsthesia, and can be used for patients whose general condition is so poor that other methods are extremely hazardous. The publicity given to the occasional complications of incontinence and perineal fistula have made many surgeons chary of this method. Radical prostatectomy for carcinoma by this route will be mentioned later.

Endourethral Resection. In this country endourethral resection of the prostate is usually reserved for the small fibrous type of gland and for carcinoma. Few attempt total removal of the larger glands. Both types of instrument used, the Thompson punch and the McCarthy diathermy resectoscope, need special training. No detailed description of the technique is given here. Hæmorrhage is checked by coagulation diathermy, and the bladder drained by in-dwelling catheter for a few days. The main complications are hæmorrhage with clot retention, incontinence, usually temporary. Stricture, due to trauma from a large endoscope or from the indwelling catheter is said to be avoided by passing the instrument and draining the bladder through the bulb— "bulbar urethrotomy". In well chosen cases the results of resection are good and may be lasting.

Carcinoma

Carcinoma of the prostate is not always easy to recognize. In some instances it is only discovered after operation on histological examination of an apparently simple specimen. At the other end of the scale it may be quite obvious on rectal examination and typical secondary deposits may be present in the bones when first seen. It is occasionally difficult to distinguish chronic inflammatory or calculous disease, but in the main it is usually found that carcinoma is more often present than not when suspicion of it is aroused on rectal examination. Biopsy may confirm the diagnosis. Fragments for examination obtained with the resectoscope will show a carcinoma which impinges on the bladder neck or urethra. Samples from the periphery of the gland may be taken by open perineal operation, or, less certainly by needle puncture through the ischio-rectal fossa guided to the suspicious area by a finger in the rectum. Early diagnosis is important. Clinically obvious carcinoma is unlikely to be suitable for radical extirpation, but the converse is also true.

Estimation of the serum acid sodium phosphatase may occasionally be a help in the diagnosis. Normally it is 2 to 3·5 units. A rise confirms the presence of prostatic cancer especially with secondary spread. A normal finding, however, does not contradict the diagnosis. It is perhaps most useful as a guide to the progress of the disease.

Treatment

Apart from the relief of retention there are two main methods—hormonal and operative. The former is applicable to those patients, the vast majority, in whom the growth is already too extensive for radical extirpation. Large doses of œstrogen are given daily and their action is sometimes supplemented by castration. This is most conveniently achieved by "evisceration" of the soft testicular tissue from within the tunica albuginea, which is then sutured to prevent bleeding. The daily dosage of œstrogen varies from 3 to 100 mg. The larger doses are used to control the disease in the early stages and improvement may be expected in a few weeks. They may be reduced but a maintenance dose must be given for the rest of the patient's life. Should the toxic effects of stilbœstrol or dienœstrol—chiefly nausea and vomiting —be troublesome, the more concentrated ethinyl œstradiol (0·5 to 2 mg.) may be better tolerated. In most cases the prognosis is good even when metastasis is present, but at the price of feminism of varying degree, and impotence. This may be of little consequence in the old, but when the disease is discovered in middle-aged patients it can be a serious disadvantage.

Radical operation is the removal of the whole gland with its capsule and usually of the seminal vesicles. It has been done by various approaches—transvesical, retropubic and perineal. None is easy.

The treatment of retention is the same whether due to carcinoma or adenoma. Suprapubic cystotomy should, however, be avoided and the early resection of obstructing tissue is indicated especially when radical operation is not possible. This, combined with indwelling catheterization will usually tide the patient over the period needed for hormones to take effect.

M. F. NICHOLLS

CHAPTER XXII

THE TREATMENT OF THYROTOXICOSIS

Antithyroid Agents

Treatment of the thyrotoxic patient has been transformed in recent years by the discovery and introduction of the anti-thyroid substances. They have ushered in a new era of safety in thyroid surgery and they have rendered obsolete in all but the most exceptional cases the need for individual ligation of arteries and multiple stage operations.

By their agency a small group of patients with thyrotoxicosis can be cured or at least controlled without resort to surgery. For the remainder, surgery following upon a course of one of the antithyroid agents may be necessary, but by enabling us for the first time to fulfil our main pre-operative objective—the conversion of a toxic into a non-toxic goitre—they have removed much of the hazard and increased the accuracy of the operation.

When we speak of the surgical treatment of thyrotoxicosis we imply treatment by combined medicine and surgery. Surgery is only the culminating act in the final phase of a combined method. In comparing the merits of the purely medical and the combined procedures it is important to bear in mind the altered circumstances in which thyroid surgery is conducted to-day. The adverse conditions which existed prior to 1943, when surgery so often had to be undertaken under the unfavourable conditions of uncontrolled toxicity, no longer exist.

This event has had its effect upon both patient and surgeon. It is now in our power to make the patient safe for surgery to a degree unknown prior to the thiouracil era. It is also in our power to make surgery safer for the patient, since there is no longer the same necessity for speed in operating as there was in the constitutionally ill and toxic subject. One great advantage which an unhurried operation affords is that it allows time for the deliberate identification of the parathyroid glands and recurrent laryngeal nerves so that the incidence of damage to these important structures has fallen. Equally important, a more accurate assessment of the amount of gland to be resected can be made—a key decision in the operation, for nothing brings thyroidectomy for toxic goitre into such disrepute as inadequate procedures.

The present satisfactory position is in part due to modern anæsthetic agents and methods; it is in greater measure due to the thiouracils. It is incumbent therefore upon all surgeons using the antithyroid drugs for the pre-operative stabilization of their patients to be familiar with their potentialities. In addition it is essential to see the patients with their physician in their original thyrotoxic state before therapy is initiated. If seen for the first time when a thiouracil effect has been obtained, an entirely false assessment of the severity of the disease may be made, and a wrong decision come to as to the need or time for surgical intervention.

The Thiouracils

Action

The antithyroid agents most commonly employed are methyl and propyl thiouracil. Their mode of action is to interfere with the synthesis of thyroxin within the thyroid gland by preventing the union of iodine and tyrosine into diiodotyrosine which is the precursor of thyroxin. The resultant fall in the production of circulating thyroxin stimulates the anterior pituitary to an increased production of thyrotropic hormone and this in turn is followed by an ineffectual hyperplasia of the thyroid gland, clinically manifested in a proportion of patients by an increase in its size. The thiouracils do not affect the thyroxin already stored in the gland or in circulation, which explains the short time lag before clinical improvement is noticed following the initial administration of thiouracil.

Complications

Thiouracil Goitre and Myxoedema. Since the antithyroid drugs interfere with the synthesis of thyroxin they take a much shorter time to produce myxoedema in hyperthyroid patients in whom the stores of thyroxin are low than in the normal person whose stocks of thyroxin stored in the colloid spaces of the gland are high. *High dosage and prolonged therapy* tend to produce *thiouracil goitres* (Figs. 1 and 2).

It is very undesirable that overdosage with anti-

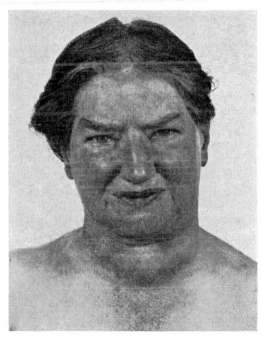

Fig. 22.1. Thyrotoxicosis: Before thiouracil therapy.

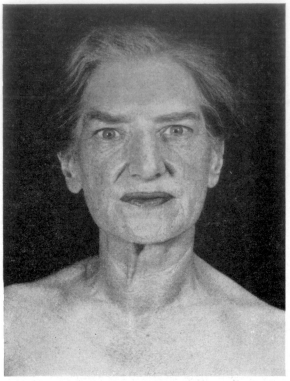

FIG. 22.2.　Thyrotoxicosis: After excessive thiouracil therapy. The patient has been treated with propyl thiouracil on too high a dosage and for too long. This has produced a "thiouracil goitre" and myxœdema with thickening of the vocal cords.

thyroid agent should occur. The resultant "thiouracil goitre" may cause pressure symptoms and force surgery while the gland is still enlarged and vascular and so greatly increase the technical difficultiés of the operation. The thickening of the vocal cords which takes place in the myxœdematous phase also constitutes a very real post-operative danger from œdema of the glottis. Tracheotomy was required in three patients operated upon at the Lahey Clinic during the myxœdematous phase (Cattell, 1949).

Furthermore in spite of what has been written to the contrary, my experience is that an irreversible state may be set up if myxœdema is produced by antithyroid agents or at least a state which takes a long time to adjust itself. In addition it complicates the surgeon's decision as to how much thyroid to remove at operation and post-operatively seriously retards the patient's return to normal health and thyroid function.

Toxic Reactions

Thiouracil is a poison to some individuals and although the mortality from *agranulocytosis* is extraordinarily low considering the widespread use of the antithyroid agents, the fact remains that any therapeutic measure that carries with it the risk of death, however remote, requires that special precautions shall be taken in its application. It cannot be too strongly urged that routine blood counts as a safety method of control are not only useless but *dangerous* as the drug may strike with dramatic suddenness. Blood counts which may be normal one day, may be seriously leucopenic the next. Fortunately this sudden and dramatic fall rarely, if ever, occurs without giving rise to warning symptoms. It is for this reason that the *clinical method of control* is recommended. For the clinical method of control to be safe, everyone coming in contact with the drug—patient, nurse and doctor—must be absolutely familiar with its side effects, and immediate action taken upon any of the well known toxic features presenting (fever, malaise, nausea, headache, sore throat, rash, etc.). This action will take the form of instantly stopping the administration of the drug, of giving a prophylactic injection of penicillin and making an immediate examination of a blood smear. In the latter connection a formal differential count —unless the polymorphs are alarmingly scanty—is unnecessary and time consuming. It is a simple matter for an experienced pathologist to tell from a smear, almost at a glance, whether the granulocytes are plentiful or not. If the *granulocytes are scanty* it will be wise to abandon thiouracil therapy altogether; after the blood count returns to normal the patient should be put on to iodine and followed up with a thyroidectomy. If the *granulocytes are plentiful* after a toxic reaction, it is sufficient to wait a week and then to switch to another antithyroid agent—for example from methyl to propyl thiouracil. Toxic effects— once they have subsided—with the exception of persistent leucopenia do not contra-indicate the continuation of treatment. In using the term leucopenia it should be borne in mind that an absolute polymorphonuclear count which is a neutropenia for one person is not necessarily a neutropenia for another. The interpretation of the term must be related to the pre-therapy normal count—hence the importance of this count for the purposes of comparison subsequently. Thus, a patient with a normal high count of, say, 5,000 polymorphs which drops to 1,500 polymorphs is to be regarded more seriously than a patient with a low normal of say, 3,000 polymorphs which drops to 1,500, the first representing a drop of 70 per cent., the second a drop of 50 per cent.

Hæmorrhage

Thiouracil produces effects upon the gland of primary toxic goitre which only occur minimally or not at all in the nodular thyroid of the older patient. It increases the size of the gland, renders its consistency hard and rigid and increases its vascularity many times.

It is important to be aware of these effects and so prepared for the very severe bleeding which can occur at operation. If this comes as a surprise it may well extend the most experienced surgeon. Much can be done to diminish the technical difficulties associated with the altered physical state of the gland, by careful preparation with iodine, by avoiding pre-operative overdosage with thiouracil and by a sense of timing in the choice of the optimum moment for the operation, but despite observing these precautions there will still be occasional cases calling for all the operator's skill if bleeding is to be controlled, an adequate amount of gland removed and no damage inflicted upon either of the recurrent laryngeal nerves.

Dosage

Growing experience shows that there is little to choose between methyl and propyl thiouracil. They both produce the same effect, in the same dosage, in the same time and with much the same reaction rate. It seems probable that the earlier doses used were too high—the maximum initial dosage should not exceed 200 mg. twice a day, and in many cases an excellent response will be obtained from half this dose. Because of its availability methyl thiouracil has been used in this country more than propyl, and perhaps for this reason acquired a reputation for having a higher toxic reaction rate; in practice there is little difference in the respective reaction rates, approximately one in five patients showing some toxic manifestation. It is, however, worth bearing in mind that a patient who is sensitive to one form of anti-thyroid agent may respond normally to another, so that after a brief interruption treatment may be continued with safety. (For example, Mercazole—1 Methyl-2 Mercaptoimidazole—average comparable dosage 2-4 mg. b.d.)

Administration

Thiouracil can be used in combination with surgery as a pre-operative agent with a view to bringing the patient to a safe operative level, or its administration can be prolonged with a view to obtaining stabilization without operation—chemical thyroidectomy so to say.

In-patient treatment is advisable for all cases at the outset but this can give way to treatment as an out-patient as soon as the patient seems well and strong enough to make the necessary journeys to attend regularly, i.e. at weekly intervals at first though this period can be prolonged as the course proceeds.

Medical Cases. The initial treatment with all patients is the same: the patient is admitted for a period of observation during which, apart from a general examination, a pre-therapy Basal Metabolic Rate and a "baseline" differential white cell count are done, the weight taken, the neck measured and X-rayed to exclude deviation or compression of the trachea and retrosternal goitre, and cardiological and other opinions obtained when in doubt. All toxic patients should, in addition, be interviewed by a mature and sympathetic Almoner, and in exceptional cases by a psychiatrist, so that we may be familiar with the home housing conditions and other relevant social and personal factors. After the first few days of the resting phase most patients should be allowed to go to the bathroom and to get up for a short time each evening.

Having weighed all the available data the selected antithyroid agent is started and continued in its initial dosage until the patient is symptom free. Progress is assessed by observing an improvement in the patient's general clinical condition—usually first noticed at the end of ten days— by a fall in the B.M.R. and sleeping pulse rate and by an increase in weight. When symptom free the dosage is halved and gradually reduced during the course of the next three months, after which a smaller or *maintenance* dose is substituted and maintained for a *minimum period* of six months. If at the end of this time the patient remains symptom free the thiouracil is stopped and the patient provisionally discharged with instructions to report for reassessment in three months' time or before if there is a recurrence of the thyrotoxic symptoms. If this regime is followed, few patients will or should be free from supervision and therapy in less than one year.

While thiouracil treatment is continuing it is usual, although not essential, to have a white cell count at fortnightly intervals. A second B.M.R. estimation during the course of therapy may also be a useful guide to the duration of therapy and occasionally may give valuable warning of impending hypothyroidism.

An initial pre therapy white cell count below 3,000 associated with neutropenia contra-indicates treatment with thiouracil.

Relapses. So far as it is possible to judge, approximately half the patients on thiouracil alone relapse following the first full course of thiouracil and a substantial number of those that relapse, relapse again following a second course. The inference is that the relapser goes on being a relapser with repeated courses, but it is only fair to say that of those that relapse a proportion only are thiouracil failures and others relapse because of the persistence of the original precipitating factor such as domestic or financial worry.

Relapses, if they are going to occur, tend to happen quickly, i.e. within two to four months of stopping treatment. *Short* courses of thiouracil are followed by a high relapse rate, so that treatment with antithyroid agents must be continued for a substantial period—not less than six months after the patient has become symptom free.

The permenancy of the remission induced by thiouracil is not yet known, nor is it known if its carcinogenic properties in certain animals will ever produce cancer in man. Time alone will decide these points for us.

Surgical Cases. The initial procedure when using thiouracil as a *pre-operative* agent is the same as for medical cases. Administration continues until the patient is symptom free or, ideally, just short of this point when the drug is stopped altogether. The B.M.R. averages a drop of a point a day in primary and a point every other day in secondary toxic goitre, so that a patient with primary thyrotoxicosis and a B.M.R. of plus 42 who is to have a thyroidectomy can be told that it will take approximately six weeks to prepare her for operation. In cases of *primary* thyrotoxicosis, if the thiouracil therapy before operation has been prolonged, iodine (minims x t.d.s. in milk) should be given pre-operatively for a period of at least three, and sometimes four weeks, or it will not produce its full *devascularizing* effect. The first two weeks of iodine therapy should overlap with the last two weeks of the thiouracil therapy. The usual short course of 10 to 12 days is sufficient in cases of toxic *nodular* goitre as they have not the same tendency to bleed. Those patients who have been receiving the terminal part of their thiouracil course as out-patients may with advantage begin their pre-operative iodine before they return to hospital, which should be not less than three days before the anticipated day of operation. Finally a post-therapy pre-operative white cell count should be carried out on the day before operation to exclude a delayed thiouracil leucopenic reaction. In calculating the optimum day for operation it is important not to forget to take into consideration the date of onset of the next menstrual period.

Definitive Treatment: The Three Groups

When faced with a thyrotoxic patient, who may be young or old, who may be with or without enlargement of the thyroid gland and with or without the classical features of the disease, it can be perplexing to make up one's mind as to the most suitable definitive line of treatment.

In practice it will be found that the majority of thyrotoxic patients when first seen can be divided into three groups:

a *Medical* group—in whom there is present a special indication for
    medical treatment;

a *Surgical* group—in whom there is present a special indication for
    surgical treatment;

and   a *Residual* group—in whom the method of treatment can only be
    decided after a period of trial with the antithyroid agents.

In arriving at a decision as to the appropriate line of treatment in an individual case it is helpful first to exclude those patients who fall naturally into a medical or surgical category. Let us consider first those in whom medical treatment is indicated.

Group 1. Medical Treatment—the indications

Mild Thyrotoxicosis. Medical treatment is indicated in all patients with mild thyrotoxicosis, that is to say, those with a B.M.R. of not more than plus 20 and a pulse rate of not more than 90. The usual methods of rest and sedation will suffice for the majority; a few will require thiouracil; *surgery is absolutely contra-indicated*.

Recurrent Thyrotoxicosis. Recurrent thyrotoxicosis might be regarded as the *cardinal* indication for the use of thiouracil; radio-iodine is now available for the same purpose. Re-operation on these patients is always hazardous because of the risk of damaging either or both recurrent laryngeal nerves. Thiouracil is also of particular value in treating patients with a unilateral recurrence associated with a recurrent laryngeal nerve palsy on the side opposite to the recurrence. If the recurrence takes place on the side of the nerve lesion re-operation can be considered with less anxiety as the underlying nerve has already been damaged.

Age—Stress and other Factors. Medical treatment should also always be employed whenever possible in *young* children and in the *elderly* and at times of exceptional physiological stress such as *puberty, pregnancy* and the *menopause*, when thiouracil cover will generally be all that is necessary. In the case of thyrotoxicosis associated with pregnancy it should be stated that it is unnecessary to interrupt the pregnancy. The danger of producing sub-thyroid babies as a result of thiouracil therapy during pregnancy appears to have been greatly exaggerated, but iodine should replace the thiouracil for the last four weeks of pregnancy. In those few cases in which the prospective mother does not tolerate the antithyroid agent, thyroidectomy during pregnancy after iodine preparation may rarely have to be carried out. The thiouracils are secreted in the milk so that it is wise either to wean the child after birth or to continue with only very small doses to avoid cretinism.

Medical treatment will also be the elective method in patients in whom thyrotoxicosis is complicated by an anxiety state, in poor operative risks and when expert surgery is unavailable or refused.

Group 2. Surgical Treatment—the indications

Surgery, as the primary definitive line of treatment, is indicated when *pressure* symptoms are present as shown by displacement or compression of the trachea, or when symptoms of pressure might be precipitated by the use of thiouracil as in a retrosternal or intrathoracic goitre.

It is also generally agreed that surgery is advisable in patients with *auricular fibrillation* or other cardiovascular disturbance attributable to the thyrotoxicosis. Surgery may also be the most desirable method of treatment in those who are unable or unwilling to attend regularly, in the unreliable and unco-operative, for social or economic reasons and for reasons of size or nodularity or because malignancy cannot be excluded. By a process of elimination it also becomes the only effective expedient in those patients in whom medical treatment has failed, i.e. the *thiouracil sensitive, the thiouracil relapses* and the *thiouracil resistant*.

There is no reason to withhold antithyroid agent in the pre-operative preparation of toxic patients in the surgical group provided that it is administered under close supervision and followed by iodine in the usual way. In many instances there may be a very satisfactory response to antithyroid agents and in approximately one-third of the cases of auricular fibrillation of thyrotoxic origin normal rhythm will be restored.

Group 3.   Residual Group

The exclusion of patients in the two previous groups leaves us with a large residual group, all of whom have moderately severe thyrotoxicosis (pulse rate 90-120) or severe thyrotoxicosis (pulse rate above 120). This is a group of mixed thyrotoxics, some primary, some secondary, in whom there is no clear-cut indication as to whether they would be best treated by medical or surgical methods. If we treat all patients in this group surgically, then we shall automatically operate upon a number who might have been cured medically. If we treat all patients in this group medically for an indefinite period of time we are going to submit a considerable proportion to a prolonged and eventually fruitless course of therapy.

The difficulty is that at the first examination we have no way of predicting which patients will be stabilized by antithyroid agents and therefore could be excluded from surgery, and which patients will relapse after medical treatment, and would therefore be better prepared for surgery from the outset. Accordingly all patients with severe or moderately severe thyrotoxicosis who do not naturally fall into the medical or surgical categories mentioned should be submitted to a course of antithyroid agents in order to determine their response to the drug.

Therapeutic Trial

The procedure recommended is as follows: Give to all patients in the residual group a therapeutic test course of antithyroid agent for a period not exceeding one month or until symptom free, whichever is the earlier.

The situation should then be reassessed. It is at this early stage that the position of all these patients should be reviewed and **not after months of antithyroid treatment,** because those who are going to respond *well*, respond *quickly*. Excluding those who fall out because they are thiouracil sensitive, two groups will be found to emerge for reassessment —a small group which responds indifferently and a large group which responds well to antithyroid agent.

The Thiouracil Resistant. This group consists of patients who respond slowly or not at all to antithyroid agents. Experience suggests that the majority of these refractory patients will never become completely symptom free on the antithyroid agents at present available, however prolonged the use of these drugs may be.

If after one month's treatment any doubt still remains a further four weeks' antithyroid therapy should be given. If at the end of this time the patient remains refactory the antithyroid agent should be stopped, iodine started and operation carried out as soon as the maximum response to the iodine has been obtained.

The Thiouracil Responsive. Patients who respond quickly to thiouracil will be found at the end of the four week period to show a marked clinical improvement. Once again it is at this early stage that a decision should be taken as to whether to continue with medical treatment or abandon it in favour of surgery. It might be argued that there is no decision to take and that all patients who show a favourable initial response should be treated along medical lines until they are stabilized or fail to respond any longer to the drug. This is the tendency in some centres but is an attitude which fails to take into consideration the varying demands of the different age groups and the influence of social and economic factors upon the course of the disease. Thoughtful surgeons operating upon the thyroid to-day are fully aware of the value of thiouracil and give it full credit, but at the same time feel that certain patients in this group should be operated upon just as some others should be encouraged to continue with antithyroid therapy only. The decision as to whether the future management of the patients in this group should be along medical or surgical lines can usually be resolved by reference to the following points: *the age, the facilities available, the patient's attitude, the precipitating factor.*

Age. PRE-MENOPAUSE. Broadly speaking the younger adult patients should be operated upon; certainly those under 30. There is a natural reluctance to interfere surgically with the endocrine system at this age yet younger patients do not tolerate well the tedium of prolonged thiouracil therapy. They are impatient of results and inclined to find the repeated visits to hospital irksome and boring, and for this reason they may not progress favourably. More important still the younger age group—because the gland reacts maximally to the antithyroid agent—are more liable to develop a thiouracil goitre and quite suddenly to slip over into myxœdema unless very frequent and time consuming visits are made to a thyroid clinic.

MENOPAUSAL AND POST-MENOPAUSAL. In menopausal and postmenopausal patients who are responding well it is wise to avoid thyroidectomy and to persist rather with antithyroid agents if these are well tolerated. Commonly a thyrotoxic flare-up during the menopause is a transient manifestation of the disease and will die down as the climacteric comes naturally to its end.

Post-menopausal patients, even if the gland is nodular, respond in my experience in a more satisfactory and lasting manner to antithyroid agents than patients in the younger age groups. Operation will necessarily be advisable in those showing displacement of the trachea, a retrosternal goitre, or with associated cardiovascular disease or if there is any suspicion of malignancy although coincidence of the latter with thyrotoxicosis is exceedingly rare.

Post-menopausal patients without these complications should be encouraged to persist with the full course of antithyroid agent and the subsequent maintenance dose for some months after they have become symptom free.

Facilities Available. If the surgical facilities available are poor, as they can be, it will be prudent to continue with medical treatment. Only if they are good does surgery become an alternative to medical methods and it should then be carried out immediately the patient has had her pre-operative course of thiouracil and iodine. The medical facilities available can also be poor—by this I mean the time and care the physician concerned is prepared or able to give to the patient. Continued supervision by one man is essential in these mixed diseases of psyche and soma and this demands both time and patience.

The Patient. Patients with thyrotoxicosis are usually intelligent and their own wishes in regard to treatment must be consulted after the advantages and disadvantages of both methods have been explained to them; for example the surgical cure is quick and permanent and removes the goitre, but involves an operation: medical treatment may produce relief of symptoms without an operation but a permanent cure is not certain and surgery may be necessary in the end. Some patients find medical treatment tedious and frustrating, others will only show improvement when told that surgery is not contemplated—and so on.

The Precipitating Agent. If a precipitating agent can be found and removed, the patient will be more than half way towards a permanent relief of symptoms without any other form of therapy. In searching for such a factor intercurrent illness or disease should first be excluded. Special enquiry should then be made, but in privacy and gently, into many supremely personal matters. Common contributing factors are married unhappiness, housing difficulties often associated with living with "in laws", exhaustion from the prolonged strain either of overwork in the home or nursing a sick relative, the emotional shock resulting from an unhappy love affair or the death of a close friend or member of the family, an unsuitable occupation or financial or domestic worries in their manifold varieties.

It should here be put on record that it is typical of the contrariness of this disease that no relevant precipitating factor can be found in the majority of thyrotoxic patients. If one is revealed which can be relieved, medical treatment alone may well be all that is necessary. It is in the cases in which there is an obvious domestic or psychological obstacle to recovery which *cannot be removed* in which the greatest judgment is required in determining the most suitable form of treatment. Such patients will almost certainly relapse if treated with thiouracil alone. Subtotal thyroidectomy in these circumstances should be reserved for the severely thyrotoxic in whom the measure of improvement produced may be sufficiently significant to enable the patient to review and assess her own problems with a fresh outlook and in a more balanced manner. No rules, however, can be laid down, each patient and each problem must be assessed and treated individually.

Iodine Preparation

There is one short rider that should be added to the subject of treatment; some of the younger patients especially do not tolerate thiouracil well and if the thyrotoxicosis is of moderate severity only can be brought to a safe operative level with iodine alone. In selected cases, this method of preparation still has a definite place.

Radioactive Iodine

It is not possible yet to assess the part radioactive iodine is ultimately likely to play in the diagnosis or treatment of thyrotoxicosis. Encouraging reports have been received from a number of centres.

The amount of radioactive iodine present in the thyroid gland itself can be measured by means of a Geiger counter. If the amount of radioactive iodine present in the plasma is determined at the same time, the thyroid iodine clearance rate can be measured and this is of diagnostic value. From here it is removed both by the thyroid and the kidneys. The rate of uptake by the thyroid is related to the activity of the gland, being rapid in toxic goitre and slow in myxœdema. In consequence during the same period there is proportionately less or more iodine available for excretion by the kidneys and this amount can be measured.

These variations form the basis of tests which can be used for diagnostic purposes to determine the presence or absence of thyrotoxicosis, and is especially valuable in those doubtful cases in which the clinical picture may be complicated by an anxiety state. It is equally useful in determining the degree of hypothyroidism in a case of myxœdema and can be helpful in circumstances when the B.M.R. is likely to be inaccurate.

For therapeutic purposes the dosage is based on the severity of the toxicity and the size of the gland. A single dose is usually sufficient but subsequent smaller doses may have to be given. The very simplicity of the treatment naturally makes it popular with patients. The clinical response normally follows a similar pattern: in the first few days the gland becomes tender, to be followed in the course of the first week by an exacerbation of toxicity. Clinical improvement follows at the end of the first fortnight and in four weeks 97 per cent. of the radioactivity is dissipated.

Until we know whether the threats of carcinogenesis, and kidney or ovarian or bone marrow damage are real or groundless it will be wise to reserve I^{131} for the treatment of patients over the age of 50, for cases of recurrent thyrotoxicosis and patients who are unsuitable for operation or who are resistant or sensitive to the antithyroid agents. In the meantime its potentialities continue cautiously to be explored.

Terminology

In view of the numerous anti-thyroid agents available the drug thiouracil (methyl or propyl) has been selected for use in the text—in the generic sense—as being the representative of the antithyroid group which has been most widely employed up to the present time.

The number of these agents is steadily increasing and their composition constantly altering in an attempt to produce a less toxic and more potent product.

VICTOR RIDDELL

References

ANSELL, G., and MILLER, H. (1952) *Lancet* **ii,** 5.
CATTELL, R. B. (1949) "Transactions of the American Goiter Association," p. 201.
DONALD, C. (1945) *Postgrad. med. J.* **21,** 41.
FRASER, R., and HARRISON, R. J. (1952) *Lancet* **i,** 382.
NEWSHOLME, G. A. (1952) *Lancet* **ii,** 805.
POCHIN, E. E. (1950) *Lancet* **ii,** 41, 84.

CHAPTER XXIII

CARCINOMA OF THE THYROID

Thyroid carcinoma forms approximately 1 per cent. of all cancers, being three times more common in women than men. The histological interpretation of the different types of malignant disease of the thyroid is notoriously difficult. There is no uniform agreement amongst pathologists on the classification of the various types of cancer in this situation and there is frequently disagreement on the interpretation of the same histological section. Confusion has been added to the study of an already complex subject by the hyperplastic effects upon the gland of thiouracil which may produce a picture closely simulating malignant disease. It is possible that this tendency on the part of the anti-thyroid agents to confuse the issue is responsible for some of the high incidence figures for cancer reported from some clinics. There is, however, a measure of agreement about the different *clinical* forms in which cancer of the thyroid may be present. The malignant process can arise *de novo* or in a previously present goitre. On this basis at least five different types can be recognized—two bilateral when first seen and three unilateral (initially).

Diffuse Carcinoma (bilateral: *de novo*)

In this variety the cancer arises *de novo* in a previously normal gland and is diffuse throughout both lobes. It is usually of bad prognosis.

Diffuse Carcinoma (bilateral: pre-existing multinodular goitre)

In this variety of diffuse carcinoma the cancer arises in a previously present multinodular goitre. It is in connection with the frequency with which cancer arises as a secondary change in the multinodular goitre that there is some difference of opinion. It seems probable that while the possibility of malignant change in multinodular goitres is unquestioned the liability is less than 5 per cent. A balanced evaluation of the position is of the greatest practical importance since if the tendency to malignant change is interpreted too radically it might lead surgeons to advise a "prophylactic" thyroidectomy in many patients who showed little more than an unevenness of the surface of the thyroid.

In practice it would seem reasonable to leave alone those patients with small multinodular goitres who are symptom free *provided* the goitre appears to be quiescent as shown by the absence of any history

264

of recent increase in size and provided that the patient is warned to report immediately any alteration in consistency or increase in size which should subsequently be noticed. In spite of exercising this kind of discrimination the majority of patients presenting with a multinodular goitre will still be operated upon for reasons of size, incipient thyrotoxicosis or uncertainty of diagnosis, but a proportion will be spared an unnecessary major operation while running a minimal risk if the precautions outlined are observed.

Malignant Adenoma (unilateral: pre-existing unilateral goitre) (Fig. 1)

In this variety—the malignant adenoma—the cancer arises in a previously present unilateral goitre. Malignant change occurs more commonly in the solitary "adenoma" than in the multinodular goitre. Its frequency in this country whether arising *de novo* or in a previously present "adenoma" is probably of the order of 7 per cent. although Hermanson, Cargill and Lesses (1952) have quoted a figure as high as 14·4 per cent.

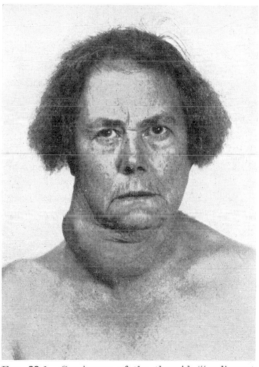

FIG. 23.1. Carcinoma of the thyroid ("malignant adenoma") with glandular metastases.

Symptomless Solitary Swelling (unilateral: *de novo*)

This variety, which is the commonest of all, is also the most favourable and the one most liable to be left alone for the reason that it presents as a *symptomless* solitary swelling of recent origin and is *indistinguishable* clinically from the innocent simple adenoma. It often occurs in young women and is usually of the papilliferous type. The thyroid with a solitary nodule must be assessed in quite a different light to the gland with multiple nodules. It cannot be too strongly urged that such a swelling should be regarded just as we regard the doubtful lump in the breast—as malignant until proved otherwise, and should therefore be excised not because it may become malignant, but because it may already *be* malignant.

The majority of unilateral goitres present with symptoms, and symptoms sufficiently striking for their removal to be advised—for example because of pressure, hæmorrhage or toxicity. It is only the few that are symptomless and it is these swellings which are so tempting to leave alone. In advising patients to have these removed it is important to bear in mind that the operation for their removal is hemithyroidectomy (not enucleation), a minor procedure compared with the subtotal operation, a small premium to pay for a high rate of insurance, for the results are amongst the best in cancer surgery.

Occult Carcinoma (unilateral)

The most fascinating and the rarest type is occult carcinoma of the thyroid. It is exactly comparable to occult carcinoma of the breast. In this variety the primary in the thyroid is too minute to be palpable; the condition draws attention to itself by virtue of the enlarged cervical lymph nodes which on biopsy are found to contain typical thyroid metastases. Until the presence of the primary in the thyroid was demonstrated to be a feature of these cases, the glandular swelling in the neck used to be referred to as carcinoma of a lateral aberrant thyroid. A lobectomy on the side on which the glands are enlarged together with a dissection of the palpable cervical glands on that side is probably the best treatment, if such a rarity should ever come one's way.

Radioactive Iodine

One of the most significant advances of modern times has been the development and use of radioactive iodine in the investigation and treatment of diseases of the thyroid gland. The use of this isotope has now passed the experimental stage and as it seems likely to play an increasingly important role in this field it may not be out of place here briefly to review the history of its development.

Introduction

Although all atoms of an element (e.g. iodine) behave in the same way chemically, they do not necessarily have the same physical properties, in particular the masses of the atoms may be different. Because the atoms of one element behave the same chemically they all occupy the "same place" in the periodic table of the elements, and are therefore called "isotopes" ($'\iota\sigma\sigma\varsigma$=same, $\tau\acute{o}\pi\sigma\varsigma$=place). Some isotopes have an unstable nucleus to the atom, and in reaching a more stable state they spontaneously emit energy in the form of alpha particles (the nuclei of helium atoms), beta particles (high speed electrons), or gamma rays (similar to X-rays), or some combination of these. The time taken for the activity of an isotope in a living creature to fall to half its initial value is known as the biological half life, and will be less than the physical half life, as biological excretion is added to physical decay.

Iodine occurring in nature has an atomic weight of 127 (written I^{127}) but many radioactive forms of other atomic weight have been prepared. The first application of radioactive iodine to the study of thyroid function was that of Hertz *et al.* in 1938, who worked on animals. They used I^{128} which had a half life of only 25 minutes, and this made any prolonged investigation impossible as the material rapidly decayed below a detectable level of activity. The first clinical studies in humans were by Hamilton and Soley (1939, 1940, 1942) who used I^{131}, of half life eight days, in their classical investigations of thyroid metabolism. Hamilton *et al.* (1940) were also the first to use radio-iodine to study cancer of the thyroid. The first demonstration of carcinomatous tissue taking up radioactive iodine was made by Keston *et al.* (1942). The extensive use of I^{131} in thyroid investigation is due in no small measure to the avidity with which the thyroid takes up iodine, the concentration in the thyroid sometimes reaching 10,000 times that of the average throughout the body.

Dosage

The isotope of iodine most commonly used at present is, as is implied above, I^{131}. In England it is manufactured at the Atomic Energy Research Station at Harwell by irradiating tellurium of atomic weight 130 with neutrons in an atomic pile. I^{131} has a half life of eight days and emits both beta particles and gamma rays. The beta particles—which are the tissue destroying particles—only travel about 2 mm. in tissue and cannot, therefore, be detected outside the body. The gamma rays are much more penetrating and are readily detected external to the body using a suitable counter.

For tracer investigations quantities of I^{131} up to about 50 μc (1 μc=1 microcurie=1/1000 millicurie) are usually employed, but for the destruction of normal thyroid function about 70 millicuries might be used (i.e. over 1,000 times the quantity used for diagnostic purposes), and for the treatment of a thyroid carcinoma as much as 250 mc. has been taken in a single "drink", comparable quantities being administered in subsequent treatments of the same patient, if these become necessary.

Administration

The isotope used is administered in solution by mouth, being given in a small and harmless dose for diagnostic (tracer) purposes and in a larger dose for therapy. It is rapidly absorbed from the intestinal tract into the blood stream, being detectable in the thyroid area within 20 minutes. It is largely removed by the thyroid and kidneys but small amounts are concentrated in the salivary glands and gastric mucous membrane. The isotope is excreted in the urine at a rate dependant upon the function of the kidneys and the thyroid condition present. In a normal person approximately 50 per cent. will be excreted in the first 48 hours and up to 90 per cent. by the end of four days. In myxœdema the radio-iodine uptake by the thyroid is small and a correspondingly larger amount will be excreted in the urine in a shorter time, and in hyperthyroidism the opposite will be the case. In cancer of the thyroid the excretion rate will depend upon whether or not the tumour is iodine concentrating.

Methods of Detection

The great value of radioactive isotopes in clinical investigation is consequent upon the extreme sensitivity of the physical methods of detecting them. Isotopes may be administered in quantities insufficient to cause biological disturbance, and their subsequent fate may be detected by (i) a Geiger counter, (ii) a scintillation counter, or (iii) auto-radiographs on photographic emulsions.

Geiger counter. This instrument, which is capable of detecting the disintegration of a single atom, was developed by Geiger while working under the late Lord Rutherford at the Cavendish Laboratory in Cambridge in the early part of this century. It was further developed by Müller in the 1920's, and to-day exists in several forms. A common type consists of a copper gauze cylinder 4 in. long and 1 in. diameter with a fine wire running along its axis, the whole being enclosed in a glass tube with a mixture of alcohol vapour and argon to about one-sixth of atmospheric pressure. A steady voltage of about 1,000 volts is maintained between the copper cylinder and the central wire. If a gamma ray falls on the counter, an electrical discharge will be initiated between the cylinder and the wire. This discharge is amplified and recorded electrically. It is important that the counter should be suitably shielded so as to receive radiations from known directions only. Such an improved counter has been described by Pochin et al. (1952) for local counting and an adaptation of this counter has been devised to determine the distribution of radio-iodine throughout the length of the body for "profile" counting.

Scintillation counter. Some materials fluoresce when alpha, beta or gamma rays fall upon them. The minute scintillation due to a single beta or gamma ray can be detected by a special light sensitive cell called a photomultiplier, and can be recorded electrically. The scintillation counter is so sensitive that only a very small dose of radio-iodine is required for tracer work. For this and other reasons the scintillation counter is likely to be used more and more in the future.

Autoradiographs. The third method of observing radiocative isotopes in biological material, is to cut a thin histological section of a biopsy specimen and place it in intimate contact with a photographic emulsion. Any particles emitted by the radioactive material cause a blackening of the emulsion (after normal development), the blackening being greatest in regions of highest concentration of radioactive material. The histological section and autoradiograph may be compared to determine the exact location of radioactive material in the specimen.

Precautions in the Use of Radioactive Isotopes

The radiation from radioactive isotopes is a potential hazard to the investigator, to the patient and, after disposal, to the general public. The precautions to be observed in their handling and disposal have been set out in a document prepared for the Medical Research Council by the Atomic Energy Research Establishment.

The Treatment

Thyroid cancer is best treated by complete surgical excision. If excision is not possible thyroid cancer should be treated with radio-active iodine, provided the carcinoma can be shown to take up the radioactive iodine sufficiently. If excision is impossible and the gland cannot be induced to take up radioactive iodine it will be necessary to resort to the third of the available methods of treatment—deep X-ray therapy.

Radio-iodine Uptake. Before deciding upon treatment with radio-active iodine it is necessary to demonstrate that the tumour concerned is capable of concentrating radio-iodine. Unfortunately all thyroid carcinomata do not take up radio-iodine, but it is now believed that more do so than was previously thought. The detection of radio-iodine uptake by a tumour is not always as straightforward an investigation as might be supposed and is particularly liable to be complicated if there is normal thyroid tissue nearby. Recently it has been shown that certain thyroid tumours, both primary and metastatic, which by external counting methods showed no initial evidence of radio-iodine uptake, were found to take up iodine *after removal* OR destruction of the contralateral lobe and all remaining normal thyroid tissue. This is an important development and has substantially increased the number of thyroid carcinomata and their metastases which can hopefully be submitted to treatment by radioactive iodine. Take-up is particularly likely to occur if the tumour is well differentiated.

The explanation of the behaviour of such thyroid tumours may be that the concentration of isotope by the tumour is greater when it is competing for radio-iodine against the kidneys alone and not against kidneys and normal thyroid (Pochin *et al.*). In addition the detection of weak uptake is technically simpler if there is no site of strong uptake such as thyroid tissue adjacent. Thus it may be that uptake in a thyroid tumour or metastases is *revealed* rather than induced by removal of normal thyroid tissue.

Metastases. Metastases distant from the thyroid gland are most readily discovered by "profile" counting. Metastases lying close to the kidneys or bladder and those near to the stomach or salivary glands may all contain radioactive iodine and so may be difficult to detect if searched for too soon after the tracer dose of radio-iodine has been taken. If metastases are present examination after a few days is likely to be more successful as by this time almost all the administered radio-iodine will have been excreted in the urine. Paradoxically the presence of metastases in thyroid carcinoma would appear to afford no contra-indication to radical surgery upon the primary growth provided that the secondary deposits can be shown to concentrate radio-iodine and so render themselves liable to self destruction.

Operability

In arriving at a decision as to the best course of treatment to pursue it is wise first to determine the local operability of the particular tumour under review.

Assessment of Operability. It is not always possible by clinical methods alone to determine whether any given case is operable or not and resort to actual operation may alone decide this point. At the same time fixation of the gland—due to transcapsular spread—with in consequence a limitation of its excursion on swallowing is a suspicious sign as also is paralysis of a vocal cord which may not always be associated with a hoarse voice and may therefore not be suspected unless the cords are *routinely examined by laryngoscopy*. Confusion in diagnosis sometimes arises between malignancy and chronic thyroiditis —which can only be settled by biopsy: occasionally a calcified nodule in the thyroid will be deceiving but its true nature will usually be revealed by a straight X-ray.

Limitations in Treatment. The following plan of treatment is an attempt to provide a practical guide in the light of our present knowledge but it should not be interpreted too rigidly in so constantly changing a sphere of therapy. It must also be borne in mind that no single surgeon has had so wide an experience of thyroid cancer that he can be dogmatic about treatment. Further it must be admitted that great as the potentialities of radio-iodine are in this field it has not so far always fulfilled our hopes. Success has been limited and disappointments numerous, in particular the behaviour of metastatic deposits may be contrary and unpredictable.

For a further account the reader will be well advised to study the comprehensive paper by Pochin *et al.* (1952) frequently and gratefully referred to in this analysis of the present position.

OPERABLE

Operable cases should be treated by thyroidectomy—inoperable cases by radio-iodine or radiotherapy according to the degree of differentiation present as revealed by preliminary biopsy. In operable cases, however, it seems doubtful whether preliminary biopsy is worth while or justifiable as material for examination will be supplied by the operation specimen, and in bulk, which will allow a more comprehensive examination by the pathologist. Only when a case is inoperable or the diagnosis is in doubt should a biopsy be done—as for example if chronic thyroiditis is a possible alternative diagnosis.

Unilateral. Unilateral operable thyroid cancer may present in two forms (excluding occult carcinoma) (i) the *suspected* (malignant adenoma) and (ii) the *unsuspected* (solitary symptomless "adenoma").

Malignant Adenoma ("type" 4). If the diagnosis is certain the treatment is total unilateral lobectomy which should include all thyroid tissue on the affected side together with the isthmus, the pyramidal lobe and any enlarged cervical glands. In an operable case of this kind there is no clear indication that there is any advantage in removing the contralateral normal lobe unless it is known that malignant tissue has been left behind or metastases are suspected of being present which might thereby be revealed and possibly induced to take up radio-iodine. In the absence of such special circumstances the normal lobe should be left undisturbed.

Unsuspected Carcinoma ("type" 5). Carcinoma occurring in the solitary symptomless swelling is usually discovered "accidentally" when the "adenoma" is cut across in the theatre after operation. As a rule the operation for its removal is a hemithyroidectomy, that is to say a partial lobectomy on the side affected, leaving a strip of thyroid tissue posteriorly as when removing a simple adenoma. A total lobectomy would, of course, be carried out if the tumour was discovered to be malignant during the course of the operation.

Bilateral. In diffuse operable thyroid cancer affecting both lobes, total thyroidectomy should be the surgical aim. The operation, in the writer's opinion, should be confined to the removal of the thyroid gland and associated enlarged lymphatic glands. It is questionable whether a standard block dissection with bilateral removal of the sternomastoid and infrahyoid muscles is any longer justifiable or beneficial in view of the availability of radio-iodine. If transcapsular spread has already occurred and the growth is involving the muscles the condition must surely be regarded as inoperable.

Following thyroidectomy the patient should be sent for radioactive iodine investigation by profile counting of any remaining areas in the body of iodine uptake.

INOPERABLE

In inoperable thyroid cancer *a preliminary biopsy* should be carried out with the object of determining the degree of differentiation of the tumour (and incidentally its thyroid origin and malignant nature), as the subsequent treatment will be much influenced by the histological picture. In hospitals which are not yet equipped with radioactive iodine facilities for investigation, the preliminary biopsy may form the basis of selection of cases for treatment.

Unilateral. If the biopsy shows well differentiated tissue the remaining normal thyroid tissue should be removed by operation or, if this is not feasible, it should be destroyed by radioactive iodine in therapeutic dosage. Following the removal of all normal thyroid tissue the tumour should be tested for radioactive iodine uptake and if this can be demonstrated, radio-iodine treatment should be instituted.

Bilateral. If the biopsy shows well differentiated tissue the remaining normal thyroid tissue scattered throughout both lobes should be destroyed by radioactive iodine in therapeutic dosage. The gland should then be tested for any residual areas concentrating radioactive iodine and if any can be demonstrated, radio-iodine treatment should be instituted.

Inoperable tumours—unilateral or bilateral—which are *undifferentiated* should be treated with radio-iodine if they can be shown to take it up but this is uncommon. In most cases in this category such uptake will not be demonstrable and treatment should be with *radiotherapy*.

Tracheostomy. Tracheostomy is sometimes necessary when respiratory obstruction is present. In these circumstances it is essential to use a rubber tube if the area is being or is to be irradiated.

VICTOR RIDDELL

BIBLIOGRAPHY

HAMILTON, J. G., and SOLEY, M. H. (1939) *Amer. J. Physiol.* **127,** 557.
HAMILTON, J. G., and SOLEY, M. H. (1940) *Amer. J. Physiol.* **131,** 135.
HARRISON, R. J. H. (1952) *Lancet* **i,** 382.
HERMANSON, L., GARGILL, S. L., and LESSES, M. F. (1952) *J. clin. Endocrinol.* **12,** 112.
HERTZ, S., ROBERTS, A., and EVANS, R. D. (1938) *Proc. Soc. exp. Biol. N.Y.* **38,** 510.
KESTON, A. S., BALL, R. P., FRANTZ, V. K., and PALMER, W. W. (1942) *Science* **95,** 362.
NEWSHOLME, G. A. (1952) *Lancet* **ii,** 805.
POCHIN, E. E., MYANT, N. B., HILTON, GWEN, HONOUR, A. J., CORBETT, B. D. (1952) *Brit. med. J.* **ii,** 1115.

CHAPTER XXIV

SURGERY OF THE ADRENAL GLAND

THE adrenal is without doubt this decade's most fashionable endocrine gland and surgeons are moving into this new and expanding field. Every surgical operation evokes a response from the adrenal even before the patient has been anæsthetized, but in this chapter the reaction of the adrenals to an injury will not be discussed and only those diseases considered which may be benefited by an operation on the adrenal gland.

Diseases which may be Benefited by an Operation on the Adrenal

I. *Cortex*
   (a) Tumours without Endocrine Symptoms.
   (b) Tumours with Endocrine Symptoms.
       i. Cushing's syndrome.
       ii. Androgen effects.
       iii. Œstrogen effects.
   (c) Hyperplasia
       i. Cushing's syndrome.
       ii. Adreno-genital syndrome.

II. *Medulla*
   (a) Tumours without Endocrine Symptoms.
   (b) Phæochromocytoma.

III. (a) Addison's Disease.
   (b) Hypertension.
   (c) Carcinoma of the Prostate and Breast.

Tumours without Endocrine Symptoms

These may arise in either cortex or medulla. There is no difference between the treatment of these tumours, whether benign or malignant, and a tumour anywhere else in the body. If diagnosed in an operable state they should be excised but no special problems are presented and they will not be discussed further.

Tumours with Endocrine Symptoms (Œstrogen and Androgen)

Because of their bizarre nature these tumours attract a good deal of attention but they are uncommon. In boys before puberty precocity will occur and occasionally the infant Hercules type is seen. In males after puberty sexual changes are rare because an increase of androgens is without any obvious effect and an œstrogen-producing tumour is uncommon. In women and girls the change is usually to the male type but precocity may occur if an œstrogen-producing tumour appears before puberty. Unfortunately many of these tumours are malignant but surgical excision for either benign or malignant growths offers the only hope of cure.

Cushing's Syndrome

At one time this was thought to be due to a basophil adenoma of the pituitary. To-day the current view is that this syndrome may be due to overaction of the pituitary but that this acts through either a tumour or hyperplasia of the adrenal cortex. In this respect it is analogous to thyrotoxicosis and like it responds to a surgical operation, not on the pituitary but on the gland affected by the abnormal pituitary, in this case the adrenal. From the practical point of view it does not matter whether the cause is in the pituitary or the adrenal. The treatment is the same for both and consists of removal of an adrenal cortical tumour if present, otherwise a subtotal (90 per cent.) adrenalectomy is required.

The clinical features of Cushing's syndrome are well illustrated in Fig. 1—the buffalo type obesity with thin limbs and a heavy trunk, the extreme muscular weakness, the skin changes which include striæ, ecchymoses and a florid face. In addition these patients have hypertension, amenorrhœa or impotence, osteoporosis, a raised blood sugar, a low plasma potassium and a high carbon dioxide combining power. Of particular value to the surgeon is an estimation of the 17-keto-steroids and 11-oxysteroids in a 24-hour specimen of the patient's urine. In Cushing's syndrome due to a tumour of the adrenal cortex the excretion of 17-ketosteroids is usually raised but when the adrenals show only hyperplasia this increase is present in only half of the patients. The 17-ketosteroids are a product of androgen metabolism, in women the normal excretion is 5 to 15 mgm. per 24 hours, and practically all comes from the adrenal, in men the normal is 8 to 22 mgm. and a proportion is derived from the testis. The 11-oxysteroid excretion, a product of a hormone connected with protein metabolism, may be raised in this syndrome.

The treatment of Cushing's syndrome is surgical; in the present state of our knowledge medical measures are at best only palliative. If a tumour of the adrenal is suspected the surgeon should explore the most likely side first; if he finds a tumour it should be removed. If he

+ which is that?

well, well,

does not find a tumour what should he do? If the gland is small and atrophic it is probable that there is a tumour in the other gland; in this case the wound should be closed and the opposite gland exposed through a separate incision either at once or at a later date. On the other hand, if the gland is normal or hyperplastic in appearance a

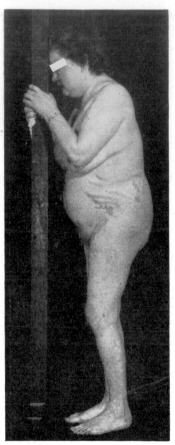
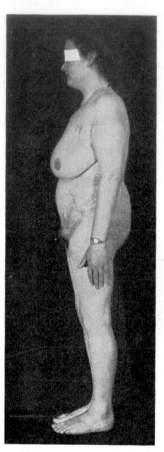

Fig. 24.1. A patient with Cushing's syndrome. Note the "buffalo" type obesity, the muscular weakness and striae.

Fig. 24.2. The patient shown in Fig. 1, six months after removal of the whole of one adrenal and 90 per cent. of the other.

90 per cent. removal should be undertaken and 2 or 3 weeks later a total adrenalectomy performed on the other side. The decision as to whether an adrenal is normal, hypertrophic or atrophic is important and experience counts. Patients with an overacting adrenal tumour, particularly in Cushing's syndrome, usually have an atrophic gland

on the other side, but most patients with Cushing's syndrome have hyperplastic glands and here a 90 per cent. adrenalectomy on the first side and a total adrenalectomy on the second is the correct treatment. Fig. 2 shows the patient seen in Fig. 1, six months after such an operation.

In Cushing's syndrome the post-operative care requires greater skill and clinical experience than the actual operation, the great thing being the management and, if possible, the prevention of post-operative adrenal insufficiency. This, curiously, is much more marked after the removal of a tumour than after the excision of all of one gland and 90 per cent. of the other. Cortisone 100 mgm. should be given on the day of the second operation and then 50 mgm. daily for three days, if the glands were hyperplastic; if the patient had a tumour cortisone in small doses, 5 to 10 mgm., may be needed for several weeks. In the immediate post-operative period the patient may become hypotensive and then an intravenous infusion containing 2 ml. of nor-adrenaline per litre administered at a rate of about 20 drops per minute will maintain the blood pressure at a satisfactory level. The diet should be low in potassium and high in both sodium chloride and sodium citrate.

Even with a regime of this type the syndrome of acute adrenal insufficiency may develop, often with great suddenness during the first 2 to 4 weeks after operation. The early symptoms and signs include: nausea, and vomiting, hiccough, loss of appetite, weakness, apathy, insomnia, a rising pulse rate and falling blood pressure. If these occur the patient should be given more cortisone and an intravenous infusion of isotonic saline started. It is important to realize that cortisone by intramuscular injection takes 18 or more hours to become effective; it is therefore useless in an acute crisis, and in these circumstances Eucortone 10 to 20 ml. intravenously should be given and repeated as necessary.

Phæochromocytoma (Chromaffinoma or Paraganglioma)

This rare tumour usually arises in the medulla of the adrenal gland but may occur elsewhere in the sympathetic nervous system. It is usually single but tumours may be bilateral or even multiple.

The classical clinical picture is of paroxysms of hypertension associated with the following symptoms which disappear when the blood pressure returns to normal: Headache which is of the hypertensive type and throbs with the heart beat; palpitations; dizziness and blurring of vision; pain in the chest and upper abdomen which may resemble angina pectoris; sweating; pyrexia up to 105° F. during an attack and sometimes present minimally between attacks; nausea and vomiting; tachycardia and peripheral vasoconstriction with pallor, numbness, tingling and cramp-like pains.

The paroxysms at first last for a few hours or less but in the classical case gradually get more infrequent and last for longer until they cease and the hypertension becomes permanent. Unfortunately many patients present an atypical picture; in some the paroxysms may be absent and the condition resembles essential hypertension; in others there may be no symptoms due to the excessive production of nor-adrenaline until an unsuspecting surgeon operates for a supposedly non-functioning adrenal tumour. I once diagnosed a phæochromo-cytoma as a carcinoma of the kidney and removed it; the pathologist told his class of students that it was a carcinoma of the kidney and both of us got a surprise when the microscopical report showed that it was a phæochromocytoma.

When one suspects that a patient may have a phæochromocytoma various tests may help to confirm the diagnosis. Repeated plain X-ray films at various depths nearly always show the outline of the tumour, and this is probably the best way of locating it. An intravenous pyelogram and the peri-renal insufflation of air help in some patients.

Benzodioxane and Dibenamine are said to lower the blood pressure in patients with a phæochromocytoma and to leave it unchanged in patients with hypertension due to other causes. This diagnostic test is not reliable and too many false positives or negatives occur. Regitin does apparently lower the blood pressure in patients with a phæochro-mocytoma and not in patients with essential hypertension; it may well prove to be a reliable test.

Probably the most reliable diagnostic test is the estimation of the amount of adrenaline and nor-adrenaline in the patient's urine. The normal is about 70 micrograms per day; in patients with a phæochromo-cytoma the level varies between 400 and 4,000 micrograms per day even when the urine has been collected between attacks.

The treatment of a phæochromocytoma is surgical. The main difficulty is to locate the tumour. If it is not in either adrenal it is usually near the abdominal aorta but it may be in the thorax. If there are no localizing signs it is best to explore the abdomen through a paramedian incision. Once located the tumour should be removed; an early step in the operation should be division of the adrenal vein because manipulation of the tumour before this step may precipitate an attack of hypertension. After removal the blood pressure falls; this should be watched carefully and controlled as already described with an intravenous infusion of nor-adrenaline. Few surgical operations give such satisfactory results as the removal of a phæochromocytoma because a really sick patient is returned to normal.

The Adreno-Genital Syndrome

This occurs in women at or just after puberty. The clinical features include amenorrhœa, masculine hirsuity, male build, a deep voice, an enlarged clitoris, failure of the breasts to develop and usually an increased level of 17-keterosteroid excretion.

The treatment is unsatisfactory. Unilateral adrenalectomy has been tried on a number of occasions; menstruation usually starts but the other symptoms remain unaltered. It is possible that subtotal removal of the remaining gland might bring about further improvement but this is unproven.

Carcinoma of the Prostate and Breast

In patients who have advanced carcinoma of the prostate bilateral total adrenalectomy offers a chance of further survival but not of cure. After the response to œstrogen therapy and castration has begun to wane a further period of palliation often lasting for 12 months or more can be achieved by this operation. It is of course essential to provide replacement therapy for the lost adrenals, and to-day this is most conveniently done with cortisone; if deoxycortone acetate is given as well the amount of cortisone can be reduced. In advanced carcinoma of the breast the results of adrenalectomy are less satisfactory but nevertheless a few patients may be improved.

Addison's Disease

A few cases have been reported of successful adrenal homografts in these patients, but the success rate is extremely low indeed and much work has to be done before this method of treatment can be of routine value.

Hypertension

The treatment of malignant hypertension by bilateral adrenalectomy may prove to be of value in selected patients. Substitution therapy with cortisone and deoxycortone acetate is essential.

C. G. ROB

Reference
WALTERS, W. (1952) *Lancet* i, 221.

CHAPTER XXV

SURGERY OF THE RESPIRATORY SYSTEM

Carcinoma of the Bronchus

WITHIN the last few years Bradford Hill and Doll (1950) have carried out an extensive research into the relation of smoking to carcinoma of the bronchus. There appears to be little doubt that heavy (over 20 per day) cigarette consumption predisposes to the disease, and that the very real rise in the incidence of carcinoma of the bronchus which is now only second in frequency to gastric carcinoma may be directly related to the increase in cigarette smoking. This finding may well account for the striking change in the sex incidence of the condition recently, for as short a time as ten years ago the male to female ratio was 20-1, but it has now fallen to 7-1. It seems likely that this change may be due in part to the increasing consumption of tobacco by women.

With the advent of mass radiography and the more general awareness of the commonness of carcinoma of the bronchus, early diagnosis is becoming more frequent and the results of treatment have improved. Two uncommon modes of presentation or concomitant features should be mentioned. The first is the development of osteo-arthropathy manifested either as finger clubbing or as joint pains, these may be the first symptoms of carcinoma of the bronchus and are more often associated with the peripheral type of tumour than with the common main bronchus lesion. Both the clubbing and the joint pains disappear rapidly after the tumour has been removed. Secondly, carcinoma of the bronchus may be associated with peripheral neuritis, and this again may be the first symptom of the disease, although it is a rare phenomenon.

Treatment

Radiotherapy. The results of resection are superior to those from any other form of treatment such as radiotherapy or the use of nitrogen mustard. A combination of resection and radiotherapy may prove to be better than either alone, but as yet patients treated in this way have not been followed up long enough for definite conclusions to be drawn.

Two techniques are in use, *pre-operative radiotherapy* which may lessen the risk of dissemination of the tumour at operation and may possibly render patients operable who previously were not, and secondly *post-operative treatment*, planned to reach the lymphatic fields in the mediastinum after the lung has been removed. The latter carries the risk that the inevitable irradiation changes in the remaining lung may lead to respiratory deficiency and death, but nevertheless may prove to be the preferable of the two techniques.

Radiotherapy is also of considerable value in alleviating the symptoms such as cough, hæmoptysis, and caval obstruction, and often the shrinkage of the tumour allows freer drainage of pus dammed up behind it. Palliative doses should, therefore, be given to the majority of patients where the tumour proves inoperable at thoracotomy, and in those who have symptoms and are found inoperable for other reasons.

Resection. It being agreed that resection is the ideal treatment, the presence or even the suspicion of a carcinoma is an indication for thoracotomy. As it has been shown that the prognosis is better in patients who have had a resection even when local metastases were known to be present (Oschner and DeBakey, 1948), than in those where no resection was undertaken, the lung should be removed wherever possible. Not only will survival be longer, but also the side effects due to the suppuration behind the growth, the osteo-arthropathy and so on, will be alleviated.

The only certain way to ascertain whether or not a lung is removable is to perform a thoracotomy. The radiologically obvious invasion of mediastinal lymph glands makes inoperability likely but the following are contra-indications to thoracotomy:

Contra-indications to Thoracotomy:

1. *General*
    (*a*) General metastases.
    (*b*) Respiratory insufficiency.
    (*c*) Other general diseases.
2. *Local*
    (*a*) *Nerve Invasion*
        (*a*) Hoarseness (left recurrent nerve invasion).
        (*b*) Diaphragmatic paralysis (phrenic nerve invasion).
        (*c*) Horner's syndrome (sympathetic nerve invasion).
    (*b*) *Visceral Spread*
        (1) Invasion of the œsophagus.
        (2)   ,,   ,,   heart.
        (3)   ,,   ,,   superior vena cava.
        (4)   ,,   ,,   pleura.
    (*c*) *Invasion of trachea or opposite bronchus.*

1. General metastases obviously preclude operation. There is still not a satisfactory method of assessment of respiratory function and the presence of a carcinoma may be a cause of dyspnœa, but a history of

dyspnœa on exercise and of chronic bronchitis, particularly when associated with expiratory spasm and emphysema, make pneumonectomy hazardous. A maximum breathing capacity below 40-50 should also contra-indicate resection.

Senility is probably the "general disease" which presents the chief problem in these cases, but advanced years alone are no contra-indication to surgery. Resection has occasionally been undertaken in patients over 80 and frequently in those in their 70's.

2. The contra-indications mentioned under this heading all suggest that the disease is well advanced and that the lung is almost certainly irremovable.

Displacement of the œsophagus by glands does not contra-indicate thoracotomy, but invasion seen either during a barium swallow or at œsophagoscopy does.

The recent onset of cardiac irregularity, in the absence of any other cause and in the presence of a carcinoma of the bronchus strongly suggests invasion of the left auricle. Superior caval obstruction is not uncommon, it is usually due to glandular pressure and precludes surgery. A blood stained pleural effusion is almost certain evidence of multiple pleural secondaries, but a simple effusion does not contra-indicate thoracotomy.

Finally, although operations for tracheal reconstruction have been undertaken the invasion of the trachea should, except in very special circumstances, preclude thoracotomy.

The invasion of the ribs and the presence of an oat cell carcinoma are taken by some surgeons to indicate inoperability, but the pain caused by rib erosions may in itself justify surgery, and although the oat cell carcinoma carries the worst prognosis (Carlisle *et al.*, 1951) long periods of survival have been recorded after removal of this type of tumour.

Pneumonectomy. The operation most frequently carried out in the treatment of bronchial carcinoma is pneumonectomy. This has a mortality in the order of 15 per cent. Recently efforts have been made to excise a wider lymphatic field at the time of resection, this has been termed *Radical Pneumonectomy*. The pericardium is opened and widely excised, and as many as possible of the regional glands, including the paratracheal nodes, are removed. On theoretical grounds, even admitting the greater likelihood of complications, this operation should give a higher survival rate than less extensive resections.

Aylwin (1951) realized the risk of the spread of tumour due to manipulation at the time of operation. He therefore decided to tie the pulmonary veins as the first step in the dissection and so to lessen the risk of tumour embolism. This modification has already shown some improvement in the late results.

Lobectomy. There is no doubt that this operation has a place in the treatment of carcinoma of the bronchus, the mortality is very much lower (2 per cent.) and it is often possible particularly in upper lobe resection to remove a high proportion of regional glands without removing the lung.

Possibly this operation should be confined to the treatment of peripheral tumours (which constitute 12 per cent. of the total) and of those patients whose respiratory reserve is low, but even when it has been employed as the operation of choice for all bronchial carcinomata (where feasible) the late results have been almost as good as those of pneumonectomy.

Results. Two major factors influence the late results, the histology of the tumour and the presence or absence of glandular metastases.

Of patients subjected to thoracotomy most series report an operability rate between 60 and 70 per cent. The expectation of life of patients found to be inoperable is very short (four to six months) whereas in those where resection has been possible the survival rate has been improving considerably in recent years and the diagram shows the percentage of patients alive at various periods after resection for carcinoma.

Where hilar glands have been found to be in-

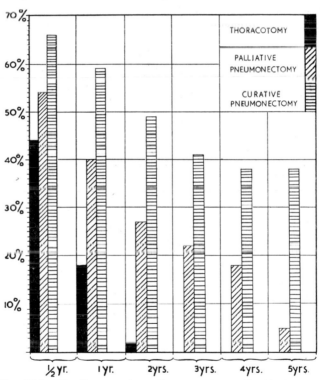

Fig. 25.1. The diagram shows the percentages of patients surviving various periods after operation. Palliative pneumonectomy implies the presence of glandular metastases at operation. In "curative" cases no such lesions were found. (Based on A. J. Moon's figures from the London Chest Hospital.)

volved at operation the two-year survival rate has been in the order of 25 per cent. Where these glands have been free from metastases it has been much better (48 per cent.).

The best prognosis of all is carried by patients with squamous cell tumours. These represent 66 per cent. of the total carcinomas of bronchus. Oat cell tumours (19 per cent. of carcinomas) are the most lethal and the rarer adeno-carcinomas (5 per cent. of total tumours) are intermediate. A five-year survival rate of 51 per cent. has been reported in patients with squamous carcinomata without glandular metastases.

Pulmonary Tuberculosis

Influence of Chemotherapeutic Agents

The introduction of streptomycin and the other chemotherapeutic agents which have been developed since, has profoundly affected the selection of patients for surgical treatment. Although at one end of the scale those patients who might have needed surgery have had their disease arrested by these drugs, at the other end, patients who would previously have been regarded as hopeless have been rendered suitable for operation. As resection in the treatment of pulmonary tuberculosis was introduced at about the same time as chemotherapy for the disease, it is impossible to estimate the value of the drugs in enabling this procedure to be carried out with so low a risk of infection, but their influence must be considerable.

Resection for Pulmonary Tuberculosis

There is not general agreement on all the indications for resection, for the late (5-10 years) results of the operation are not yet available and comparisons with the known results of thoracoplasty are not always valid. However, the number of resections being carried out is rapidly increasing and the mortality and early results are very similar to those of thoracoplasty. Where the disease has been sufficiently extensive to have led to involvement of the bronchus at the site of section in the tuberculous process, the rate of development of bronchopleural fistulæ after resection has been high (8 per cent.). As this complication causes a great deal of morbidity and often calls for thoracoplasty in its treatment, many surgeons still prefer to reserve resection to patients who fall into the categories listed below. The large discrepancies which exist in the complication rate in published series occur because the rate of tuberculous infection at the site of bronchus section also varies within wide limits (15 to 60 per cent.) according to the type of case which has been subjected to the operation.

Indications. With these provisos, the following list gives the chief indications for resection in pulmonary tuberculosis:

1. *Pneumonectomy:*
   (a) Destroyed lung.
   (b) Bronchostenosis.
   (c) Pyopneuomothorax.
   (d) Disease in which cavities are so placed that thoracoplasty would be ineffective and lobectomy inadequate.
   (e) Failed thoracoplasty.
2. *Lobectomy:*
   (a) Lower lobe cavities.
   (b) Tuberculous bronchiectasis.
   (c) Solid tuberculous foci unsuitable for segmental resection.
   (d) Ruptured or leaking cavities.
3. *Segmental Resection:*
   (a) Tuberculoma and tuberculous cold abscess of bronchus.
   (b) Some isolated cavities.

Pneumonectomy

The mortality of this operation is high (20 per cent.) as the majority of the patients have advanced disease, and tuberculous endobronchitis is common (no resection should be carried out where the process is active). The development of a bronchopleural fistula complicated as it must be by a total empyema is almost invariably fatal. If, however, the resection is uncomplicated the end results are excellent.

Pleuropneumonectomy has been advocated in every case (Sarot, 1949). It appears to be unnecessary except in patients where a pyopneumothorax is present prior to operation, as post-operative empyemata are very rare unless a bronchopleural fistula develops.

Thoracolysis four weeks after, or at the same time as the pneumonectomy, is widely practised. The operation usually consists of the removal of decreasing lengths of the ribs above that removed to enter the chest and excluding the first rib, i.e. the second, third, fourth and fifth ribs are removed. This procedure has two purposes: by centralizing the mediastinum, over distension of the opposite lung with the theoretical risk of reactivation pre-existing disease, is prevented, and secondly the size of the empyema which may develop is reduced, as also possibly is the actual risk of fistula formation.

Lobectomy

This operation carries a much lower mortality (3 per cent.) as it is often an operation of election and is often unassociated with endobronchitis at the site of bronchus section, also if a fistula and an empyema develop in these patients they are seldom fatal.

After this operation the risk of over-distension of the remaining lobe also exists. Where a lower lobectomy has been carried out a phrenic crush and a pneumoperitoneum enable this residual space to be obliterated, where an upper lobe has been removed a *thoracolysis*, that is removal of lengths of three or four ribs, may be undertaken either at the same time as the lobectomy or four weeks later. Whether these procedures are in fact necessary is debatable.

Segmental Resection

Tuberculosis may start as a segmental lesion, but soon transgresses the intersegmental planes, hence the scope of this operation is limited. However, for solid lesions it is often possible and is ideal. Where segmental resection is undertaken for cavitating disease, the risk of development of pleuropulmonary fistulæ is considerable unless great care is taken to close any possible sources of leakage in the remainder of the lobe after the segment has been removed. The mortality of this operation is low.

Collapse Operation for Pulmonary Tuberculosis

Thoracoplasty

Since the introduction of the principle of apicolysis in thoracoplasty by Semb (1936), and its development by Price Thomas (1942), the results have been excellent both in early sputum conversion and in the absence of late breakdown of the disease. The mortality of the operation necessarily depends on the type of patient under treatment, but 3 per cent. probably represents the overall figure. The sputum conversion rate which approaches 90 per cent, sets a high standard which other collapse operations must achieve before thoracoplasty is superseded.

At present it may be said that seven rib thoracoplasty remains the standard "collapse" operation for pulmonary tuberculosis. Its disadvantages are two-fold; it has to be done in two, three or even four stages and secondly, although with adequate physiotherapy the deformity caused may be negligible, it remains a mutilating procedure.

Extrapleural Pneumothorax and Lucite Plombage

In these operations all, or nearly all the ribs are left *in situ*, the apex of the lung is "stripped" from inside the bony cage and off the mediastinum down to the hilum, the remaining space is then dealt with in a variety of ways.

The filling of this extrapleural space with air had a vogue in Britain for some time and is in widespread use on the Continent, but the complication rate was high, due to hæmorrhage and infection, and the late results were uncertain. These factors more than outweighed the doubtful advantage of the possibility of abandoning the extrapleural pneumothorax when the disease was judged to be arrested. For these reasons modifications have been sought to lessen the risk of hæmorrhage and infection and maintain collapse permanently. The most successful of these has employed the principle of lucite plombage.

In this operation an apicolysis is carried out, the intercostal bundles are detached from the ribs and fall in with the lung. The space remaining is filled with inert material (lucite) in the form of balls or packs.

This procedure lessens the risk of infection as the necessity for "refills" is avoided, and the musculoperiosteal layer over the apex decreases the area of potential tuberculous contamination of the extra-pleural space. The results of this operation *qua* sputum conversion approach those of thoracoplasty, but late tuberculous infection of the space does occur in a proportion of these cases.

Tuberculous Empyema and Decortication

The incidence of tuberculous empyema and pyopneumothorax has fallen sharply within recent years; since chemotherapy has been intro-duced and since artificial pneumothorax therapy has been used with greater discretion.

Eighty per cent. of the tuberculous empyemas complicate pneumo-thorax therapy and the prognosis in untreated cases is bad, but when the complication is adequately dealt with it should not unduly influence the outlook of the patient.

There are two essentials for success in the treatment of tuberculous empyemas. (1) The pleural cavity must be obliterated, (2) the under-lying pulmonary lesion must be controlled. The complication is invari-ably due to communication of a pulmonary lesion with the pleura. The onset may be acute, when a cavity ruptures into the pleura, or insidious, when a small pulmonary lesion breaks through the visceral pleura.

Three factors have recently altered the treatment of this condition—*chemotherapy* which has already been mentioned, the introduction of *resection* and, thirdly, the conception of *decortication*.

Obliteration of the Pleural Space

Where no bronchopleural communication is present, and uncom-monly where there is one, it is often possible to obliterate the space by *aspiration* even where the empyema is long standing. The aspirations have to be frequent and thorough, and should be combined with local and parenteral chemotherapy.

In other cases the lung, which is prevented from expanding by the thick walls of the empyema, may be enabled to expand by *decortication*. This operation consists in the removal of the parietal pleura as well as the visceral layer. The empyema may be removed intact or it may be opened and stripped from the lung and chest wall in turn. In either event if the underlying lung is healthy it will expand rapidly and obliterate the pleural cavity.

Treatment of Underlying Disease

Where the empyema space has been dealt with by the methods already referred to, the treatment of the remaining pulmonary disease differs little from that in cases where no empyema has been present; however, where collapse therapy or resection are indicated the first stage of the thoracoplasty or the resection may be carried out at the same time as decortication.

The major difference in patients with tuberculous empyemas occurs in those with persistent pleuropulmonary fistulæ. In these cases resection is essential and removal of both infected visceral and parietal pleura is ideal. Where the underlying lung is diseased throughout, *pleuropneumonectomy* is performed. Where only one lobe is involved, lobectomy combined with decortication of the residual lobe is indicated.

Where there is no fistula, thoracoplasty may be the operation of choice, but its extent should be considerably diminished if aspiration or decortication have enabled the healthy lower lobe to expand.

Schematic Representation of Treatment of Tuberculous Empyema

	Tuberculous Empyema No Fistula	*Tuberculous Pyopneuomothorax Persistent Fistula*
Upper Lobe Disease	Aspiration or Decortication and Seven rib thoracoplasty	Lower lobe decortication and upper lobectomy.
Lower Lobe Disease	Upper lobe decortication and lobectomy.	Upper lobe decortication and lower lobectomy.
Destroyed Lung	Pneumonectomy or total thoracoplasty.	Pleuropneumonectomy.

Surgery of Trachea and Bronchi

The lesions of trachea and main bronchi which may be suitable for operation are seldom encountered, for the changes which are caused in the lung beyond the damaged bronchi usually dominate the clinical picture. However, the following conditions have been successfully dealt with:

(1) Adenoma of the trachea and bronchus.
(2) Carcinoma of the trachea.
(3) Fracture and accidental division of the bronchi.
(4) Stricture of the bronchus.
(5) Tracheal and bronchial deficiencies following pulmonary resection.

End to End Anastomosis

This has been successfully carried out after complete, or almost complete division of a bronchus either in the treatment of a fracture of the cartilage, of adenoma of the bronchus where the intrabronchial tumour or its extrabronchial extension have been removed, or of accidental bronchial division during lobectomy. In each case primary healing took place with almost no stricture formation.

Simple suture of the trachea has also been successfully performed after the removal of a small wedge of its circumference which contained a benign tumour.

The Use of Autografts

Where a greater deficiency has been made than could be dealt with adequately by simple suture, it has been necessary to bridge the gap either with some form of prothesis or with an autograft.

The materials used had to have the properties of elasticity and of rigidity; a graft was first successfully used by Belsey (1946, 1950) who used wire and fascia lata to bridge a gap in an excised trachea. This was repeated later by Rob and Bateman (1949) in the treatment of deficiencies of the upper trachea and oesophagus.

More recently Gebauer (1950, 1951) has perfected a technique of autografting which is more flexible and has, in consequence, a wider application. He uses skin from the back stripped of fat and epithelium, and strengthened by steel wire threaded through it.

This technique enabled him to treat strictures of the bronchi and trachea successfully, the strictures being opened and the graft being inserted between the cut edges. This method also can be applied where large tracheal or bronchial deficiencies have to be bridged following resection.

The Use of a Prosthesis

This method has recently been employed with success by Cotton after the excision of a carcinoma of the trachea, when a stainless steel tube was used. The technique has the objection, however, that it is very liable to cause strictures.

Acute Empyema

With the advent of chemotherapy and its early use in the treatment of pneumonia, acute empyema has become less common. Once the condition has advanced to the stage where thick pus is present, its treatment is as it always has been, that is, adequate dependent drainage after rib resection and debridement of the cavity. Alternatively, decortication may be undertaken; that is excision of the walls of the empyema allowing early expansion of the lung and obliteration of the pleural space.

In the early acute stage of an empyema, however, it may be possible to avoid operation if vigorous conservative treatment is applied. This consists of *daily complete aspiration* of the empyema with the use of local and parenteral penicillin and regular breathing exercises. This regimen may be supplemented by the injection of *Streptokinase-Streptodornase* into the empyema space, this has the effect of dissolving the fibrinous exudate and so allowing the essential complete aspiration to be achieved 24 hours later. By these means surgical drainage can often be avoided.

Lung Abscess

The whole picture of lung abscess has altered in recent years, not only has the condition become less common, due in part to improvements in anæsthesia and chemotherapy, but also it appears to be less malign when it does develop, and drainage operations are now rarities in the chest hospitals.

Apart from the unusual examples of lung abscess due to infection with Staphlococci or Friedlander bacilli, lung abscess is almost always due to bronchial embolism. The factor which led to the necessity for external drainage was the development of large sloughs in the putrid lung abscess, these could not be expectorated and effectively prevented adequate bronchial drainage. With the advent of chemotherapy this problem no longer appears to exist.

Treatment

By conservative treatment a high proportion of lung abscesses are now enabled to heal. Sutherland and Grant (1950) showed that if the two principles of high dosage chemotherapy (2 million units of penicillin daily) and postural drainage were insisted on, over 75 per cent. of acute lung abscesses could be cured without surgery.

Where chemotherapy fails, extensive irreversible damage is almost invariably present in the lobe involved, resection becomes the treatment of choice.

There remain cases of the hyperacute type where early drainage may be a life saving measure, but these are few and far between.

Thymectomy and Myasthenia Gravis

The exact relation of the thymus gland to myasthenia gravis is still not clear, but the operation of thymectomy is well established in the treatment of the disease, Blalock (1941) and Keynes (1946, 1946a) having both done large series. This operation is also performed in the treatment of thymic tumours. When malignant these may be or may not be associated with myasthenia, but benign tumours are more often associated with the disease.

The results of thymectomy have two aspects, first, in the improvement of the myasthenia and, second and quite separately, the reduction in the prostigmine dosage. The majority have their symptoms improved by the operation, but quite a high proportion have to continue with their prostigmine although they are considerably improved subjectively.

J. R. BELCHER

References

AYLWIN, J. A. (1951) *Thorax* **4**, 173.
BELSEY, R. (1946) *Thorax* **1**, 39.
BELSEY, R. (1950) *Brit. J. Surg.* **38**, 200.
BLALOCK, A. (1941) *Amer. J. Surg.* **54**, 149.
BROCK, R. C. (1951) "Lung Abscesses." Oxford, Blackwell Scientific Publications.
CARLISLE, J. C. *et al.* (1951) *J. Thorac. Surg.* **22**, 74.
COTTON, B. H. *et al.* (1952) *J. Thorac. Surg.* **24**, 231.
DOLL, R., and HILL, A. B. (1950) *Brit. med. J.* ii, 739.
GEBAUER, P. W. (1950) *J. Thorac. Surg.* **19**, 604.
GEBAUER, P. W. (1951) *J. Thorac. Surg.* **22**, 568.
KEYNES, G. (1946) *Brit. J. Surg.* **33**, 201.
KEYNES, G. (1946a) *Proc. R. Soc. Med.* **39**, 600.
OSCHNER, A. *et al.* (1948) *J. Thorac. Surg.* **17**, 573.
PRICE THOMAS, C. (1942) *Brit. J. Tuberc.* **36**, 109.
REID, H. (1949) *Brit. J. Surg.* **36**, 271.
ROB, C. G., and BATEMAN, G. H. (1949) *Brit. J. Surg.* **36**, 202.
SAROT, I. A. (1949) *Thorax* **4**, 173.
SEMB, C. (1936) *Acta. chir. Scand.* **76**, 1.
SUTHERLAND, A. W., and GRANT, L. J. (1950) *Lancet* i, 350.

CHAPTER XXVI

PROGRESS IN CARDIAC SURGERY

UNTIL 1939 the only cardiac condition for which surgical treatment was widely used was constrictive pericarditis. Since then a whole new field of surgery has been opened up. The first landmark was in the closure of patent ductus arteriosus (Gross and Hubbard, 1939), then the war came and great developments were made in the treatment of cardiac wounds. In 1945 Blalock and Taussig showed that certain forms of cyanotic congenital heart disease could be improved by surgery. But perhaps the most important step of all was the relief of mitral stenosis by direct operation on the valve. The importance of this operation lies in the fact that in England alone there are several thousand mitral stenotics who would benefit from the operation, in contrast to the few hundred cases of congenital cardiac abnormalities suitable for surgery.

The conditions which can now be considered for surgical treatment are:

Congenital Abnormalities
1. Patent Ductus Arteriosus.
2. Certain cases of Cyanotic Heart Disease.
3. Acyanotic Pulmonary Stenosis.
4. Coarctation of the Aorta.

Acquired Conditions
5. Constrictive Pericarditis.
6. Mitral Stenosis.
7. Cardiac Wounds.

To these might be added a number of conditions in which surgery has been attempted occasionally with success, but the operations devised can hardly be considered to be past the experimental stage. These will not be considered here. They include:

Mitral incompetence.

Transposition of the aorta and pulmonary artery.

Aortic Stenosis.

Coronary Insufficiency, and other conditions.

The surgery of the heart is likely to make important new advances once a technique is developed by which the circulation by-passes the heart, which can then be operated on in a dry state. An extra-corporeal pump, which will maintain the body circulation has been used in animal experiments, but its use is fraught with difficulties, so far only partly overcome. The great vessels near the heart must be canalized to deflect the blood to the artificial heart in such a way that they can be immediately and completely repaired. The maintenance of the coronary circulation throughout the operation presents another problem. The aortic orifices of the coronary arteries must be unimpeded by the aortic canalizing technique. Since the large blood flow through these vessels returns directly to the heart, mostly by the coronary sinus, either this vessel, too, must be canalized or an equivalent volume of blood to that lost by this route must be constantly added to the circulation. The blood must be heparinized to prevent clotting in the extra-corporeal pump, with the inevitable consequence that hæmostasis becomes difficult to secure. Yet another difficulty is to exclude air bubbles from the circulation especially when the empty heart is finally connected up.

Theoretically it is possible to by-pass either the right side of the heart or the left or indeed both may be put temporarily out of use if an artificial lung preparation is connected with the artificial heart. This adds further technical difficulties, but creates the best conditions for operation and is essential if the operation is for the repair of a septal defect in the heart.

Another experimental technique which seems to offer real possibilities and may prove very valuable in cardiac surgery is that of cooling the patient's body temperature to a level at which the basal metabolic rate is so low that the heart only beats very slowly. At suitable temperatures animals are found to go into a condition similar to hibernation, which allows fairly extensive operations to be performed on the heart without the use of an extra-corporeal pump. In some centres the technique is being tried on human beings.

Patent Ductus Arteriosus

Normally the embryonic ductus between the aorta and the pulmonary artery becomes obliterated in the first few days after birth, but occasionally this closure does not take place. When unassociated with other congenital abnormalities it represents about 10 per cent. of all cases of congenital abnormalities of the heart. The physical signs in babyhood are equivocal; it is not until the age of 3 or 4 that the classical machine-like murmur, extending through the whole cardiac cycle, becomes audible in the pulmonary area. The X-ray appearances may help to substantiate the diagnosis (see Fig. 1). Uncomplicated patent ductus may cause no disability.

If the ductus is large and allows a considerable portion (sometimes over half) of the blood flow from the left ventricle to pass into the pulmonary circulation, pulmonary hypertension will be present and the right ventricle will hypertrophy. Such degrees of shunt are not uncommon and cause breathlessness on exertion, palpitations and sometimes retardation of growth. The expectation of life in patients with patent ducti is, as would be anticipated, less than in the normal. It is not, however, right sided heart failure which is their greatest danger, but the occurrence of infective bacterial endocarditis. A third of the cases of patent ductus coming to post mortem before the days of modern antibiotics and surgery died as a result of endocarditis.

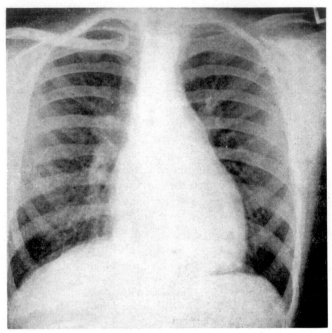

FIG. **26**.1.   Patent Ductus Arteriosus.   The heart shape is characteristic with the filling of the "pulmonary bay" on the left side.

Gross and Hubbard (1939) showed that the relatively simple operation of ligature of the duct not only corrected the disadvantage at which the heart was working, but removed the risk of bacterial endocarditis supervening. Since on rare occasions the ductus appears to recanalize, they later recommended division of the ductus with suture of the pulmonary and aortic ends, but this is a much more hazardous procedure in most surgeons' hands and is not widely practised.

Tubbs (1940) was the first to tie a patent ductus successfully in the presence of infective endocarditis. Once endocarditis has developed the operation carries a very much greater risk than in the uninfected case when the operative mortality should be well below 5 per cent. However, the infected case should be treated with antibiotics in an attempt to control the process and then operated on. Once the ductus is closed the endocarditis is unlikely to persist.

The safest time to operate in uninfected cases is between the ages of 5 and 12. There is rarely an indication for surgery before five as the condition is usually symptomless and bacterial endocarditis extremely rare before this age. Patients much over 20 without disability or infection must be considered individually. The operative risk is rather greater and the chances of developing infective endocarditis less, but it is worth operating in some cases.

The ductus can be approached across the left pleural space by either an anterior or postero-lateral approach; the latter gives the better access. The ductus is friable, especially in adults when there may be atheroma of the adjacent aorta. The recurrent laryngeal nerve must be isolated and gently retracted before dissecting round the ductus. There is often a fold of pericardium overlapping the ductus which can be retracted downwards. If any difficulty is experienced in identifying the limits of the ductus, the pericardium should be opened to facilitate the exposure. A fine suture material is not recommended as it may cut through the ductus; floss silk is suitable. It is preferable to apply several ligatures in order to separate the aorta from the pulmonary artery in the hope of preventing recanalization. It is essential that the ligatures be tied tightly.

It must not be forgotten that patent ductus is sometimes associated with cardiac abnormalities and in some of these cases its patency is essential to life. If there is any question of such related abnormalities it is wise to open the pericardium and inspect the heart before proceeding to ligate the ductus.

Congenital Cyanotic Heart Disease

Only some of the many types of congenital cyanotic heart disease are amenable to surgery. In recent years several careful studies of these cases have been made, and it can be said that in the majority a fairly accurate diagnosis can now be made on clinical grounds. It must be emphasized that an accurate diagnosis is essential not only in order to select the patients suitable for surgery, but also to determine which of the several operative procedures is most suitable for the individual case.

Angiocardiography and cardiac catheterization go a long way to supply more accurate information than can be obtained on clinical grounds alone; but as neither of these procedures are devoid of risk, they should not be used routinely.

Angiocardiography presents such technical difficulties from the radiographic point of view that its usefulness is limited. Serial X-rays taken at intervals of 1 second after intravenous injection of an adequate quantity of radio-opaque dye will show each individual chamber of the heart, and whether there is a right to left shunt. Interpretation is difficult owing to the fact that there is no single view which will show the heart chambers without overlapping.

Cardiac catheterization is at present a more widely practised procedure. A catheter introduced into a large vein and pushed up to the heart will show the pressure changes in the chambers of the right side of the heart, the pulmonary artery and the pulmonary capillaries. (When the catheter is jammed into a small pulmonary arteriole the pressure which is read there can be shown to be closely related to that in the pulmonary capillaries.) Blood can be withdrawn from various sites at which the tip of the catheter lies; estimation of its oxygen content may reveal a mixture with arterial blood indicating a left to right shunt. While this procedure is being carried out the position of the catheter is determined by X-ray screening.

If an exact diagnosis is not reached before operation, it is sometimes wiser to omit these procedures and open the pericardium to inspect the heart. The experienced cardiac surgeon will gain much information in this way and can introduce needles into the various chambers of the heart and read the pressures within them. It must be admitted, however, that even after all these methods have been employed mistakes can be made.

It will be appreciated that the surgeon undertaking such surgery will require to work with an experienced cardiologist; indeed, there is no other branch of surgery in which a team of workers, each as expert in his aspect of the subject (surgeon, cardiologist, radiologist, anæsthetist, etc.), is more essential. The surgeon cannot become as expert in diagnosis as the cardiologist, who will also see the patients not suitable for surgery. For this reason the clinical picture of only the commonest group of these patients will be described. This is Fallot's tetralogy and represents about 20 per cent. of all the patients with congenital heart disease.

The tetralogy consists of pulmonary stenosis, patent interventricular septum, overriding of the aorta, and enlargement of the right ventricle. By overriding of the aorta is meant dextroposition so that it communicates with both ventricles. The pulmonary stenosis may be at the valve itself or more commonly in the pulmonary outflow tract of the right ventricle, when it is termed subvalvular or infundibular. The pulmonary artery is usually smaller than normal, and in 20-25 per cent. of cases the aorta descends on the right side. When the stenosis is at the valve itself it is always short and strictly confined to the valve ring. The orifice is often very narrow: 2 or 3 mm. in diameter being common. When the stenosis is infundibular it may, however, be quite long. In these cases the wall of the outflow tract is grossly thickened proximally, and beyond it is a dilated chamber with thinner walls (the infundibular chamber). The level of the stricture in the outflow tract is variable and, with it, the size of the infundibular chamber. Owing to the obstruction to the pulmonary outflow, much of the blood from the right ventricle enters the aorta resulting in cyanosis. The cyanosis is augmented by polycythæmia in response to the anoxæmia which results from the poor blood supply to the lungs.

Infants with this condition are usually noticed to be cyanosed at birth, but it becomes increasingly marked and is later associated with clubbing of the fingers. Breathlessness is the predominant symptom. As they grow older they often squat in a characteristic posture; growth is usually stunted and they are mentally backward. The essential feature of poor pulmonary blood flow can be demonstrated with X-rays.

Operative relief of Fallot's tetralogy is achieved by increasing the reduced pulmonary blood flow. It can be done by indirect methods or by dilating the narrowed pulmonary outflow tract. In the indirect operations a systemic artery is anastomosed to a pulmonary artery. Blalock (1945 and 1946) described an operation making an end to side anastomosis between the subclavian and a pulmonary artery. When the pulmonary artery is too small for this but not completely atresic, he does an end to end anastomosis sacrificing thereby a branch of the pulmonary artery. Potts (1946) described a similar operation using the aorta instead of the subclavian artery, doing a side to side anastomosis.

Blalock's Operation. Before planning this procedure one should know on which side the aorta descends. This is not always obvious on straight X-ray but can be determined with the aid of a barium swallow. It is usual to operate on the opposite side to the descending aorta, but the final choice depends on this and three other factors: the age of the patient, whether it has been decided before opening the chest which operation would be most suitable, and the size of the left and right pulmonary arteries. Some indication that one pulmonary artery is atresic can be obtained from straight X-rays and if so this should be confirmed by angiocardiography. The subclavian artery is dissected up to the point at which it gives off its branches. Each of these is ligated, the artery controlled proximally by a simple arterial clamp and then divided as far distally as possible. The blood supply to the arm is adequate via collateral channels. In a very few cases the subclavian artery proves to be too short to allow a satisfactory anastomosis; a more common difficulty is poor development of the pulmonary artery. These difficulties can usually be predicted if an angiocardiogram has been done.

Before incising the pulmonary artery it is necessary to occlude it proximally and distally; a special clamp has been devised for the proximal part of the artery. It is easiest to control the artery distal to the site of anastomosis by slipping ligatures round the divisions and applying gentle traction.

The anastomosis is made with very fine silk. The everting suture should be interrupted at least three times as it is probable that the size of the lumen increases subsequently with the child's growth and this would be limited by continuous stitches. The vessels' walls should not be handled with forceps or they will be damaged and the danger of thrombosis increased. In suitably chosen patients, the pulmonary artery pressure is so much below that in the subclavian that there is a rapid blood flow through the anastomosis which undoubtedly helps to prevent its occlusion by thrombosis.

These children stand blood transfusion badly; they are at the onset polycythæmic and cannot stand an increase in blood volume. However, should there be considerable blood loss, infusion is essential. Saline and glucose will suffice unless the loss is gross.

Potts' Operation. This is essentially similar in principle, a side to side anastomosis being made between the aorta and adjacent pulmonary artery. The approach must be on the side of the descending aorta. As the aorta cannot be occluded for the length of time necessary to perform the anastomosis, it is essential to use a specially devised clamp which allows some flow along the aorta whilst the area of the anastomosis is shut off. The operation can be used as an alternative to Blalock's and is especially useful when the subclavian artery is too short to allow its use.

Direct Operations on the Pulmonary Valve. Brock (1948) and Sellors (1948) both described operations on the pulmonary valve for relief of stenosis. This operation is indicated not only as an alternative to the indirect operations in cyanotic heart disease, but also in pulmonary stenosis unassociated with cyanosis. This condition will be considered below.

If the direct operation is to be done it is essential to know whether the stenosis is at the site of the valve or below it. When the stenosis is valvular there is nearly always a post-stenotic dilatation of the pulmonary artery. This may be discernible on straight X-ray, but will be more clearly visible on angiocardiograms. It may, however, be confused with the infundibular chamber which may be quite large when the stenosis is subvalvular. When the heart is exposed it is possible to feel the valve from outside, and when the stenosis is valvular the jet of blood coming through it is palpable through the wall of the pulmonary artery.

The heart is usually approached through a left anterior thoracotomy incision. The pericardium is widely opened anterior to the phrenic nerve and the heart inspected. If there is doubt as to the nature of the stenosis, a catheter may be introduced through the right ventricular wall and the pressures recorded as the tip of the catheter is moved up and down the pulmonary outflow tract. It is possible also to insert the little finger into the ventricle and palpation will give some further information, especially regarding the size of the interventricular septal defect and the degree of overriding of the aorta.

If the stenosis is infundibular it is essential to choose a site fairly low down for incision into the right ventricle or one may not be below the stenosis itself. Before incising the ventricular wall a few ml. of procaine 1 per cent. is injected into the heart muscle. Abnormal cardiac beats must be anticipated at this stage, and stimulation of the very sensitive ventricular endothelium cut down to the minimum. The initial incision into the ventricular wall need not enter the heart as less blood is lost if the cutting and dilating instruments are gently insinuated through the remainder of the wall. Bleeding is best controlled by gentle finger pressure.

The first instrument to be introduced is a curved probe with which it is possible to feel the degree of stenosis and localize it accurately. Many instruments have been devised for cutting and stretching valvular stenoses and individuals will choose their own. It is probably wise to commence with a flat cutting instrument to make an initial incision in the valve and subsequently extend it with dilators. Brock has devised dilators with a patent lumen allowing some pulmonary blood flow while they are *in situ*. No harm appears to result from the pulmonary regurgitation which must result from the operation.

The nature of the infundibular stenoses makes them much more difficult to relieve. As a stenosis at this site may be much longer than that at the valve, and as its walls are of a thicker and more fibrous nature it is essential to punch out some tissue. Various techniques for this are in use but none can as yet be considered to be established. There would seem to be a greater danger of the stricture reforming in infundibular stenoses than in the valvular ones, but there is as yet no evidence on this point.

After the intracardiac manipulations have been completed, the ventricular wall is sutured, and the pericardium closed with interrupted sutures placed at least 2 cm. from one another as it is essential to allow any fluid collecting in the pericardium to drain out into the pleura and so avoid cardiac tamponade.

Our knowledge of the prognosis in various types of congenital heart disease is unfortunately limited. In any individual child with the condition it is not possible to forecast accurately the risk of operating and the prognosis with or without operation. It must, however, be on balancing these forecasts that the advisability of operating must be determined. Campbell (1948) finds that 1 in 5 children with cyanotic heart disease reach the age of 12 and only 1 in 10 the age of 24. If the particularly bad risk cases are excluded the operative mortality may be about 10 per cent.

The severely disabled infant requires early operation if it is to survive; but clearly the risk will be greater in the more disabled, and the technical difficulties below the age of 3 or 4 become almost prohibitive. The most suitable age for operation for most cases is between 4 and 10.

In selecting patients for operation, Taussig's dictum that the only cases suitable for operation are those in which the disability is due to too little blood reaching the lungs must always be kept in mind; neither the direct nor the indirect operations restore normal conditions. There will be some cases of Fallot's tetralogy in whom surgery will offer too little to justify its risks.

The choice between the direct and indirect operations is a matter of controversy. The direct operation does not increase the load on the right ventricle as is done by the indirect operations, all of which lead to an increased flow into the aorta to allow for the blood lost to the pulmonary circulation via the artificially created ductus. On these theoretical grounds the direct operation seems preferable and when the stenosis is valvular is the method of choice. Owing to the technical difficulties of the direct relief of subvalvular stenosis it is probable that indirect operations will continue to be done for at least some of these cases. In severe cases the manipulations of the heart itself during the direct operation carry perhaps an added risk, but the operative mortality for the two operations is comparable.

Some immediate improvement in colour follows successful operations but further improvement over the first few post-operative weeks can also be expected. This is dependent both on the post-operative recovery of the heart muscle after it has been subjected to the strain of operation, and also to the correction of the polycythæmia which is greatly reduced and may disappear if a good blood supply to the lungs is achieved.

In at least half the cases that survive operation there is a very marked improvement in exercise tolerance. The child who was previously confined to home and guarded by parents as a precious but almost useless individual will often recover sufficiently to go to school and enter into life in the outside world. The mentally and physically retarded will develop rapidly and be able to lead full lives.

Acyanotic Pulmonary Stenosis

Though pulmonary stenosis is usually associated with other cardiac defects, especially of the interventricular or interatrial walls, it occurs alone in about 10 per cent. of congenital abnormalities of the heart. As there is no defect to allow a right to left shunt there is no cyanosis unless it be due to peripheral vascular failure. In most of these cases the stenosis is valvular. They suffer from breathlessness, have a limited exercise tolerance and their end is usually due to congestive heart failure. The average age of death is about twenty.

The condition is suitable for the direct operation on the valve described above and it should be done in all cases with a gross degree of stenosis unless the condition of the heart makes the risk prohibitive.

Coarctation of the Aorta

This congenital abnormality of the aorta consists of a stricture, most commonly set just beyond the origin of the left subclavian artery. However, it is sometimes found more proximal to this, when it is usually associated with gross abnormalities of the heart. Very rarely it lies more distal along the course of the aorta. It may be associated with aneurysmal dilatation beyond the site of the stricture.

The condition may give rise to early death owing to cardiac failure; but, if the child survives for a few years, the greatest hazard is that of hypertension which is manifest only in the upper part of the body and may lead to death from cardiac failure, a cerebral hæmorrhage or rupture of the aorta. Perhaps a quarter of the patients with coarctation of the aorta suffer no material symptoms from it; indeed, it may never be diagnosed until it is found on the post-mortem table. However, should the condition be associated with hypertension the prognosis is poor, and most patients die between 20 and 40.

The important clinical feature which is so characteristic of the condition is the absence of palpable pulses in the legs associated with hypertension in the upper part of the body. The diagnosis should not be difficult if the condition is thought of; for hypertension, especially in a relatively young person, should lead one to feel for the pulse in the legs.

These patients develop grossly dilated arteries which bypass the stricture and may be visible on the surface of the body; these dilatations in the intercostal arteries may give rise to a characteristic notching of the ribs which may be seen on straight X-rays. Other radiological features are the absence or reduction of the aortic knuckle and changes in the appearance of the heart due to its dilatation or hypertrophy. On the whole the X-ray appearances are not sufficiently characteristic to allow a purely radiological diagnosis to be made. Angiocardiography is also somewhat disappointing. It does show the level of the stricture, but from the surgeon's point of view its length is of even greater importance, and this technique rarely gives valuable evidence on this point.

The condition can be successfully treated by excision of the stenosed portion of aorta and end to end anastomosis. It is only possible if the stricture is of limited length and the aorta above and below is adequately supple. It is a hazardous procedure and, as might be expected, the greatest difficulty lies in the excessive bleeding which is encountered from the anastomotic vessels throughout the operation and in particular from the dilated intercostal arteries coming off the aorta just proximal to the stricture.

In recent years some success has been achieved by inserting homogenous grafts to bridge a gap too great to allow the two ends of the aorta to be brought together.

Operation for this condition must be expected to carry a mortality of 10 to 20 per cent. but the result after a successful operation can be anticipated to be very good in nearly all cases.

Constrictive Pericarditis

The relief of constrictive pericarditis by surgical excision of the pericardium is the oldest of cardiac operations and was first practised over thirty years ago. The basic principles remain those suggested by Delorme in the last century, but modern development in anæsthesia and surgical technique enable the operation to be done with greater safety.

The condition is nearly always the result of tuberculous pericarditis. In some patients the acute phase passes unnoticed, while others are severely ill with pericardial effusion and tamponade. At this stage there is no place for surgery, apart from aspiration of fluid which may be a life saving measure. Thickening of the pericardium develops slowly: only after months or years does it contract sufficiently to interfere with heart action. The mechanical effect which produces symptoms is the interference with diastolic expansion, particularly of the right ventricle.

The clinical picture which results is that of a raised venous pressure giving enlargement of the liver, ascites, pleural effusions and engorged neck veins. The pulse volume is low and the cardiac pulsation as seen on the X-ray screen diminished. Breathlessness is not a marked symptom and, unlike right sided cardiac failure from mitral stenosis, the lungs remain dry. In more than half the cases some calcification in the pericardium can be demonstrated radiologically.

Once the condition has been diagnosed the problem becomes one of when, rather than if, one should operate. There is a tendency to operate earlier than used to be done, but if the tuberculous process is active in the pericardium or indeed elsewhere in the body, the danger of lighting it up is real. If, however, the patient is not improving with rest and aspirations of the pleural and peritoneal back pressure effusions, it may become necessary to operate relatively early.

Operation should be preceded by aspiration of effusions in order to minimize the mechanical disadvantage under which the lungs must work. It has already been emphasized that relief of constriction of the right ventricle is the most important aim of the operation; the left ventricle, too, is better freed, but clearance of the atria and the venæ cavæ is too hazardous and their continued encasement in fibrous tissue does not appear to maintain the symptoms. Both layers of the pericardium must be removed; they are usually fused. As a general rule the more extensive the decortication the more satisfactory the result. The fibrous tissue may actually invade the heart muscle, in which case its removal is time consuming as the utmost care must be taken not to damage the coronary vessels. Occasionally fibrillation is present before operation but this is not a contraindication to surgery. During the dissection abnormalities of rhythm are to be expected.

Some favour approaching across the left pleura, others by a median sternotomy. The latter method allows more satisfactory exposure of the right ventricle and is to be preferred for that reason. A really adequate removal of the pericardium cannot be completed without working round to the posterior surface of the heart, and therefore one or both pleural cavities are likely to be opened in the course of dissection. In the early stages of the operation, when only a small portion of the pericardium has been removed, it is remarkable how the heart may bulge out through the aperture, demonstrating very vividly the restriction of normal diastolic enlargement.

Mitral Stenosis

Mitral stenosis is nearly always the result of rheumatic infection and is the commonest valve lesion resulting from this disease. It has been estimated that a quarter of a million of the population of this country have mitral stenosis. A significant proportion of these patients can be relieved surgically. How to make cardiac surgery available to this large number of patients is an immense problem.

Pathology. It has been estimated that it takes two to eight years for the pathological process of rheumatism to cause stenosis of the valve. The valve is affected in the acute phase together with the myocardium, but the late effect of the disease is on the valve only, and it is entirely mechanical. The reparative fibroblastic proliferation seriously interferes with the function of the valve, causing sclerosis, often followed by calcification.

The edges of the valves become thickened in the earlier stages and as the process progresses the commissures between the valves are obliterated, thus narrowing the valve aperture. It is at this stage that surgical separation of the valves at the commissures re-establishes free movement and restores a functioning valve.

If the sclerosing process advances, the valves themselves become rigid and their chordæ tendinæ are involved in the thickening, becoming shortened and bound together. Once this stage is reached no known surgical procedure can restore a functioning valve (see Fig. 2).

In some cases the pathological process produces rigid valves without gross stenosis; in such cases incompetence predominates in the clinical picture. Simple division of the commissures in these cases will not overcome the incompetence. There is often some incompetence associated with a tight mitral stenosis but the small size of the aperture itself does not allow sufficient regurgitation of blood for it to become a serious mechanical factor. It might be thought that the freeing of the stenotic valves by operation would inevitably result in a serious degree of regurgitation. Fortunately this is not the case; provided adequate mobility of the valves is restored they come together satisfactorily when the valve closes.

The other unhappy sequel to the operation that might be anticipated is the reformation of the stenosis. Provided the acute rheumatic process is no longer active this is unlikely and, in fact, so far no cases have been reported of recurrence of stenosis after satisfactory operative relief. It is not safe to operate until some years after an acute rheumatic phase owing to the danger of lighting up the disease process, which results in rheumatic myocarditis and post-operative failure.

The Mitral Valve

| Normal. | Mild Mitral Stenosis. | Advanced Mitral Stenosis. |

2A.
Viewed
from
the
atrium.

2B.
Viewed
from
the
ventricle.

2c.
In
section.

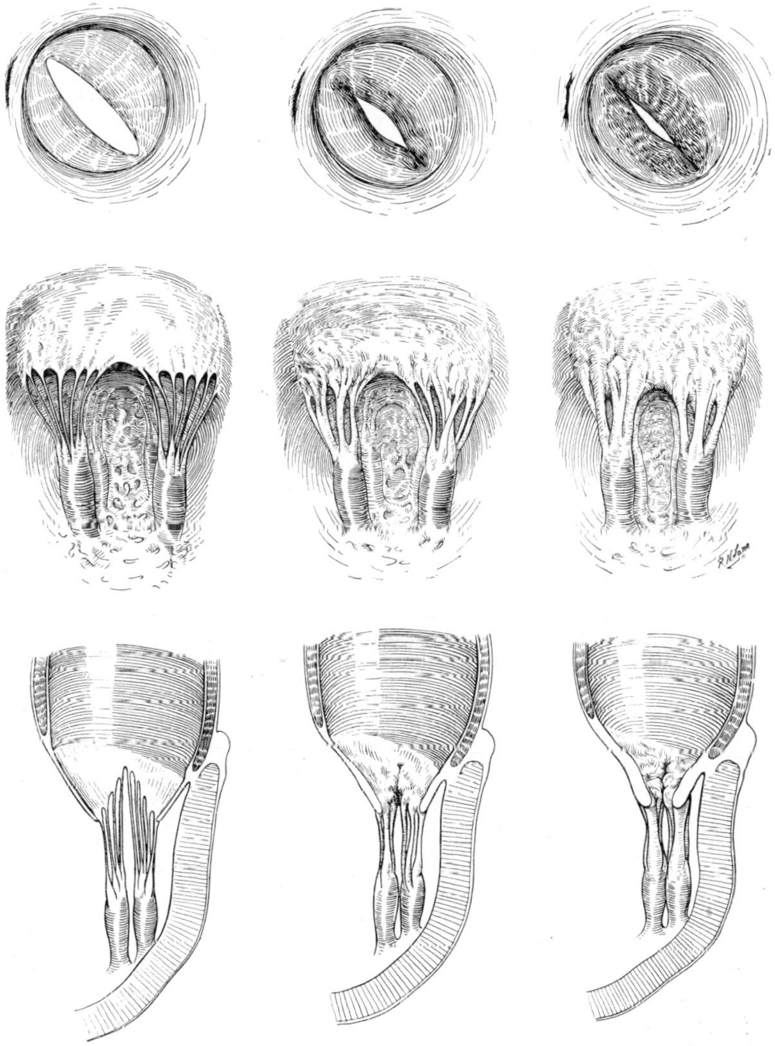

Fig. **26**.2. The normal valve is depicted in the left hand pictures. The central column of pictures depicts a valve suitable for operative relief of the stenosis. Note the reduction in size of the orifice, the puckering and thickening of the edges of the cusps. There is some thickening and shortening of the chordæ tendinæ.

The valve depicted in the right hand column shows a more advanced pathology and at this stage valvotomy is unlikely to give a satisfactory result. The puckering involves the whole of both cusps, which are thickened and rigid; the chordæ tendinæ are so shortened that they would prevent even a supple valve reaching a satisfactory closed position.

The cases to be considered for surgery are therefore those with a tight mitral stenosis in whom the rheumatic disease process is no longer active. Some patients with rheumatic heart disease do not outlive the active phase of the disease; but those that do frequently have little or no disability for a period of years after which time their exercise tolerance diminishes and the heart may go into failure as a result of the mechanical disadvantage under which it has to work. It is at the time of the onset of this later deterioration that the operation is now most frequently done. In future years the operation may become safe enough to recommend when there is little disability and before the deterioration has started, but as yet the risks of operation are too great.

Clinical Selection. The clinical selection depends especially on the following points:

1. Lesions of other valves.
2. Mitral incompetence.
3. Rheumatic activity.
4. Absence of cardiac failure.
5. The disability.
6. The size of the heart.
7. Calcification of the valves.
8. Systemic emboli.
9. Auricular fibrillation.
10. Hæmoptysis.
11. Paroxysmal cardiac dyspnœa.
12. Cardiac catheterization.

1. *Lesions of other valves.* The disability must be primarily due to mitral stenosis. It is often associated with other valve lesions especially of the aortic valve. The cardiologist must be satisfied that these, if present, are not of major clinical significance and also that the disability is not largely due to myocardial damage.

2. *Mitral incompetence.* This condition is now believed to be comparatively rare, whilst in the past it was thought to be more common than stenosis. Its diagnosis is not easy as mitral systolic murmurs can be caused by many other conditions. Diagnosis is based on the nature of the mitral systolic murmur, an accompanying thrill, enlargement of the left ventricle and of the left atrium and diastolic distension of the left auricle. At operation the regurgitant stream can be felt with the finger as it approaches the valve. The presence of gross incompetence contraindicates operation.

3. *Rheumatic activity.* There is no simple method of determining this; the greatest reliance must be put on the absence of any history of

fever associated with swelling of joints or other clinical manifestations of the condition for at least two to three years. The erythrocyte sedimentation rate if raised may suggest activity, but it is raised in many other conditions including cardiac failure.

4. *Cardiac failure*, of mild degree, at the time of operation is not an absolute contraindication, but makes the patient a bad risk. The prognosis following operation is better in those cases that have recovered from cardiac failure and best in those that have never been in this state.

5. *The disability.* Clearly it is not justifiable to submit patients to a major surgical procedure when they have minimal disability unless their prognosis is known to be bad. The most experienced cardiologist will have great difficulty in giving a prognosis in these cases, but increasing disability as shown by a falling exercise tolerance over recent months is undoubtedly a bad sign. It is probably safer to operate before this deterioration sets in, but as yet the operation cannot be considered safe enough to offer patients known to have mitral stenosis but in whom the disability does not prevent a full and enjoyable life.

6. *The size of the heart.* If the heart is enlarged it is necessary to determine which chamber is affected. Gross dilatation of the left atrium is a contraindication to operation whether or not it is due to mitral regurgitation. Enlargement of other chambers indicates conditions other than mitral stenosis and the cause must be sought and assessed as a cause of the patient's disability and prognosis.

7. *Calcification of the valves.* When the valves are calcified it may make the operation technically more difficult and it may not be possible to fashion a good functioning valve, but it is not a bar to operation.

8. *Systemic emboli.* Provided these have not resulted in incapacitating disability themselves, they are regarded as an indication for more urgent operation. The risks of surgery are undoubtedly increased, but once a systemic embolus has occurred the outlook without surgical relief of the stenosis is very bad.

9. *Auricular fibrillation.* This common complication also adds to the risk of operation and likewise carries with it a worse prognosis for the patient without operation. For this reason fibrillation will probably rarely influence the decision whether or not to operate.

10. *Hæmoptysis.* In mitral stenosis it may be due to rupture of an engorged vessel in the lung or, especially when there is associated fibrillation, to pulmonary infarction. The former cause indicates pulmonary hypertension and is a factor in favour of operation.

11. *Paroxysmal cardiac dyspnœa.* Represents pulmonary hypertension and carries with it a poor prognosis; it is considered an important factor favouring operation.

12. *Cardiac catheterization.* Will show the pressures in the right ventricle, pulmonary artery and pulmonary capillaries. It allows, in fact, an accurate assessment of the pulmonary hypertension, but cannot show the pressure in the left atrium. The procedure is as yet so new that no final assessment of its value in mitral stenosis can be given. However, in the light of our present knowledge it can be said to help to confirm the diagnosis and with extending experience may prove valuable in the selection of cases for operation (Fig. 3).

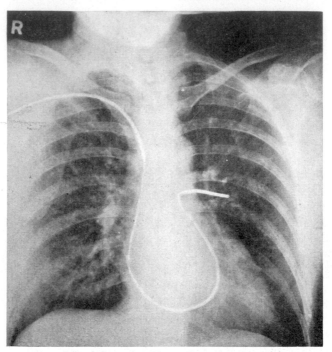

FIG. 26.3. Mitral Stenosis. The catheter has been introduced through the subclavian vein and right heart so that its tip lies in the left pulmonary artery.

The operation. It is usually performed through a left posterolateral or anterolateral thoracotomy incision, the pericardium being widely opened to expose the left auricular appendage. The valve is reached with the index finger through the appendage, but if there is a history of emboli or if thrombi can be felt in the atrium a brisk flow of blood is allowed through the incision in the appendage before inserting the finger in the hope that any loose thrombi will be washed out. Occasionally the appendage is fibrosed or the site of a massive thrombus, when it will be unsuitable for the insertion of the finger. The valve can be approached through the pulmonary veins and through the left ventricle, but in the presence of a large thrombus it may be wiser not to proceed with the operation.

It is possible in most cases to split the valve ring at the commissures with the finger with considerable accuracy. If there is gross thickening or when the ring is found to be of elastic consistency, a knife must be used to cut the commissures. Various types of knife are in use, their common feature is that they lie along the index finger and that the cutting edge can be controlled by palpation with the pulp of the finger. It is essential that the valve cusps themselves are not damaged or serious incompetence will result. The larger anteromedial or aortic cusp is the important factor in maintaining efficient function of the valve.

On removing the finger from the heart the auricular appendage is clamped with a specially designed instrument and then sutured. The left coronary artery lying in the groove in front of the appendage must be unimpeded.

Anæsthesia in these patients presents many special problems, but, in particular, there is a danger period shortly after induction which may be associated with a drop in blood pressure and serious cardiac embarrassment. For this reason anæsthetic agents which cause vaso-dilatation must be used with great caution.

The other major problem which has to be met by the surgeon and anæsthetist together is irregularity of the cardiac rhythm and in particular ventricular fibrillation. Some extra and abnormal beats appear to be inevitable during the cardiac manipulations. However, it must be appreciated that displacement of the heart from its normal position is never well tolerated and this should and can be avoided. The ventricular endothelium appears to be the most sensitive part of the heart to direct stimulation. Fortunately in this operation this endothelium can be left untouched, but some abnormal beats must be anticipated from manipulation of the valve ring itself. Various drugs might be expected to reduce this sensitivity; on the whole they have proved disappointing. Quinidine has been used as a prophylactic, but it is of doubtful value. Procaine can be used locally in the pericardium and intravenously. In the pericardium it is found to be an irritant. Intravenously it undoubtedly helps to control or prevent abnormal rhythm, but causes marked vasodilation, which has been already mentioned as dangerous. A new procaine derivative, procaine amide, which can be taken by mouth or injected, has not yet proved itself much superior to procaine hydrochloride.

If the operation is only performed on patients who have a considerable disability from their mitral stenosis a marked improvement in exercise tolerance can be expected in most cases after operation. The mortality of the operation will largely depend on the selection of cases. If the obviously bad risk patients are not operated on, an operative mortality of under 10 per cent. can be expected.

A. H. M. SIDDONS

References:

BLALOCK, A. (1946) *Ann. Surg.* **124,** 879.
BLALOCK, A., and TAUSSIG, H. B. (1945) *J. Amer. med. Ass.* **128,** 189.
BROCK, R. C. (1948) *Brit. med. J.* **i,** 1121.
CAMPBELL, M. (1948) *Guy's Hosp. Rep.* **97,** 1.
GROSS, R. E., and HUBBARD, J. P. (1939) *J. Amer. med. Ass.* **112,** 729.
KEELE, K. D., and TUBBS, O. S. (1940) *St. Bart's. Hosp. J.* **1,** 175.
POTTS, W. J., SMITH, S., and GIBSON, S. (1946) *J. Amer. med. Ass.* **132,** 627.
SELLORS, T. H. (1948) *Lancet* **i,** 988.

CHAPTER XXVII

PERIPHERAL VASCULAR SURGERY

In the eyes of history, the last decade may well prove to have been one of the most creative and formative periods in the development of Peripheral Vascular Surgery. But progress rarely comes as the spectacular accident; like the incoming tide it gains here an inch, there an inch, until suddenly we see it in its full flood. Between the two wars, Thomas Lewis set himself and his co-workers the task of examining closely the very foundations of our knowledge of the fundamental behaviour of blood-vessels. His philosophy was that of the great—an innate curiosity to understand and to seek knowledge for its own sake. The proper place for the study of mankind was man, and with simple tools, which are so often the mark of a man of genius—frequently but a syringe and needle, or blood-pressure cuff—he clarified for us the mechanisms of vascular pain and of the skin responses to trauma, cold, heat and œdema—to name but a few of his contributions.

In the thirties, an observation by Royle and Hunter in Australia on the effects of nerve section led to the "rebirth" of sympathetic surgery; even now the indications for and—more important—the contra-indications to, such surgery are still in dispute. The significance of the discovery of Heparin at this time received but slow appreciation; it may well prove to have been a therapeutic landmark as significant as penicillin. Only now is it being used with full vigour, and its other effects on the serum lipids and arterial clot recanalization may prove as important as its anticoagulant properties.

Then came the Second World War. War has so often been the spur to new thoughts and ideas in Vascular Surgery. But this was a stern test, for the modern missile meant mutilation and disruption of the main vessel and of the collaterals wide in its wake. It was soon evident that the surgeon's role, as the mere ligator of vessels, spelt almost certain catastrophe for the limb. The call for new methods was answered first by Blakemore and Lord, when they introduced their technique of vein grafting with the aid of vitallium cannulæ. The method itself was a failure, for the vessel lumen was narrowed and clotting followed, but it stimulated research into methods of vessel suture, and the use of vein grafts to bridge the arterial gap. Blalock then demonstrated the feasibility of joining the subclavian to the pulmonary artery, and thereby opened up an entirely new field of cardiac surgery. Gross and his team showed that an arterial homograft, suitably stored, could be

311

used in large-vessel surgery, and this added impetus to the application of this method to the peripheral vascular tree. Restoration of continuity of the vessel path became the aim and pursuit of the progressive surgeon.

Antibiotics made much of this surgery safe and, indeed, possible, even though we now accept this advance as something quite as natural to surgery as the gloves which the surgeon dons. In fact, we often overlook that this made it possible to observe and watch with safety the toe gangrene, previously so often the harbinger of a high amputation or death.

Vein surgery was not neglected. There was a change in attitude to the problem of varicose veins. Injection therapy, undertaken for decades without question as correct and without hazard, was shown to be futile as regards ultimate results, dangerous in its sclerosant damaging effects on the deep vein valves, and responsible for pulmonary embolism. Post-operative deep venous thrombosis was accepted as a challenge; high vein ligation, or anticoagulant therapy were introduced, and the problem was studied with much energy and thought. Even the process of ageing has not been neglected, for search has continued for a causal agent related to arteriosclerosis, and the blood lipids have been shown to be an important factor in its genesis. All in all, this is indeed a proud and remarkable story to tell.

The Arterial Tree

Anatomico-physiological Considerations

From the functional point of view, the peripheral circulation may be divided into three parts:

First, the proximal major vessels which are essentially passive conducting tubes, their calibre remaining unchanged, except in special circumstances.

Second, the small muscular arteries and strong arterioles which truly regulate the local blood-flow changes by means of a triple mechanism of control—local chemical (metabolites), nervous, and hormonal.

Third, the "minute vessels", as Lewis termed them, which include the small arterioles, the capillaries proper, and the venules. (There is no sharp line of distinction as the one passes into the other.) Their influence on limb blood-flow is negligible; locally produced metabolites regulate their calibre.

Tissues require a basic minimal blood-flow, per unit time, to survive; for the skin the minimal metabolic need has been estimated as 1 c.c.

per minute per 100 c.c. tissue (Burton, 1939). The toe gangrene, therefore, commonly does not mean local digital vessel disease, but a proximal major vessel block that has reduced the blood-flow below the local needs. It is not enough for the blood to arrive, it must flow, i.e. circulate; thus an extensive local venous thrombosis will halt arterial flow and may lead to skin or muscle death.

Blood-flow. A few simple hæmodynamic facts need to be appreciated. The rate of flow in a vessel depends on two factors, (*a*) the local arterial blood-pressure, (*b*) the size of the vessel lumen. The latter behaves in accordance with Poiseuille's law,* and slight increase in calibre thus speeds the blood-flow. On the other hand, the wall resistance of the small vessel is high, and the local blood-pressure falls and so does the flow in direct proportion to the length of such vessel. The resistance of these vessels has been shown to have an important bearing on the flow of the collateral circulation. The collaterals are best pictured as by-passes joining one segment of the vessel to the other, and distributing at the same time branches to the skin and muscles. With a major vessel block, such collateral blood-flow has to overcome the resistance of the small collateral vessels—"collateral resistance", and, in addition, the "peripheral resistance"—now known to be particularly important—of the distal main arterial tree. Sharpey-Schafer and Dornhorst (1951) have devised a method for calculating these resistances and have shown, for example in a subclavian artery ligature, that the peripheral resistance, as distinct from the collateral resistance, accounted for some 65 per cent. of the total resistance at the end of 24 hours. The relaxation of vessel tone in the collaterals and skin vessels (the foot and hand are classed as skin in such studies) should lower the peripheral resistance and increase blood-flow; such is the purpose of sympathectomy procedures. But this can be a double-edged weapon, for if the collateral head of pressure is feeble and the initial flow slow, such sympathetic denervation has been shown to result in a fall of pressure in the distal main tree. The distal blood-flow is thus slowed and clotting may occur. Moreover, as the sympathetic supply is distributed in the main to the skin vessels, such feeble flow shunts into the skin rather than the main tree; this further favours clot extension. On such reasoning, a sympathectomy before the collaterals have had time to develop, may thus do harm. We should not readily label Nature as irresponsible and ignorant of her own mechanisms, when she chooses to keep the avascular limb pale and cold, and only allows blood and

---

* *Poiseuille's law:* The rate of flow of blood through a tube varies directly with the fourth power of the radius. For example, if the flow through a vessel 1 mm. be 10 c.c. per minute, an increase of the vessel radius to 2 mm. (all other factors being unchanged) will raise the flow 16 times, *i.e.* 160 c.c./min.

warmth to spread to the skin as the deep flow becomes established.

Vascular Spasm. The peripheral arterial tree is maintained in a state of alertness—tone—to meet the changes in environmental demands. This physiological state has been much abused in recent years by regarding it as morbid and labelling it as "spasm". As an Editorial (*Brit. med. J.*, 1952) comments, "spasm has in fact become a medical cliché, and is often invoked as an explanation of the otherwise inexplicable". The effects of such loose language have been by no means innocuous, for treatment came to be based on such theoretical speculations. It may be said forthwith, therefore, on scientific basis, that firstly organic vascular disease does not induce "spasms" in the major vessel; if it did, sympathectomy could not release it, for the calibre of the main vessel is in no way influenced by such procedure. The corollary follows that a calcified main artery is not a contra-indication to sympathetic surgery, for the worth of such surgery lies in its influence on the collaterals and skin vessels only. Secondly, diseased or injured vessels do not induce reflex spasm in the collateral arteries. The practice of excision of vessel segments—arteriectomy—to sever theoretical reflex arcs has no physiological sanction (Cohen, 1944) and is to be condemned; if there is any associated collateral vessel damage, death of the limb is hastened.

Rise of distal temperature after sympathectomy or reflex heating does not indicate a release of "spasm" either—if it did, the greater rise obtained in a normal limb would lead to the absurd conclusion that such a limb is also in greater spasm. Pickering (1951) advocated instead the term "vasoconstriction" and has well emphasized that vessels are not "whimsical" in their behaviour and do not go into protracted spasm without special reason, i.e. a particular type of stimulus or trauma is required. Such traumatic arterial spasm will be discussed later. In many cases diagnosed as "spasm", unsuspected emboli or thrombi can be demonstrated by arteriography.

The Vasomotor Nerves. The sympathetic impulse traverses two sets of nerve fibres different in their humoral mechanism of nervous transmission—pre-ganglionic (cholinergic) and post-ganglionic (adrenergic). This has a bearing on the problem of post-operative sympathetic nerve regeneration and will be discussed subsequently. The vasomotor nerves accompany the somatic nerves and, as is well known, later leave in segmental fashion to join the peri-arterial plexus. No ganglion cells exist in this mesh, and peri-arterial nerve-stripping measures will neither denervate the limb nor influence the local artery calibre. The vasomotor fibres are distributed mainly to the skin vessels, and the muscle collaterals are but poorly supplied, but Barcroft and his co-workers (1943) have shown that sympathectomy definitely increases the muscle blood-flow. The relative increase is, however, slight and only about one-thirteenth of that achieved by the local metabolites of exercise. Sympathectomy cannot, therefore, be expected to cure claudication. But if the arterial block is suitably placed and the distal re-entrant collaterals are large, the increased blood-flow may be sufficient to relieve the mild claudication or, more usually, increase the walking distance.

Vasodilator fibres to the limbs in man are still a matter of speculation. As far as is known, too, there are no afferent sympathetic fibres. The dramatic relief of "resting" ischæmic pain after sympathectomy is held to be due to the improved blood-supply, and not the cutting of any sensory path. Some vessels are painful on direct puncture or handling, but this is related to accompanying somatic nerve fibres.

The "head ganglion" of the sympathetic nervous system is the hypothalamus. Within it lies the thermostat controlling body temperature, and by varying the impulse rate discharge (there is constant machine-gun barrage of sympathetic impulses) the circulation in the limbs is adjusted to conserve or to increase heat loss and thus maintain a constant body temperature. In the normal skin the range of blood-flow may vary from 94 c.c. per minute per 100 c.c. tissue with full dilatation to 3 c.c. with maximal vasoconstriction (Goetz and Ames, 1949). Warmed blood from a heated extremity, on arriving at the thalamus, inhibits sympathetic tone and leads to reflex vasodilatation in all other limbs. After adequate sympathectomy, reflex heating should cause no further rise in temperature or blood-flow; the limb remains dry and does not sweat. The cortex maintains a controlling (inhibiting) influence on the thalamus. Emotion, fear, and pain can cause intense peripheral vasoconstriction. During sleep sympathetic tone is inhibited and maximal peripheral vasodilatation results (Ingram, 1930). Every effort must be made, therefore, to relieve the patient of his pain and to induce sleep. "Sleep is the diastole of life." The hypothalamus also influences the pituitary, and this close liaison accounts for the sympathetic effects in many endocrine disturbances.

Clinical Considerations

Nature is lavish in her blood-supply to the limbs, and Kunkel and Stead (1938) and Abramson (1944) have shown by plethysmograph studies in cases of arteriosclerosis and thromboangiitis, that the maximal blood-flow in a limb may be reduced 50 per cent. without any symptoms or signs. *Skin surface temperatures* should not be accepted as an accurate guide to the state of the deep vessel circulation, and indeed, very little reliance is placed these days on temperature responses in the decision regarding sympathectomy. There may be "normal" temperature readings, though the blood-flow is only half normal, as judged by plethysmography (Goetz, 1950). A limb with blockage of the femoral artery and severe claudication symptoms may yet show a normal rise on reflex heating. On the other hand, a good sympathectomy result may be obtained, even though the skin temperature rise to reflex heating has been poor. This has been difficult to understand, but the work of Bazett and co-workers (1948) provides an explanation. They showed that in organic arterial disease much of the heat of the sluggish stream is absorbed in the proximal limb segment; as a result of such "pre-cooling", especially liable to occur in multiple arterial blocks, the blood reaches the toes at extremely low temperature. A slight rise of distal temperature in such a limb on reflex heating thus implies a significant increase in peripheral blood-flow.

Reflex heating, by immersing one upper extremity or both feet in water at 110° F. (45° C.) is now accepted as the most practical, certain, and safe method for such skin temperature studies. Spinal anæsthesia is no longer employed; paravertebral blocks are uncertain and an unnecessary ordeal for the patient; sympatheticolytic drugs are better used as a form of therapy.

Limb inspection is often casual, but can be instructive. In the horizontal position, vein filling on the dorsum of the foot is reasonable evidence of a good circulation; this does not apply after sympathcetomy, for vein tone will have been abolished and vein filling may be seen, even up to an area of gangrene. Rubor of the foot and toes, especially "cold" rubor, on limb dependency is an indication of a grimly deficient circulation. The dusky red appearance is due to capillary paresis, and these sunset colours truly paint the fading life of the limb.

Undue significance is still attached to absent dorsalis pedis, or even posterior tibial, pulses; it is still not appreciated that in some 14 per cent. of normals the dorsalis pedis is congenitally absent, and in 5 per cent. the perforating peroneal artery replaces the posterior tibial.

Oscillometry is of particular value for detecting doubtful pulsation. The actual figure of the oscillometric swing is an individual variation, and depends on factors such as blood-pressure, limb œdema, and muscle thickness, and also varies with the cuff level and make of instrument. The relative swing, as compared in the two legs, is the important consideration. Oscillometry figures are, however, some guide in prognosis; for example, a swing of 0·5 divisions at the ankle (using a Collens oscillometer) is a reasonable assurance that, provided no further thrombosis occurs, immediate gangrene is not a threat. In assessing the collateral circulation, too, the higher the blood-pressure at which the oscillometric swing comes through, the better the circulation. At times the oscillometric swing may be reasonable, and yet the symptomatology suggests vascular disease. The oscillometric response to exercise is then a valuable test. In the normal, after exercise there is an immediate rise in oscillometric swing at calf level; with a deficient circulation, the swing falls. The pulse wave is absorbed in the dilated vascular tree of the calf. This is known as "paradoxical reaction to exercise" (Ejrup, 1948). Oscillometry, however, has its limitations, and undue significance should not invariably be attached to low readings. As Dornhorst and Sharpey-Schafer (1951) have shown, with a good collateral circulation there may be negligible oscillometric swing, but the measured resting blood-flow be reasonable.

Plethysmography is, of course, the best method for assessing the blood-flow, but is time-consuming, and its clinical use is, therefore, restricted. It, too, has its limitations in that it records resting blood-flow; the metabolites in an ischæmic limb lead to maximal vasodilatation, and higher blood-flows than in the unaffected limb may be found.

Arteriography is the most reliable and certain of all methods for providing information as to the state of the main arterial tree. Above all things the surgeon is seeking information as to the presence, and extent of, any arterial blocks. The method is now in general use in this country, and the modern organic iodine media have proved without risk. "Diodone" (Pyclosil-(Glaxo)) 35 to 50 per cent. is to be preferred, and "Arteriodone" (Glaxo) 42·5 per cent. gives excellent pictures. The technique is well known, but a recent advance for the lower limb is the use of a large X-ray plate on which the knee is flexed to a right angle (Mackenzie and Hamilton, 1953). General anæsthesia is preferable, for the injection can be unpleasant and the patient is often tremulous. For the beginner and, indeed, for the assured picture, exposure of the artery by small transverse incision is to be preferred. The technique of direct vessel puncture should be mastered, for this is essential in the follow-up studies of patients after vessel grafting. For common femoral artery injection, the vessel is fixed between the index and middle fingers of the left hand and the needle slowly introduced directly perpendicular to the skin. The state of the higher vessels can only be determined by an aortogram, which is obtained by piercing the aorta just below the 12th rib, three fingers from the posterior midline (Semple and Whiteside, 1951). The method has proved safe and has given valuable information as to the presence of aortic blocks and the possibilities of high vessel grafting.

Arterial Disorders and the Sympathetic Nervous System

The Limb Vasomotor Supply

The Upper Limb. The pre-ganglionic fibres stream out from T2 to T7 or sometimes down to T9 or T10 and pass via the stellate ganglion to the brachial plexus. Barcroft and Hamilton (1948) have shown conclusively that *no* sympathetic fibres to the hand emerge through the roots of C8 or T1. No possible advantage is, therefore, to be gained by including stellate ganglionectomy in upper limb denervation. Indeed, it has been demonstrated that not only is the resultant Horner's syndrome ugly, but such stellate ganglionectomy leads to nasal vaso-dilatation (Guttman's sign), and if bilateral, the patient is saddled with permanent nasal blockage, recalcitrant to vasoconstrictors or nasal surgery (Jepson, 1951). Theoretically, upper limb denervation could be achieved by section of the chain below the stellate ganglion. However, inconstant sympathetic neural pathway may be provided by a branch from the second thoracic ganglion to the lowest trunk of the brachial plexus (Kuntz's nerve); another ramus also runs from the third thoracic nerve to join the second (Kirgis and Kuntz, 1942). A thorough sympathectomy, therefore, demands division of the chain below the third ganglion and removal of any rami associated with the second.

The Lower Limb. Sympathetic fibres stream out from T10 to L2 and form synapses in the paravertebral ganglia. Excision of the upper three lumbar ganglia cuts off all the vasoconstrictor impulses passing down via the fourth lumbar ganglion and its upper three sacral ganglia to the leg and foot; it also ablates the grey rami to the lumbar plexus. The anatomical pattern of the chain varies. Usually there are four lumbar ganglia, sometimes five; frequently the second and third ganglia fuse, and on exceptional occasions one enormous ganglion only may be present. The first ganglion may be difficult to identify, and one can never be absolutely sure of its removal at operation. Usually it lies on the crus of the diaphragm, but at times passes through the crus and lies buried. The direction of the rami may be helpful to identify the ganglia; in the upper two the rami are long and pass in cephalic direction; the third ganglion rami run transversely, and the fourth runs in caudal fashion. The intervening chain is at times but a thin thread. Theoretically, excision of the second and third ganglia is adequate, but the author invariably removes the fourth ganglion (identified by its constant caudal splitting into two or three divisions), for on several occasions a large independent ramus has come across from the third lumbar nerve.

Boyd and his co-workers (1949) have urged that the ganglionectomy should invariably include removal of L1. At first such more thorough procedure commends itself for two reasons: (*a*) there seems obvious advantage in removing, especially for the high arterial block, the tone of the large collaterals of the thigh, (*b*) theoretically, denervation of a wide strip of skin on the medial side of the leg in the area of distribution of the saphenous nerve is assured—an important consideration in sympathectomies for varicose ulceration. Northfield and Monro (1953), however, have shown that after any degree of paravertebral lumbar sympathectomy the thigh tone and the sweating pattern on the inner side of the calf skin continues. Such sympathetic tone, they declare, is maintained by "untouched" accessory ganglia (to be discussed) which contain at least half of the sympathetic ganglia to the thigh. Moreover, in the male bilateral removal of L1 may be followed by paralysis of the ejaculatory mechanism— not impotence—and the subsequent sterility has led to legal procedures. Rose (1953), however, maintains that seminal anorrhœa rarely follows the high purely lumbar ganglionectomy, and requires, in addition, T12 ganglionectomy.

It is evident, therefore, that no particular advantage is to be gained by the removal of L1 ganglion. Certainly there need be no such endeavours in the average arteriosclerotic case, where superficial femoral artery block is the problem. The removal of L1 ganglion may entail strong deep retraction, and this has precipitated aortic thrombosis (Learmonth, 1950).

Auxiliary Ganglia

Accessory (ectopic) sympathetic ganglia, whose pathways do not follow the sympathetic trunks, have been described by Skoog (1947) for the upper limb, and by Boyd and Monro (1949) for the lower limb. These ganglia are inaccessible to the surgeon. In the upper limb they may lie in the spinal canal and by means of a small nerve, the vertebral nerve of Wrete, pass and link up to the higher brachial plexus nerve roots. Each small ganglion receives a white ramus and the grey ramus proceeds from it. In the lower limbs the ganglia lie deep to the psoas muscle, on the tips of the transverse processes of the vertebrae, or on the anterior nerve roots themselves. The significance of their continued function after high lumbar sympathectomy has been discussed. Only actual division of the anterior roots would ensure their destruction, and this has been advocated by Ray and his colleagues (1943).

The further importance of these ganglia and their connections lies in the fact that they may provide an alternate pathway for sympathetic impulses after the usual sympathectomy. It is now known (Haxton, 1947; Barcroft and Hamilton, 1948) that after sympathectomy the vasomotor and sudomotor reflexes are completely absent six months after operation, whereas a year or more after operation they have in many cases returned. The new paths are functionally inferior to the original, and in the cases examined clinical improvement has been maintained. Regeneration has been the explanation put forward, and special precautions have been taken to prevent reunion of the divided chain by burying the ends in muscle or encasing them in silk or tantalum cylinders. Re-exploration has failed to demonstrate any such regeneration (Jepson, 1951; Cohen, 1953). Indeed, "after ganglionectomy it is necessary to postulate the growth of pre-ganglionic (cholinergic) medullated axons down the degenerated remnants of a post-ganglionic (adrenergic) non-medullated fibre" (Kinmonth and Hadfield, 1952). There is no evidence that this is possible. The most likely explanation for such apparent regeneration is re-routing via the accessory sympathetic paths. Experience in poliomyelitis teaches that, whatever the explanation, re-routing of nerve impulses takes time.

Post-ganglionic Sensitization

It is now known that in man a post-ganglionic sympathectomy does not cause any excessive rise in sensitivity to adrenaline-like substances circulating in the blood. After any sympathectomy the vessels regain much of their tone, but, though in animals the return of tone is four times as great after a post-ganglionic as after a pre-ganglionic sympathectomy, this does not apply to man (Barcroft and Walker, 1949). Pre-ganglionic section has not improved the results, more particularly in Raynaud's phenomenon. Most surgeons now prefer to do a full ganglionectomy, as it is likely to eradicate all stray fibres that may be present.

The return of tone after any type of sympathectomy does, of course, influence the blood-flow. In the hand, at the end of a week the maximal post-operative blood-flow has fallen to a quarter, and after a fortnight to an eighth (Barcroft and Walker, 1949). In the feet the flow does not fall so greatly, and in the diseased lower limb the normal flow may be expected to be doubled by sympathectomy (Lynn and Barcroft, 1950). An interesting finding is that the high temperature of the toes or fingers is usually maintained, despite this fall in blood-flow.

The Place of Sympathectomy

A sympathectomy achieves many things:

(1) The blood-flow of the limb, especially to the skin, is finally doubled. Such a warm limb can withstand minor traumata far better.

(2) The limb is no longer affected to the same extent by changes in environmental temperature or emotion.

(3) The dry limb, after sympathectomy, does not lose heat by sweating. In addition, higher distal temperatures continue, despite the return of tonus and the fall of blood-flow. This influences healing, which is a chemical process and is stepped up by higher temperatures.

(4) The relaxation of vein tone reduces the resistance to arterial inflow.

(5) Sympathectomy abolishes the peripheral vasoconstriction produced by smoking (Rapaport *et al.*, 1950).

Two further facts may be noted about sympathectomy:

(*a*) The patient with a high block, e.g. at the common iliac bifurcation or external iliac, gets the better result with sympathectomy. Larger collaterals are opened and can sweep a good flow of blood into the distal major vessel. The blood-flow per minute is the important factor. Their claudication, at times sciatic or of the buttock, frequently improves.

(*b*) The patient with absent distal pulse and yet a warm foot, as for instance in popliteal block, does well with a sympathectomy. This obviously means that a good collateral circulation has developed, and sympathectomy will improve it.

Intermittent Claudication

John Homans (1939) has said, "*if you take the trouble to ask any patient with gangrene, you always obtain a history of intermittent claudication*". I, therefore, tell all patients with claudication: "Sympathectomy will improve your skin circulation and is the best measure available to protect you against the development of gangrene. Your claudication is unlikely to be cured, but you will find your walking distance certainly doubled or trebled; very exceptionally, claudication is all but cured. You will have a warm foot." A persistently cold foot sorely bothers these patients and prevents them falling asleep.

The grading of patients with claudication by Boyd and his co-workers (1949) is a notable advance. There are three grades:

Grade 1. The patient develops pain on walking, but the pain clears as the walking continues. The metabolites of exercise are here able to invoke a blood-flow response adequate to sweep away the P-substances produced by exercise.

Sympathectomy should not be rushed in this type of case, for as Learmonth (1950) points out, it is well to allow patients to develop a natural collateral circulation to metabolite stimulus. Operation may, indeed, precipitate further thrombosis.

Grade 2.   Pain develops on exercise and continues, but the patient can, with effort, still walk. The collateral circulation is here still fairly good, but not adequate. Sympathectomy usually leads to improvement.

Grade 3.   These patients are compelled by the pain to halt absolutely. Sympathectomy will not improve their claudication, but may be necessary for skin nutrition reasons. Two operations have been introduced to relieve such claudication pain: (*a*) popliteal neurectomy, i.e. division of the gastrocnemii nerves of supply. The operation has proved a failure, for claudication pain in the soleus muscle group now developed; (*b*) tendocalcaneus section. In this procedure, the tendon is divided by tenotomy knife two inches proximal to its insertion, and the calf muscles are thus placed on slack. Before this is done, the hips, knees, and ankles should be X-rayed to exclude any latent osteo-arthritis, which is liable to be flared by the foot-slapping action after tendon section. Ankle œdema is another troublesome complication. Few patients, except working men, are prepared to change their claudication for a quite unpleasant limp.

Replacement of the thrombosed arterial segment by a homograft —vein or artery—is a new hope for some of these cases and is now on clinical trial. A failed graft may be a tragedy; and vein grafts certainly, and indeed arterial grafts do clot months after operation. Before undertaking such an operation, the effect of a sympathectomy should be observed. Only a small group of cases have proved suitable, and at the moment it is well for the average surgeon to be the candle holder and look on. Sir Henry Cohen's saying about heroic surgery can here be well applied, "the feasibility of an operation is no indication as to its desirability".

Sympathectomy for Skin Ischæmic Lesions

It should be borne in mind that in the arteriosclerotic the collateral and smaller vessels are usually remarkably free of disease, despite the changes in the major vessels. Sympathectomy can, therefore, influence them. In diabetics with arteriosclerosis, only the digital vessels tend to be involved and there is good proximal blood-supply; local foot amputations, without sympathectomy, thus often succeed.

Obviously, a sympathectomy cannot improve an already gangrenous area, but certainly the formation of a line of demarcation appears to be hastened. When such gangrene reaches and involves the metatarsal heads, a high amputation becomes necessary. Transmetatarsal and partial foot amputations for such gangrene have been well tried out in the last decade. Although occasionally successful, flap sloughing, persistent sinuses, and painful stumps have proved troublesome complications. Experience indicates that a gently performed below-knee amputation usually succeeds, even in the aged. Even such a failed below-knee amputation is not a tragedy, for with antibiotics re-amputation is readily feasible and the patient's life has not been jeopardized.

It is remarkable how the vascular status of a foot with amputated toe or toes improves after sympathectomy, and further amputations are rarely necessary. Edwards and Crane (1951) followed up for a period of at least two years 89 sympathectomized local foot amputations; only one case required further amputation in the affected leg.

The essential indication for a sympathectomy is intolerable "resting pain". Typically the patient sits up in bed at night, rubbing his foot or letting it hang out of bed, and usually arrives in hospital with the limb markedly œdematous. The dramatic relief of pain is often difficult to explain purely on a basis of improved blood-supply to the affected foot; the shunting of blood by the sympathectomy to the vasa nervorum may be a reasonable alternative explanation (i.e. the pain has been due to an ischæmic neuritis). Often, however, the pain is due simply to bad management of the gangrene. Gangrenous toes should be soaked in soapy water, rather than kept dry; the contraction of the mummified area is responsible for much of the agony. Aureomycin ointment (3 per cent.) or glycerine are suitable dressings.

At times the single mottled toe develops complete gangrene, or the apparently small lesion spreads after sympathectomy. This is due to the fact that sympathetic action is a mass action and opens up the vessels to all the digits; the sluggish stream takes the easier path rather than the partially obstructed ones, with the result that the affected toe suffers. This can, in fact, be predicted on occasions by preliminary reflex heating tests; the temperature of the toe likely to suffer after sympathectomy will be found to fall, as de Takats (1944) first pointed out. This is especially true in the thromboangiitis obliterans case, where the digital vessels are diseased in varying degree.

Contra-indications to Sympathectomy

First, *the ischæmic limb of acute onset*, i.e. following a sudden thrombotic episode. Sympathectomy may then apparently precipitate a massive gangrene or lead to marked extension of a localized gangrenous area. The pale limb is of advantage at this stage, for the blood is kept flowing within the deeper vessels. Operative interference, and not the sympathectomy *per se* also encourages clotting, as in the venous stream, and may account for the distal extension of the fresh arterial thrombotic process.

Various other theories have been put forward. Freeman and his colleagues (1947) suggest that the opening of the arteriovenous shunts by sympathectomy drains the capillary tree. Learmonth (1950) considers that increased œdema around the doubtful ischæmic area, after sympathetic denervation, is the precipitating factor. As already mentioned, Dornhorst and Sharpey-Schafer (1951) have demonstrated after sympathectomy, a fall of local blood-pressure in the vessel distal to the block, and this will favour clot extension. We conclude that it is better in the acute case to allow the natural collateral circulation to develop for several months before doing a sympathectomy.

Secondly, *the very septic limb*; the dilatation of all the vessels to the foot or hand may lead to shunting of blood away from the septic area, and the gangrene may spread. Extensive septic involvement of the sole or forefoot is a contra-indication, but a superficial dorsal involvement is not necessarily one.

Thirdly, *the limb with marked cold rubor or deep sunset cyanosis* should not be early sympathectomized. The capillary flow continues to be paretic, with subsequent tendency to gangrene spread. It is better to tide over these patients with natural vasodilatation and anticoagulant measures, unless severe resting pain demands operation. In old patients such limbs are often dry, and Shumacker (1942) has suggested that ischæmic interference with nerve conduction performs its own "spontaneous" sympathetic denervation.

Fourthly, *for old patients* with diffuse generalized arteriosclerotic disease and cardiac and respiratory involvement, sympathectomy obviously is a "senseless sword". In these cases Haxton (1949) does a chemical sympathectomy by paravertebral injection of phenol; the method requires good experience of paravertebral blocks, and in his hands the results are good. For patients in poor condition and in agony from, say, gangrene of the heel, White's (1953) multiple neurectomies in the leg are a useful procedure; all the sensory nerves are divided by incisions placed six inches above ankle level. The anæsthetic foot is in this fashion desympathectomized at the same time. Such patients subsequently wear fleece-lined boots, get about perfectly well, and are not a burden to themselves or their families. In many patients, however, the disease is widespread with multiple or diffuse blocks and the surgeon's task is hopeless.

Operative Technique

Cervico-Dorsal Sympathectomy

Three anatomical approaches are available: (*a*) anterior; (*b*) dorsal; (*c*) peraxillary.

Anterior (Cervical) Approach. This route is now commonly favoured in this country. The small incision heals with a fine scar, both sides can be done at one sitting, and the patient is out of hospital in five days. In the modern technique, the ganglia are approached by going below the subclavian artery arch; ligature of the thyrocervical trunk is then unnecessary, and hæmorrhage from small vessels on the superior border is also avoided. Moreover, the vertebral artery does not come into the field; injury or thrombosis due to retractor pressure of this vessel have been responsible for the rare tragedy. A rubber strip sling should be passed around the subclavian artery to ensure control of accidental hæmorrhage; in stripping down the diaphanous apical pleura, dissection at first proceeds in an upward direction. Ample room is obtained for sympathetic chain dissection to well below the third ganglion. At this stage a head lamp avoids the use of cumbersome lighted retractors in a small field. The heads of the first and second ribs lie close together, and the third sympathetic ganglion is often mistakenly counted as the second. Both the second and third ganglia, with their rami, are excised. Occasionally, the pleura is opened, and catheter suction before final wound closure will then avoid surgical emphysema. Clips only are required for the skin; they should be removed not later than the second or third day (Figs. 1-6).

In some 40 per cent. of cases the sweat and vasoconstrictor fibres to the face emerge from below T1 and are destroyed by T2 ganglionectomy; occasionally this produces also a mild degree of Horner's syndrome. "Gustatory sweating" may be a post-operative complaint; on eating spiced foods, beads of sweat develop on the forehead, and this is associated with tingling and warmth of

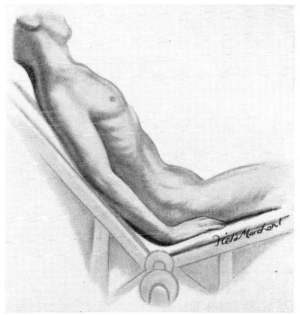

FIG. **27**.1. Cervical sympathectomy. Semi-sitting position assists venous drainage, and minimizes bleeding.

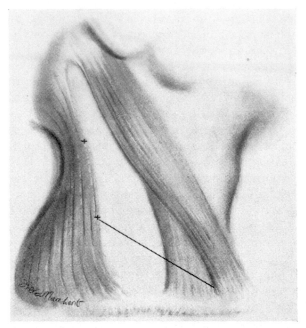

FIG. 27.2. Oblique incision avoids scar adherence to clavicle. Clavicular fibres of sternomastoid muscle are divided.

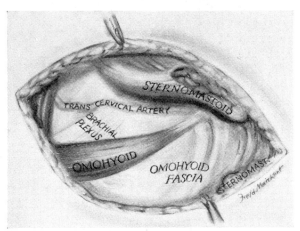

FIG. 27.3. First operative step—omohyoid muscle exposure. This muscle is the "flag" marking the lateral limits of dissection.

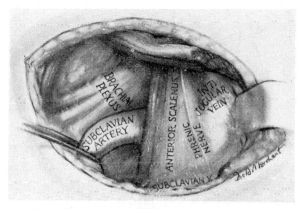

FIG. 27.4. The anatomy. Sling passed around subclavian artery. Scalenus anterior fascia is incised at latter border; its medial retraction protects the phrenic nerve from injury or retractor pressure.

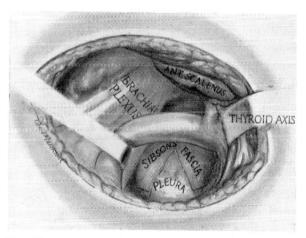

FIG. 27.5. Shows approach below subclavian artery arch. Scalenus anterior muscle and its deeper fibres have been divided. Sibson's fascia is cleared and incised ; to avoid pleura damage stripping proceeds medially, and ascends to the apex.

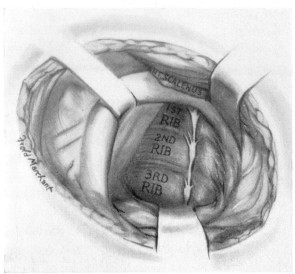

FIG. 27.6. Sympathetic chain exposed. Observe close proximity of first and second rib heads; the third sympathetic ganglion is often mistakenly identified as the second.

the face. A more serious complication is severe shoulder or arm pain particularly at night. This is more frequent after the dorsal approach and is akin to the intercostal neuritis so common after the Smithwick hypertension operation. This neuralgic pain usually clears within three weeks, but may last several months and be very unpleasant.

Dorsal Approach. This is preferred by American surgeons. After resection of the third rib and associated transverse process, a good exposure of the sympathetic chain is obtained. A more thorough type of preganglionic section, including removal of second and third intercostal nerves and their roots can be performed. This latter, as has been stressed, is no longer considered an advantage. The dorsal approach excludes search for thoracic inlet abnormalities—often an important consideration. There are other disadvantages; the greater liability to severe post-operative neuralgia, the strain of the prone anæsthetic position, and the need for two operations, as only one can be done at a sitting. This route is to be preferred for re-operating on cases where the previous cervical operation has been incomplete.

Per-axillary Approach. Atkins (1949) has developed this approach, though Goetz and Schulze were the first to use it. The second intercostal space is entered by transverse incision across the axilla, the pleura is opened, and the lung allowed to collapse. A good exposure of the third ganglion, but not of the stellate, is obtained. This operation has not proved popular in this country.

Lumbar Ganglionectomy

An anterolateral extraperitoneal approach is now the commonly accepted route (Figs. 7-12). The posterior approach (Royle's incision) along the edge of the erector spinæ and then sweeping the iliac crest,

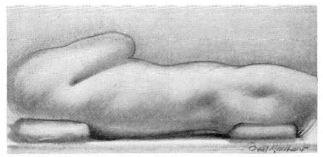

FIG. 27.7. Lumbar sympathectomy. Position of patient. Sandbags are placed beneath buttocks and shoulder.

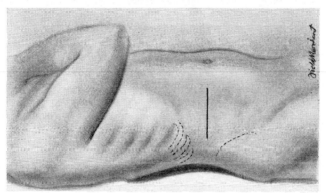

FIG. 27.8. Transverse incision extends to lateral edge of rectus muscle.

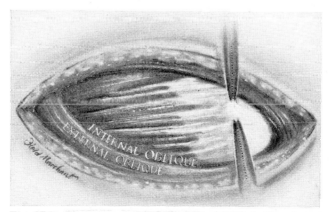

FIG. 27.9. The external oblique has been divided. The edge of rectus sheath is grasped with hæmostats, prior to incision.

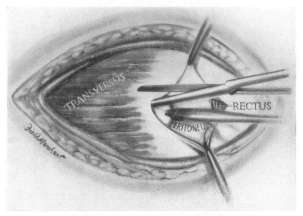

FIG. 27.10. The peritoneum is stripped from the transversus abdominis muscle and fascia by a small gauze swab.

is still favoured by Smithwick and other American surgeons. The sympathetic chain lies close to the midline, and in this incision the chain is exposed at considerable depth. The transperitoneal approach necessitates bowel packing, may be followed by ileus, and disturbs the patient quite un-necessarily. For sympathetic denervation in the aortic thrombosis it is the route of choice; damage to the collaterals in the muscles of the flanks is thus avoided.

Operation by the extraperitoneal approach is safe. In an extensive experience the author has had only one death, and that was due to cerebral embolus from a silent coronary infarction in an old man. Both sides can be done at one sitting, and the author has operated on patients at the age of 80-85. Why not, if femurs are pinned at that age? Coronary thrombosis, if of long history, does not appear to add to the operation hazard. A good anæsthetic is required, preferably with curare to relax the psoas muscle; high spinal anæsthetics are dangerous in these older patients. Learmonth (1950) has said, "My greatest regret now is that I used to refuse the possibility of help from sympathectomy, to too many patients in the older age-groups."

Post-Sympathectomy Pain. Severe pain, located deep in the groin or the medial

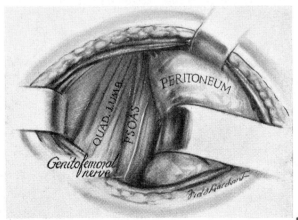

FIG. 27.11. Peritoneum being retracted. The psoas fascia is incised medial to the genito-femoral nerve; this ensures clean medial retraction of fat and lymphatic glands overlying the ganglia.

part of the thigh, is an all-too-common complaint after operation. It first comes on about the tenth post-operative day, is most marked at night, and may be associated with hyperæsthesia of the thigh or meralgia paræsthetica. It seems related to rami traction on the lumbar nerves, for it has become more common with high sympath-

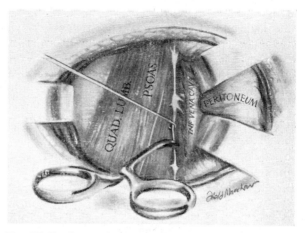

Fig. 27.12. Sympathetic chain exposed. A curved hæmostat grasps the chain; this facilitates dissection of upper ganglia.

etic ablations and the associated stronger chain traction. The condition almost invariably clears within three to six weeks, but occasionally lasts several months; analgesic drugs should not be withheld, for the pain is most distressing.

Vessel Repair and Grafting

The main principles of vessel suture may be summarized.

(*a*) Some trimming of the adventitia is always essential. In the annular repair it should be stripped up one inch. The adventitia prevents the suture sliding through the wall and fractures the stitch; its interposition in the suture line interferes with healing. It should be replaced after suture, for this will enable the fine vasa vasorum to take part in the repair.

(*b*) The sutures need to be 1 mm. apart, if the suture line is to be blood tight; silk 00000 on an eyeless curved needle should be employed.

(*c*) It is now agreed that the suture bite should include the intima. The suture material lies in a tucked-away fold, and with the swift stream does not encourage clotting.

(*d*) Eversion of the walls should be aimed at, even though that does mean some vessel narrowing. The type of stitch to be used is still open to some argument. Experimental work indicates that the simple running stitch gives as good results as any. A continuous mattress eversion stitch is favoured by most surgeons. Shumacker prefers interrupted mattress sutures, which have proved very satisfactory in his hands. The mattress suture has the advantage that a firm grip is obtained, and at the same time satisfactory eversion.

In the traumatic lesion, the longitudinal slit tear may be readily repaired, with such mattress sutures. The transversely divided vessel is a more difficult problem. Elastic retraction opens the gap, but if less than one-quarter of the vessel lumen has been divided, suture is still possible. The partially divided vessel angulates and a wide gap appears between the lumina. Such a vessel should be completely divided and then end-to-end suture undertaken. It is customary now in such repair to use two stay sutures only and to complete the anastomosis with a running mattress stitch (Fig. 13). This tightens as the flowing stream expands the suture line, but oozing points after release of the clamps may require the additional stitch. The suture line commonly holds well without aneurysm formation; occasionally arteriography shows a mild bulge in the anastomosis line, not unlike a "plumber's joint", as termed by Mason-Brown (1946).

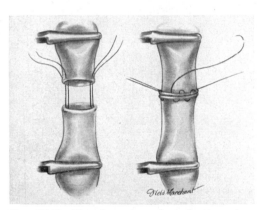

FIG. 27.13. Vessel anastomosis—using two stay sutures only (Eastcott). Observe continuous everting sutures.

Probably the greatest advance in recent years has been the development of *homovessel grafting*. A well organized vascular team set-up is required for such work. The *venous graft* is commonly taken fresh from the patient, i.e. the autogenous graft. Such venous grafts withstand arterial pressure with little subsequent dilatation and have their main application in arterial injuries or disease involving the femoral-popliteal system. The long saphenous vein is of adequate size, and the vein of choice; the superficial femoral vein is too large, but has been used when the saphenous vein has been affected by phlebitis or previously "stripped". Julian and co-workers (1952, 1953) have placed 34 such vein grafts for arterial blocks with 12 failures (many such "failures" being "experimental"). They have introduced a useful refinement in technique for the arteriosclerotic case. The artery is transected above the obstruction and anastomosed to the lower cut end of the saphenous vein, thus forming an A-V fistula. This overcomes vein spasm, prevents graft rotation, and makes certain that the valves are not obstructing blood-flow. The lower end of the artery is in the meantime prepared; the vein is then transected and the anastomosis completed.

There are no "spare" arteries in the body, except the splenic artery. *Arterial grafts* are thus used, after storage in special vessel banks. The grafts need to be taken within six hours after death, under sterile conditions, and the donor must be free of transmittable disease. Gross *et al.* (1949) and Pierce *et al.* (1949), whose preliminary work has made such grafting feasible, prefer the graft stored in nutrient solutions and kept at temperatures of 2-4°C. Hufnagel and Eastcott (1950, 1952) have shown, however, that equally good results can be obtained by the use of quick frozen grafts. They are collected into sterile tubes, rapidly frozen, and subsequently stored at −70° C. in solid carbon dioxide. More recently, dehydrated grafts, kept in hermetically sealed tubes, have been introduced and may prove to be the storage of choice. Great credit is due to Professor C. G. Rob and his colleague, Mr. H. H. G. Eastcott, in this country for their stimulus and direction of this type of work.

The method of suture for such grafts is the eversion mattress stitch, as outlined above; preservation of the collaterals is important in the event of graft failure. Systemic heparinization begins with the anastomosis and continues post-operatively; no advantage comes from local intra-arterial heparin drips, for the solution is swept rapidly into the general circulation. With such heparinization post-operative oozing and large wound hæmatomas have been a problem; Rob (1953) has advocated an excellent method of leaving the wound open and performing a secondary suture, some four to five days later.

The elastic layer of such grafts alone survives. By a process of creeping substitution the intima is replaced from the vessel ends. Aneurysm formation of the graft has not developed in man, although it has been observed in long-term studies with animal arterial grafts. The selection of suitable cases will be discussed.

Anti-coagulant Therapy

Anticoagulants are finding increasing application in peripheral vascular surgery for the acute arterial thrombotic episode, arterial embolism, ischæmic resting pain, frostbite, the venous thrombosis, and after vessel repair or grafting. The recent experimental work of Wright and Kubik (1953) indicates that anticoagulants can assist absorption of the acute arterial clot, and this may have far-reaching significance. Heparin, too, has been shown to influence the blood lipid metabolism and is now being used for such purpose in arteriosclerotic conditions.

Heparin is the anticoagulant of choice. Spontaneous hæmorrhages from the kidneys or mucous membranes are not precipitated, as with other anticoagulants; and diseases of the liver, kidneys, or parenchymal organs are in no way adversely influenced by its use. Control clotting times are usually not essential; but if necessary, the blood sample should be taken one hour after the last heparin injection. An intravenous dose of 10 ml. of 1 per cent. Protamine Sulphate will abolish the heparinized response within 10 minutes. The contra-indications to heparin are few:

(*a*) Associated brain or spinal cord surgery, or lesions. In the case with multiple arterial emboli, this is a particular consideration. Such brain infarction leads to colliquefactive necrosis, and heparin may induce bleeding into the area.

(*b*) Associated chest surgery; severe bleeding into the pleura may follow.

(*c*) Associated fractures. A post-heparin bleed into the fracture hæmatoma, in a limb encased in tight plaster, may compress and completely obstruct the muscle arterial inflow and cause the Volkmann lesion.

For the arterial lesion high dosage is advisable; it does not add any appreciable risk and insures against the spread of the thrombotic process. Heparin is always to be preferred to the uncertain action of oral anticoagulants. The only disadvantage is the intravenous route of administration but the use of a Gordh needle enables therapy to be continued by the nursing staff. Subcutaneous and intramuscular injections are now seldom employed, even though satisfactory blood-clotting levels can be obtained; extremely painful and large local hæmatomas are common complications. The arterial case requires effective heparinization for a minimum period of five days, and anticoagulants by mouth should then continue for a total period of 14 days. Weight is an important factor in assessing the dosage, and heavy patients require, say, 20,000 units instead of 15,000, as the primary dose.

Heparin Dosage (1 mg. equals 100 units).

For the *arterial lesion* the following schedule has proved satisfactory: Day 1: 15,000 units, 4-hourly; days 2-5: 15,000 units, 6-hourly; days 6-14: "Tromexan" or "Dindevan".

Prolonged clotting times may be obtained by such heparin dosage, but this is of advantage in the arterial lesion.

The Swedish routine (Bauer, 1950) may be followed for the *venous* thrombosis:

15,000 units at 8 a.m.; 10,000 units at 12 noon;
10,000 units at 4 p.m.; 15,000 units at 8 p.m.

When there are symptoms of pulmonary embolism, Bauer administers 15,000 units of heparin 6-hourly. With the "catastrophic" pulmonary embolus 25,000 units heparin should be administered forthwith.

Dicoumarol. This is a dangerous drug and few surgeons now use it. Patients vary in their susceptibility to the drug and hæmorrhages, in particular frank hæmaturia, have occurred in some 11 to 28 per cent. of cases.

"Tromexan" (Ethyl biscoumacetate). This coumarin product has replaced Dicoumarol. It is four to five times less active (toxic); there is an action lag of only 18 to 24 hours, and prothrombin times do not fluctuate quite to the same extent; complications, such as hæmaturia, have been rare. The wide individual variations in response to the drug, however, makes the regulation of dosage difficult.

Tromexan Dosage.

1,200 mg., *first day*; 1,200 mg., *second day*; 300-600 mg., *third day et seq.*, according to prothombin times.

A standard time of administration should be followed. The drug is given in divided dosage at 1 p.m. and 10 p.m. and the prothrombin concentration estimated the following day at 12 noon. A prothrombin concentration of 15 to 20 per cent. is the aim. In patients with cardiac failure, hepatic or renal insufficiency, and those who have been taking aspirin or salicylates, the initial prothrombin concentration may be low. The commencing daily dosage should then not be higher than 600 mg. Intravenous Vitamin K, 100-300 mg., has now been shown to be an effective antidote, and has proved harmless and without evident toxic effect in such large dosage. Fresh blood transfusions may be necessary.

"Dindevan" (Evans)—Phenylindanedione. The clinical use and advantages of this new prothrombinopenic drug have been well described by Toohey (1953). A therapeutic response is obtained in 18 to 24 hours, and there is a rapid return to normal of the prothrombin time, even if the drug has been maintained for weeks. Once the prothrombin level is established, there are no considerable fluctuations, and prothrombin times at seven-day intervals only are necessary. This is of particular advantage in a long-term policy of anticoagulant therapy, as may be necessary for recurrent arterial emboli, migratory thrombo-phlebitis, and the flare episodes of thromboangiitis obliterans. Defective renal function leads to delayed excretion of the drug and calls for smaller dosage. Complications such as hæmaturia have not been encountered with the usual dosage; the pinkish-orange colour of the urine with this drug is regarded as of no significance. Vitamin K_1

given orally, is the antidote and has dramatic effect in 8 to 20 hours; the water soluble Vitamin K is not as effective. Heparin interferes with the estimation of prothrombin clotting times, and the blood sample should be taken at least six hours after the last intravenous injection. A therapeutic level of 10 to 20 per cent. is aimed at, and is commonly achieved in 36 to 48 hours; the average maintenance dose is 75 to 100 mg.

Dosage Schedule:

First day, 200 mg. in divided dosage (at 1 p.m. and 10 p.m.).
Second day, 100 mg. (divided dosage). *Third day et seq.*,
75 mg. according to prothrombin times.

This drug is likely to be extensively used.

Vessel Injuries

The surgeon may find himself confronted with three types of vascular catastrophe: (*a*) Division—complete or incomplete; (*b*) Contusion—major or minor; (*c*) Occlusion—by spasm, or local pressure.

Vessel Division

In the *complete division*, the wide arterial gap makes restoration of continuity by suture, or the use of an autogenous vein or stored arterial graft, the obvious ideal for pursuit. Frequently, however, the patient arrives grossly exsanguinated, is in no state for a prolonged procedure, and the surgeon may lack experience in such technique. In civil life, two injuries in particular call for some form of repair: (*a*) the dislocated knee, with popliteal artery damage; experience has shown that the collaterals are extensively disrupted, and limb survival is thus rare; (*b*) the compound fractured femur, with femoral artery injury; this commonly ends in limb gangrene, if ligation procedures only are adopted. In some cases the local conditions may permit the use of a plastic or glass cannula, with heparinization as a temporary measure, for three to four days; the patient's general condition will then have improved, and grafting surgery can be undertaken. War experience indicates that it is dangerous to restore main arterial continuity, if there has been complete arrest of arterial flow for more than six hours (Muskart, 1945); dead muscle products swept into the blood-stream may lead to sudden death.

Vessel ligation need be no hurried affair, for this may cause unnecessary collateral vessel damage. With local pressure, the wound incision can be extended, proximal control obtained, and the bleeding point accurately visualized. To control the severe buttock hæmorrhage, temporary clamps on both the common iliac and external iliac arteries may be necessary. Lateral wounds, especially of large veins, should not be treated by ligation, for they fail to bunch for the ligature and slip; the vessel wall, if held by forceps, should be underrun by sewing-machine stitch. Triple ligation, i.e. of the main artery and its branches, is to be avoided; a short vessel stump at the bifurcation should be sutured so as to avoid narrowing of the bifurcation crutch. For the ligature, thin non-absorbable suture material, such as silk or thread, is to be preferred.

Vein Ligation

Opinion is not settled as to the need for ligature of the companion vein after primary arterial ligation. War experience statistics (De Bakey and Semione, 1946) suggest that it made no difference to the limb mortality. There is, however, something to be said in favour of it. The vein is often found contused, later clots, and even pulmonary embolism has followed. The onset of such venous thrombosis in an ischæmic limb may be sufficient to tip the scales against recovery; the resistance to arterial inflow is increased, and the capillary circulation may be halted. During the last war, limb arterial ligations were often nursed with the head of the bed blocked, so as to retard vein flow. This position favours stagnation in the venous tree, encourages thrombosis, and is therefore dangerous. Moreover, in this position leg œdema follows; this may compress the collateral vessel flow, often running at pressures as low as 40-50 mm. Hg.

Sympathectomy Procedures

A number of surgeons still favour repeated sympathetic blocks. War statistics proved inconclusive but certainly showed that in the crucial test—the popliteal artery injury—the march of events was not reversed. The hæmodynamics of collateral flow have already been discussed, and ablation of sympathetic tone argued as inadvisable for the acutely avascular limb. The Vascular Committee of the Medical Research Council (Memo. 13, 1944) did not support such sympathectomy procedures.

Partial Vessel Division

This is commonly associated with a large hæmatoma, which many hours later may first begin to pulsate; with an A-V fistula, of aneurysmal varix type, there may be but little swelling. Two findings are a help in the diagnosis of the partial lesion: (a) the presence of peripheral pulses, even though reduced in volume; this means continuity.

Oscillometry will confirm such pulsation. (*b*) A bruit on auscultation. At first, this may be a faint systolic whisper only, and develops fully some hours later.

The surgeon's function is that of the alert bystander, for he knows that the development of an aneurysm will be a life-saving event for the limb. Small entrance and exit wounds, and no fracture, will limit bleeding, assist clot compression, and favour such aneurysm sac formation. Surgical interference may, however, become necessary, owing to hæmatoma rupture or deterioration of the vascular status of the limb. Recorded clinical observations are thus particularly important. To be noted are the limb colour, digital warmth, sensation, muscle texture, and especially full details of muscle power.

Arterial Contusion

The *minor* contusion does not need surgery. If found in the course of wound exploration, it should be oversewn with adjacent muscle and fascia; in the event of wall necrosis, bleeding will be limited and aneurysm formation encouraged (Maybury, 1944). The vessel bruise is no longer regarded as an "irritant", firing reflex spasm of the main collateral vessels. Arteriectomy for such contusions has, therefore, been abandoned (Cohen, 1944).

The management of the *major* contusion is still a problem. The vessel appears red and swollen, and pulsation is absent or feeble; beyond the thrombus the distal segment is often in tight spasm, which prevents re-entrant collateral flow as in the embolus case. It is a dangerous lesion, especially if there is in addition a local fracture; wide collateral vessel damage may then be assumed.

If the distal limb nutrition has been maintained, and no major ischæmic muscle palsies have developed, local vessel measures may be unnecessary; secondary hæmorrhage is, however, a hazard, and the contusion should be oversewn with muscle and fascia. Heparinization is obviously desirable, but the risks of bleeding from associated local injuries frequently contra-indicate its use. Thrombectomy, i.e. removal of the clot, usually fails, for without heparinization clotting rapidly recurs. If the collaterals are extensively damaged, vessel grafting is essential, and the autogenous vein graft is to be preferred. Gentle packing, and leaving the skin wound open, may then enable heparinization to continue. The patient's general condition takes precedence over the limb. If this is unsatisfactory, a glass or plastic cannula should be inserted for three to four days, heparinization maintained, and grafting surgery then undertaken.

Occlusion by Arterial Spasm

This phenomenon is called into account rather glibly for all manner of vascular catastrophes. Only exploration can decide as to whether the absent pulse is due to vessel disruption, thrombosis, or spasm.

Two types of spasm may be distinguished (Cohen, 1944); (*a*) Segmentary (benign) spasm, (*b*) Reflex (malignant) spasm.

Segmentary Spasm. The vessel itself has been subjected to trauma, and there is a purely local response to a local vessel injury. The collateral vessels are not involved in such spasm. This is a myogenic response, and is initiated by stimuli, such as surgical handling, twanging of the vessel by the fractured bone or the dislocation, the stretch of the "near miss" of the bullet missile.

Such spasm is frequently associated with supracondylar fractures of the humerus or femur. It is wise and desirable to explore some of these cases, for so often the distal absent pulse and ischæmia are due to mechanical obstruction, e.g. trapping of the vessel between the bone ends, or angulation over a fracture spike. Clinical experience has taught that such spasm is not influenced by periarterial sympathectomy, sympathetic blocks, or local procaine injections. Local warm saline packs and vessel fiddling sometimes result in abrupt spasm release. Kinmonth (1952), on experimental work, advocates the local application of a solution of $2\cdot5$ per cent. papaverine. If, after 10 to 15 minutes, no relaxation follows, the wound is closed and via a small polythene tube leading to the vessel wall, 1 per cent. papaverine injections are continued. Intravenous papaverine does not work, for the spasm throttles the fine vasa vasorum, and the drug cannot reach the arterial muscle wall. A feeble blood-flow often continues through the spastic vessel segment, and as previously stressed, arteriectomy has no place in treatment.

Reflex Spasm. Here the cushioned vessel has received no direct injury, but there has been brutal "insult" to local tissues. The strangling tourniquet, masonry crush, the severe blow, as to the back of the knee —these are some of the particular stimuli. Such spasm is wide in the extent of vessel involvement, intense and unremitting, and malignant in its obstinacy unto the death of the limb. The collateral vessels are extensively involved in such spasm.

The condition is regarded as a reflex shock response with the arc passing through the spinal cord. Procaine blocks of the local major nerves should be tried first; this will block both afferent impulses and vasomotor nerves passing down within the somatic nerves. Brachial plexus blocks and spinal anæsthesia are alternative methods, and have worked. Should the spasm persist, heparinized saline should be injected under pressure into the spastic segment. Plain muscle is thus forced to assume a new posture, which will be maintained by the flowing stream. No harm seems to accrue from such forcible vessel distension, and the method has been successful on a number of occasions.

Occlusion by Local Pressure

The rising pressure of the hæmatoma or œdema may be sufficient to embarrass blood-flow to the collaterals, vasa nervorum, and the muscular branches. A local pressure of 50-60 mm. Hg. will obliterate flow in the vasa nervorum and, as Lewis showed, nerve conduction will cease in 30 to 60 minutes with such ischæmia. A progressive loss of nerve conduction, therefore, points to mounting vascular compression. As Parkes (1945) showed, these effects are first evident in the sensory cutaneous nerves; the proximal (cephalic) spread of limb anæsthesia, therefore, indicates a need for surgical decompression.

The tight plaster will increase such œdema or hæmatoma compression, and indeed it is a rule that any form of plaster splinting (even though split) is absolutely contra-indicated in the avascular limb; the fracture fixation can wait till another day. Decompression for œdema only is seldom called for; bed blocking (below heart-level) will reduce it. The elbow and popliteal hæmatoma commonly require evacuation. The tight calf hæmatoma too needs surgery, but the skin incision should be short and the fascia split by fasciotome; muscle bulging into the wound otherwise makes skin suture impossible, and infection frequently follows in such avascular limb.

Ischæmic Nerve Effects. Nerve fibres vary in their vulnerability to asphyxia; for example, fibres subserving slowly conducted pain are more resistant. Such nerve ischæmia may be due not only to local compression, but also follow reduced blood-flow after the ligature, embolus, or thrombus. The clinical features of such disturbed nerve conduction can well be observed in the leg. (*a*) *Slipper anæsthesia* of the foot; often there is an associated tongue-like extension on the outer side of the leg. (*b*) *Slow pain response.* On squeezing for example a toe, there is a delay of one or two seconds, and then the patient abruptly withdraws his foot and complains of a particularly unpleasant type of pain. (*c*) *Paresis* and wasting *of the intrinsic muscles* of the foot. A characteristic finding, too, is *"big-toe drop"*, due to paresis of the extensor longus hallucis muscle; the flexor longus hallucis also shows some loss of power. Recovery from a severe ischæmic nerve lesion is slow, and may take eighteen months; the sole of the foot may remain anæsthetic.

Volkmann's Ischæmic Muscle Contracture

Ischæmia may lead to death of the musculature only. The muscle cell withstands poorly lack of blood-supply and dies within six to ten hours; skin may survive 24 to 48 hours ischæmia. Nerve will recover, after a time, from even 24 hours ischæmia, but failure of nerve conduction is evident in 30 minutes. Progressive inability to move either fingers or toes is thus evidence of serious ischæmia, and often the earliest indication of impending muscle death.

Until 1940, it was held that venous obstruction was solely responsible for the Volkmann lesion. Griffiths then showed that arterial obstruction was the true *causa causans*. This could be brought about either by vessel disruption, thrombosis, spasm or embolism. Mechanical vessel obstruction, i.e. trapping between the bone ends, is in my experience the commonest finding in the supracondylar fracture. Later, Bowden and Guttman (1945) brought evidence that extensive venous blockage can cause muscle death. There is an arterial pulse wave, but no circulatory flow. The muscle microscopical picture after venous obstruction differs from that of the arterial infarct; there is no clear-cut boundary zone, but extensive fibrous tissue infiltration leading to complete muscle replacement fibrosis. The end result is the same. Muscle blood-flow may also be directly obstructed by the tight plaster or splint; the muscular branches of supply run at pressures as low as 60 mm. Hg. A radial pulse may thus be present, and yet the plaster compression be sufficient to throttle the muscle vessels. The state of the skin is no guide to the muscle flow; there may be a warm-skinned limb, and yet the muscles beneath may be dead.

It is evident that to operate on woody hard muscles, in rigor mortis, is to operate too late. Decompression of the venous obstruction lesion demands wide splitting of the fascia (from mid-arm to mid forearm); the fascia is left unsutured. Delayed secondary suture (fourth day) is often advisable, too, for the grossly swollen skin. Vigorous early attempts to correct the contractures by, for example, finger traction are inadvisable; the response is more fibrous tissue. These measures are for later consideration. Arthrodesis of the wrist is a useful measure for the late forearm case; for the crippling deformity of the leg an amputation may be preferable to a multitude of orthopædic procedures.

Peripheral Aneurysm and Arteriovenous Fistula
The Traumatic Lesion

Probably the most glorious chapter in the management of vascular injuries in the last war is the story of the remarkable results of surgery for aneurysms and A-V fistulæ; loss of limb or life was rare.

Aneurysms

The march of events in the formation of an aneurysm sac was well described by Maybury (1944). The aneurysm does not develop from the fluid centre of the hæmatoma, but is pounded out by the pulsating stream in the solid plugging clot. In the loose tissues of the neck, axilla, and superficial femoral triangle, such clot has at first but frail attachment and is readily dislodged. The bruit and reduced distal pulses have been discussed; occasionally the clot may temporarily block distal flow. Arteriography will define the sac and demonstrate the proximal collaterals likely to be injured at operation. The arteriogram, however, is not an absolute guide to the collateral circulation; few distal collaterals may show and yet the limb survives. It is indeed difficult to find any suitable clinical test for the assessment of the collateral circulation. The Henle-Cœnen test at operation is the best; after clamping the proximal vessel, the sac is opened—distal vessel bleeding or pulsation indicates an adequate collateral flow (Fig. 14, G). Time, as Shumacker (1946) showed, does not seem to promote an increasing collateral circulation, although this happens in the A-V fistula. A pre-operative waiting period of six to eight weeks is nevertheless

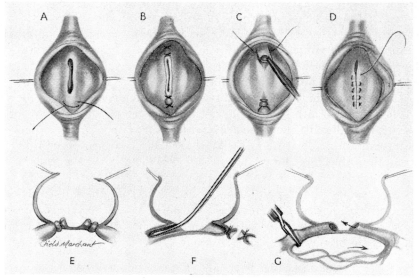

FIG. 27.14.

A-E Intrasaccular ligation for traumatic aneurysm.
F   Extrasaccular ligation.
G   Henle-Coenen test at operation for adequate collateral circulation, indicated
       by bleeding from the distal vessel after clamping the proximal.

desirable, for after the local hæmatoma absorption the surgeon has a clearer anatomy and healed vessel walls favourable for suture.

A lateral suture repair of the vessel wound is rarely feasible; Shumacker in his extensive experience (360 aneurysms) found only two suitable cases. End-to-end suture, after excision of the sac, is rarely possible in the lower limb—the vessel gap is too wide; but in the upper limb was accomplished successfully by Shumacker in nine cases. The *obliterative endo-aneurysmorrhaphy of Matas* has come to be the operation of choice and necessity. Except when associated nerve repair has to be undertaken, the empty sac is left undisturbed; the walls adhere in the fashion of peritoneal surfaces and leave no local thickening. There are two methods:

(*a*) *Intrasaccular ligation.* This carries least risk of damaging collaterals. After opening the sac, the vessel mouths are transfixed with figure-of-eight sutures, or obliterated by a running suture along the gutter leading from inlet to outlet (Fig. 14, A-E).

(*b*) *Extrasaccular ligation.* The sac is opened and a bougie passed to guide the dissection of the artery outside the sac (Fig. 14, F). This method is to be preferred when adjacent nerves are likely to be caught by the blind deep intrasaccular stitching, as for example in brachial, axillary, and subclavian artery aneurysm. Companion vein ligation is unnecessary; the limb is post-operatively nursed in slight elevation, for, as Goetz (1950) showed, this position lowers the vein resistance and facilitates arterial inflow.

The A-V Fistula

The wide propagation of the *bruit* (from the umbilicus to the toes in a femoral lesion) and its continuous character (machinery murmur with systolic intensification) differentiates it from the aneurysm, which has but a locally confined systolic bruit. Eddy turbulence as the blood swirls through the fistula, sets the vein wall dancing and accounts for the thrill and continuous bruit; halting of venous flow will thus abolish them. Cardiac output studies (Cohen *et al.*, 1948) have shown that the fistula imposes a considerable load on the heart; the output may be doubled or trebled, depending on the size of the communication. If the pulse rate slows markedly on shunt closure (Branham's bradycardia), a large fistula can be assumed. The remarkable collateral circulations that develop in long-standing fistulæ, are well known. Blood-flow studies indicate, however, that the distal limb flow is not found increased in a fistula of under two years' duration. The deliberate production of fistulæ to increase the distal limb blood-supply, as for impending arteriosclerotic gangrene (Szilagyi *et al.*, 1951) or for cerebral ischæmic lesions, thus has no physiological basis.

Skin marking of the probable fistula site is a help at operation. The area of maximal intensity of thrill and bruit is a guide. Location of the maximal sound intensity can be assisted by using the index finger as a pointer and tracing it along the vessel course, whilst auscultation on the dorsum of the hand continues. The test is now referred to as "auscultation à distance" (Maybury and Learmonth, 1946). Arteriography will only demonstrate the fistula, if the communication is small. Retrograde arterial filling by vein injection is then a useful alternative method; with the arterial circulation arrested by cuff inflation, the vein is injected and the dye can be traced as it flows through the fistula and outlines the adjacent arterial tree (Cohen, 1952).

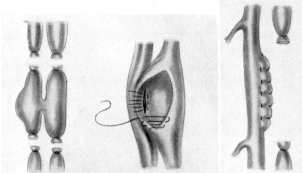 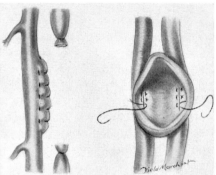

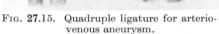

FIG. 27.15. Quadruple ligature for arterio-		FIG. 27.16. Restorative procedure for
venous aneurysm.				arterio-venous aneurysm.

Ligation procedures, i.e. the "quadruple ligature" (Fig. 15) are commonly dictated by the local pathological changes. The vessels are matted together, the proximal enlarged artery is thin-walled and readily injured, and an almost invariable associated aneurysmal bulge makes fistula excision necessary. *Restorative procedures* (Fig. 16) are only occasionally feasible; for the arterial gap is frequently wide, and the rim of the fistula calcareous and unsuited for suture. For the small fistula such surgery should be considered, a transvenous approach is used for the aneurysmal varix, and the trans-saccular route for the varicose aneurysm. Haile (1946) and Paterson Ross (1946) have pointed out that such arterial repair with coincident vein ligation may be followed by obstructive venous effects, i.e. bursting pain on standing or walking.

Sympathectomy procedures are unnecessary in operations for

aneurysms or A-V fistulæ. Deliberate proximal vessel control is essential in these operations; the common femoral and gluteal lesions require temporary clamps on *both* the common iliac and external iliac arteries. Adequate exposure of the subclavian or axillary lesion requires resection of a segment of clavicle (with Gigli wire saw). The resected segment should not be replaced. Lesions of the popliteal bifurcation and its branches are best exposed by resection of the upper end of the fibula (Elkin, 1946).

Post-operative limb death is exceptional; but in the lower limbs intermittent claudication and sensory effects have followed (60 per cent. of cases) ligation procedures. Arterial grafting is, therefore, now on trial.

Pathological Aneurysms

In the limb, arteriosclerosis is the commonest cause of the true aneurysm. The popliteal artery is the site in 70 per cent. of cases; bilateral popliteal involvement is common, and thorough search frequently demonstrates multiple aneurysms. Most of the patients are old, and the vessel wall proximal to the aneurysm is in no condition for graft surgery. The ruptured aneurysm, however, strongly requires such consideration, for experience shows that the collaterals are then disrupted and ligature only ends in limb death. Fortunately, such rupture is not a common complication. The fusiform aneurysm—a diffuse wall bulge—stays unchanged in size for years, and surgery is not required, except for pain or pressure effects (Allen *et al.*, 1946). The saccular aneurysm will, however, continue to enlarge and thus requires operation. Reconstructive and restorative procedures usually fail. The Matas type of intrasaccular obliterative endo-aneurysmorrhaphy is to be preferred, and is a simple, safe procedure. Proximal ligation only, such as the Hunterian ligation, is to be condemned for the limb mortality is higher than commonly imagined—13 per cent., and aneurysm recurrence is common. The important consideration is reduction of the sac mass, for otherwise pressure on the collaterals continues. The *mycotic aneurysm* is a dangerous lesion, for infection leads rapidly to rupture; present experience suggests that immediate operation on diagnosis is advisable.

Congenital A-V fistulæ are still a problem, particularly in the limb hypertrophy case or the angiomatous lesion with "hot ulcer" on the foot or hand. Careful arteriographic studies fail in many cases to demonstrate the multiple fistulæ. Because of their small size, such fistulæ rarely lead to cardiac complications, there is no reflex slowing of the heart on proximal vessel compression, and bruits and thrills may be absent. Proximal main artery and vein ligation will not cure and may be followed by limb gangrene. The best method of attack appears to be exposure of the main artery and ligation of the fine branches passing to the angiomatous area. It often works in temporary fashion only. Careful dissection and excision of the veins within the area is then an alternative method for dealing, in retrograde fashion, with such fistulæ; it has been effective especially in hand lesions (Cohen, 1952).

The Venous Tree

Two problems have received particular attention—varicose veins and venous thrombosis.

Varicose Veins

The last decade saw an end to the glib acceptance of sclerosant injection therapy with or without fossa ovalis ties, as the only line of management of varicose veins. Some surgeons still cling to this method. Not only is the recurrence rate high, but venography studies (Boyd and Robertson, 1947) demonstrated that the sclerosant rapidly flowed into the deep veins, adding possible damage of the vein valves, and at times producing deep vein thrombosis, and even pulmonary embolism and death. The surgeon could observe for himself the flow into the deep veins by injecting "Pentothal" into a varicosity and noting the swift induction of anæsthesia.

All are agreed that a thorough Trendelenburg ligation is a *sine qua non* in most cases. Stripping of the distal veins has of late come into use again, but these strippers are traumatic and difficult to thread through the really tortuous varicosities. The method commonly favoured is interruption and ligature of the varicosities at multiple points. Pre-operatively the skin incisions should be marked (with Biro pen) and particular attention paid to blow outs and the often neglected small saphenous vein; the gross varicosity bunch can be gently avulsed or excised. Small incisions only, rarely more than 0·5 cm., should be used. The "slipped" vein tie should not be energetically pursued; with local pressure and the Trendelenburg position bleeding soon ceases. Injection therapy, not more than 1-2 c.c. is permissible occasionally for the local cosmetically ugly vein. Sodium morrhuate solutions should never be employed, for there have been fatal anaphylactic reactions.

It is now recognized that such varicosities are frequently secondary to deep vein thrombosis. These veins do not form a compensatory mechanism; their flow is retrograde. Venous thrombosis is thus no longer regarded as a contra-indication to such surgery; indeed the need for operation is more specific and important, for they add to the local venous stasis. A word of warning is necessary as to the varicose vein "thrombophlebitis". These patients must not be kept in bed, for this encourages spread of the thrombosis to the deep circulation. Heparin will relieve their pain within six hours, and further anticoagulant therapy, preferably "Dindevan", may be necessary. The leg should be bandaged firmly with elastic strapping, and the patient kept ambulant.

Venous Thrombosis

Post-operative venous thrombosis remains as the small dark cloud over the surgeon's thoughts as he advises operation or observes the convalescence. Two factors are essential for the intravascular clot: (a) Some change in the normal clotting—anti-clotting equilibrium; (b) slowing of the venous flow.

Blood Coagulant Factors. The reasons for some patients being "clotters" are not yet fully understood. Massing of the platelets is a factor, but this is a physiological response to any trauma. Payling Wright (1947) showed that from the fourth to the eighth post-operative days the platelets become sticky, may adhere to the vein wall, and form the starting point of thrombosis. Various tests have been tried to detect such thrombotic state; daily clotting times, prothrombin activity, fibrinogen B estimations (Cumminc and Lyons, 1948); the results were variable and unreliable. Antibiotics have been suggested by Ochsner (1949) as a possible clotting factor; prothrombin studies, however, have proved reassuring. Alterations in the blood itself may not be necessary, for the distinguished physiologist Drinker (1953) is of the opinion that the local anoxia of venous stasis can lead to endothelial breakdown and clot formation in consequence.

Certain patients can be spotted as "clotters". The risk of embolism is twice the average figure in the obese; "cardiacs" are likely "clotters", especially the old case of myocardial infarction; the cancer patient, especially with necrotic growth of stomach or bowel; polycythæmia, whether primary, or secondary to emphysema or heart lesions; anæmic patients. Vein thrombosis in one leg is frequently followed by clotting in the other, on further surgery.

Hæmodynamics of Venous Flow. Over-emphasis of the importance of muscle action has led to neglect of the other mechanisms which speed vein flow. These may be summarized as (a) suction action of the expanding chest; (b) muscle action—the booster pump, or the "peripheral venous heart"; (c) the *vis-a-tergo* thrust of arterial flow; (d) gravity.

Impaired chest action, as Holman (1950) showed, will affect femoral vein flow; abdominal distension will further throttle it, for as Gatch (1950) demonstrated, the pressure in the large veins of the abdomen varies directly with the intra-abdominal pressure. The abdominal operation, owing to the restriction of respiratory movement, is thus more liable to venous complications; the dilated stomach, ascites, pregnancy, will all hamper vein flow. The importance of muscle action is now well appreciated, and early ambulation (still too often but a passive slumping in a chair) is the general routine after operation. Early walking has not solved the problem, for statistics (Loewe *et al.*, 1951) show that the incidence of post-operative thrombosis has been but halved. A neglected and important method of speeding vein flow is the assistance of gravity flow by foot bed blocks; seriously ill patients and most abdominal cases, should be thus nursed during their entire convalescence, unless there are definite contra-indications (Allen, 1953).

Early diagnosis is of the utmost importance. Bauer (1950) contends that this is possible in 99·6 per cent. of cases, but even in "clot-minded" clinics fatal pulmonary emboli occur "out of a blue sky" (six deaths per year in a General Hospital with 800 beds is an average figure). For early diagnosis, calf muscle tenderness is a more reliable sign than Homan's test (Murley, 1950). In my experience, slight pitting œdema behind the medial malleolus comes on early; this skin area drains into the soleus vein group, where such thrombosis commonly starts.

On diagnosis, vigorous anticoagulant therapy should be started. The purpose of early treatment is to prevent spread of the thrombosis to the thigh veins; this long clot is the danger both to limb and life. Heparinization does not loosen or affect clot fixation. Heparin is to be preferred for the ill patient. Oral anticoagulants should be used with caution in the older age group, and Allen (1953), who is an authority on the subject, believes that it is not safe to reduce their prothrombin time below 50 per cent. of normal.

Sympathetic blocks are inadvisable as a line of immediate treatment. Their action is evanescent, and the march of a spreading thrombosis will continue. Goetz (1950) has shown that unless muscle action is vigorous, the ablation of deep vein tone may even lead to blood pooling. The method should never be used in association with anticoagulants, for extensive hæmatomas have followed. Reflex arterial spasm from the thrombosed veins is not accepted by many in this country; nor should undue emphasis be laid on the distinction between phlebo-thrombosis and thrombophlebitis. The active "outspoken" thrombo-phlebitis is not necessarily safe; the clot may spread, and anticoagulant therapy should be instituted to prevent pulmonary embolism and to limit involvement of the collateral vein channels.

Femoral vein ligation to trap the thigh clot has never proved popular in this country. The operation, which should be bilateral, has, however, a very definite place: (*a*) when anticoagulants are contra-indicated; (*b*) as a prophylactic measure—in fat patients likely to lie flat and inert, after major abdominal procedures; in old patients with fractures of the femur, and in selected "cardiac clotters". The ligation should be performed at the end of the operation; (*c*) repeated pulmonary emboli. The latter is a particular consideration, for statistics show that of cases which have had one pulmonary embolus, 30 per cent. will have another and 20 per cent. a fatal one. The site of election for the ligature is the superficial femoral vein, just distal to the profunda join. Anticoagulants are still necessary to keep the collateral veins clear of clot. Common iliac vein ligations are now rarely undertaken; on the left side, the vein lies behind the artery, and hugs the pelvis, and ligation is difficult. Inferior vena cava ligation after a short period of popularity, has been almost completely abandoned. The late result may be appalling; some cases have been completely incapacitated, and in many marked œdema and ulceration have proved formidable problems. Repeated septic infarcts, secondary to pelvic vein thrombosis, is the only indication for this operation.

The Post-phlebitic Leg

Surgical exploration (Linton and Hardy, 1948) and phlebography studies (Lockhart-Mummery and Smitham, 1951) indicate that invariably the vein clot becomes canalized, and commonly the original vein lumen is restored. The valves are, however, destroyed, and retrograde flow leading to local venous hypertension is the problem. Deep vein disease will be confirmed by finding a venous pressure above 50 mm. Hg. in the foot on exercise, and patent, though often irregular, venous channels on phlebography. Injection of Diodone into a vein on the dorsum of the foot, with venous flow held by tourniquet above the knee, gives good pictures. The interpretation of such "ascending phlebograms" is often difficult; as Murley (1951) points out, failure of valves to show on a phlebogram does not mean that they do not exist, for the ampullary bulges near the valves, which are necessary to show them in radiography may not be present even in normal cases. Retrograde flow on femoral vein injection too is not conclusive evidence of valve incompetence.

Venous pressures can now be readily determined by the simple method of Walker and Longland (1950). Polythene tubing, filled with heparinized saline, is inserted into a dorsal vein of the foot and con-nected with a mercury manometer. In the normal limb at rest, and on standing the pressure is about 90 mm. Hg., i.e. from heart level to the point of measurement. On exercise this may fall to 18 mm., which is less than the normal colloid osmotic pressure of blood (25-30 mm.); this means that capillary reabsorption can occur during walking. In a patient with varicose veins, on walking the pressure falls to 30-80 mm., depending on the extent of the incompetent varicosities; if reflux down the varices is prevented by a below-knee tourniquet, the pressure on exercise falls to the normal range.

In contrast, the fall of pressure on exercise is small in patients with old deep vein thrombosis; certainly this never falls below 50 mm. Hg, and may even rise. The extent of the pressure fall, Walker (1950) considers, is a guide to the advisability of deep vein ligation; if the fall in pressure on exercise is slight, the case is unsuitable. Bauer (1950) introduced popliteal vein ligation to reduce the venous pressure by halting retrograde flow on standing; the muscles then pumped their blood via the collateral veins. The nigger in the woodpile is the assumption that such collateral veins retain competent valves; but it has been found that as these veins dilate, their valves, too, become incompetent. Post-operative studies indicate that the hæmodynamics are not improved for a rise in the venous pressure on exercise is com-monly found. The clinical reports in this country also have been disappointing; the leg œdema has often increased, and the rate and persistence of ulceration healing not improved. Pain, especially bursting pain on exercise, Walker regards as the best indication for vein ligation, but venous pressure studies are essential in case selection. This type of pain, it may be added, is often readily relieved by com-pression bandaging, for as Boyd and his team showed, on exercise with tight bandaging a further fall in venous pressure occurs. Popliteal vein ligation, after fairly extensive trial, is no longer favoured in this country. High femoral vein ligation, too, has proved unsatisfactory; Linton and Hardy (1948) in a review of their results—their operations included eradication of superficial varicosities—found 30 per cent. failures in operations for ulceration.

An important consideration is the finding of Barcroft and Dornhorst (1948) that high venous pressures are quite compatible with normal function, and the muscle pumps of the lower leg can work efficiently against pressures as high as 90-100 mm. Hg. We may learn a lesson from the heart with incompetent aortic valves: it hypertrophies to deal with the overloading. Building-up of the calf musculature, especially by walking, is the keystone of treatment.

Chronic Ulceration of the Leg

For practical purposes, three types of leg ulcers may be distinguished: (*a*) *Varicose*, secondary to varicose veins; (*b*) *Post-phlebitic*, secondary to deep vein thrombosis; (*c*) *Arteriosclerotic*. Ulceration may also occur, secondary to ulcerative colitis, polycythæmia rubra vera, Cooley's anæmia, and erythrocyanosis frigidorum.

The Simple Varicose Ulcer. According to Anning (1949) these account for only 11 per cent. of cases. They are superficial to the deep fascia (Boyd *et al.*, 1952) and rarely exceed one inch in diameter; large feeding veins are evident, or can be felt as "gutters" through the indurated tissue. A local patch of superficial thrombophlebitis involving the skin is the common precursor of the ulcer. Healing is readily achieved on eradication of the varicosities and subsequent compression support.

The Post-phlebitic Ulcer is a more serious problem. The ulcer penetrates the deep fascia, is often heavily infected, œdematous, and there is widespread avascular scarring, which may shackle the limb. The characteristic ulcer-bearing site—never on the foot—has been given explanation by the anatomical studies of Cockett and Jones (1953). The venous drainage of this skin area, they point out, empties directly into the deep veins of the leg via two or three easily definable perforating veins; the saphenous vein drains only the foot and the upper part of the leg. Valvular incompetence of these perforating veins will lead to reversal of flow and local skin venous hypertension. They have named it the "ankle blow-out syndrome". They advocate eradication of these perforators, i.e. "applying the principle of the Trendelenburg operation to the lower third of the leg". By longitudinal incision down to deep fascia behind the medial malleolus, and commonly including excision of the ulcer area, the perforating branches are exposed and ligated. Their early results are encouraging; but skin incisions in this area heal badly, and there has been reluctance to adopt this procedure. Linton (1952) has for a considerable time stressed the importance of these perforating branches and has employed an even more extensive procedure in the lower leg. By vertical incision extending from the tibial tubercle to below the medial malleolus, the perforators are cleanly dissected and divided, and the ulcer is left untouched; in addition the saphenous veins are stripped, and the deep femoral vein is ligated. Linton's carefully observed results show permanent healing in the majority. Deliberate procedures to expose these perforating branches may, however, be unnecessary. Operation experience indicates that such "blow-outs" are commonly found, either just above or under the ulcer area. With ulcer excision, now common practice, these perforators come within the sweep of the knife.

As already emphasized, the aim in ulcer management is reduction of the state of ambulatory venous hypertension. Elastic adhesive bandaging and walking will partially reduce it and heal the ulcer; but this breaks down again. These measures do not deal with the mechanical problem of the strangling scar tissue mass, which requires wide excision down to muscle, tendon, and periosteum, and then skin grafting. Preliminary cleansing of the ulcer is essential; streptomycin solution (1 in 500) is the most effective local antibiotic. Application of the razor skin grafts is preferably delayed a few days, for bleeding will interfere with the skin-take. Lumbar sympathectomy is a valuable additional measure for improving the local skin texture; saphenous neurectomy may be necessary to complete the denervation of the medial side of the calf. Boyd (1950) found that with excision of the ulcer area only, 50 per cent. of cases relapsed, but 90 per cent. were cured if sympathectomy was done as well. Main vein ligations, femoral or popliteal, have proved disappointing for such ulceration.

Arteriosclerotic Ulcers. These commonly occur in association with hypertensive disease. A painful red plaque, which later becomes blue, appears on the extensor aspect of the leg, or on the calf, and breaks down to form a superficial ulcer; several plaques may coalesce to form a large ulcer. The local skin arterioles are found thrombosed; they heal slowly, with rest. In thromboangiitis obliterans, similar ulcers may develop secondary to local thrombophlebitic skin involvement.

Organic Vascular Lesions

The Arteriosclerotic Limb

Recent studies indicate that a disorder of lipid metabolism may be the mechanism in the genesis of arteriosclerosis. The influence of Heparin, dietary measures, and hormones on such metabolism is now undergoing clinical study. It may be well to point out that cholesterol levels cannot be used as an indication of the total blood lipid levels.

An unsung advance is the popular recognition of the segmental nature of peripheral arteriosclerosis; an isolated toe gangrene commonly means a major arterial block high up the limb. In 1940 Leriche showed that the thrombotic obliteration may indeed be at the aortic bifurcation. Such cases are being increasingly recognized: all the pulses are absent, the limb is pale, fatigues easily, and claudicates, and in the male there is commonly impotence. A remarkable collateral circulation develops and gangrene may not occur for years. Aortography confirms the diagnosis. Extension of the thrombus may block the renal vessels.

To prevent this resection of the aortic bifurcation has been advocated but the proximal grossly arteriosclerotic stump is difficult and dangerous to suture. Sympathectomy by transabdominal approach is the most useful measure. Oudot (1953) and Brock (1953) have successfully excised and grafted such aortic bifurcations. Intensive periarteritis binds the aorta to the adjacent structures; Oudet therefore advises that dissection begins with the division of the common iliacs, and the aortic stripping proceeds upwards; bleeding from damaged collaterals is thus avoided.

In some 10 per cent. of cases the block is in the iliac arteries; a large gutter plaque is found in the common iliac, and the thrombosed external iliac is hard-walled and contracted to the size of a goose quill. The superficial femoral artery is the most frequent site of the arteriosclerotic block. Arteriography studies suggest that this commonly starts and spreads upwards from the adductor hiatus level. The block may also be found in the popliteal artery at the level of the knee-joint and tends to spread downwards to the bifurcation; the prognosis is thus more serious. In the aged, multiple blocks are a common finding; thrombotic spread to the anterior and posterior tibial arteries blocks the re-entrant collaterals and is responsible for many of the limb deaths.

Dos Santos (1949) was the first to attempt removal of the thrombus by vessel incisions and clot milking. Reboul (1951) improved on this by his operation of "disobliterative endoarteriectomy"; the vessel is widely opened, intima and adherent thrombus are stripped, and the patient is heparinized after vessel repair. Forty (1953) has recorded some good results, but in other hands severe heparin bleeding and even limb gangrene have followed. This operation, better termed "intimectomy" or "thrombectomy", has, however, a place for the very local thrombus in a large vessel, such as the iliac artery. Arterial graft replacement of the block, as already discussed, is the ideal procedure. But the generalized nature of the disease makes few cases suitable; the vessel-wall suture holding qualities are poor, multiple blocks may be present, and the general condition frequently will not permit a prolonged procedure. Rob (1953) has found that of cases with suitable radiological appearances, only 15-20 per cent. are clinically suited for surgery. The grafting result may be marred later by fresh thrombotic episodes in other segments of the arterial tree.

The prognosis of the arteriosclerotic as regards life and limb is far better than was formerly believed. Their miseries need not be added to by discussing arterial calcification findings; the vessels may indeed be pipe-stems on the X-ray plate, and yet there be little evidence of defective arterial inflow. Nor should patients be burdened with measures unlikely to improve them. Buerger's exercises are tiring and time-consuming, and may indeed be harmful (Wilkins *et al.*, 1950). Scientific studies indicate that the pressure-suction boot is dangerous, and intermittent venous occlusion machines may lead to venous thrombosis and spread of gangrene.

Thromboangiitis Obliterans

The ætiology is still obscure. The disease varies in extent and severity; it may be fulminating in onset, with rapid involvement of several limbs, or months and years may elapse between thrombotic episodes. Associated segmental fleeting phlebitis occurs in some 50 per cent. of cases, and in the "old" case often heralds a fresh arterial thrombotic attack. A skin nutritional lesion, rather than claudication, is the presenting symptom in 70 per cent. of cases, and ischæmic neuritis often dominates the picture. Three types, according to Boyd's classification, may be recognized: proximal, distal, and mixed types. Kinmonth (1948) in a follow-up study showed that sympathectomy achieves most in the distal types; in the mixed type, with both small and large vessels involved, the results are not as good. In the author's experience, the proximal localized group also do well after sympathectomy; many of these cases are, however, really early arteriosclerotic blocks rather than true Buerger's disease. "Prophylactic" sympathectomy will not affect the spread of the disease to the unaffected limb, although the onset of symptoms may be delayed.

In the upper extremity, as Learmonth (1952) observes, tissue loss never extends proximal to the metacarpophalangeal joint, and that is comforting information to the patient. Continued resting pain in the lower limb after sympathectomy is of serious prognostic import. If associated with marked cold rubor, a below-knee amputation is necessary to obviate months of misery and agony. To make this decision is difficult. Smoking, whether the patient is sympathectomized or not, definitely is an aggravating factor in this disease. Increased stickiness of the platelets after smoking has been demonstrated as characteristic of the true Buerger's disease. In a follow-up of 100 cases, Silbert (1945) found that in every case, where smoking had been given up for ten years, the disease was arrested.

Arterial Embolism

It is a paradox of this decade that with arterial technique in its finest hour, embolectomy has to a large extent been abandoned. The poor surgical results dictated it, and Learmonth (1948) led the crusade against it. Consecutive thrombosis—the "tail clot"—in the main vessel distal to the embolus accounts for the limb death. The reasons for this are as yet not fully understood. Certainly, the distal vessel, empty of blood, assumes a posture of clam-like tight contraction, and the resistance to collateral inflow is thus high. Vessel fiddling in such operations, and a low systemic blood-pressure (except in the aortic embolus), appear to increase and hold such spasm. Clot extension into the collaterals may be another reason. The years to come should bring the answer. Be that as it may, at the moment anticoagulant therapy yields better results. For the upper extremity embolus, anticoagulants almost invariably succeed. Some surgeons begin treatment with a stellate ganglion block, but this seems inadvisable; subsequent heparin-ization has been followed by hæmoptysis, extrapleural hæmatomas, and pleural effusion. Intravenous heparin in high dosage is advisable and should continue for five days, by which time the fate of the limb will have been decided.

For the lower extremity embolus, surgery may become necessary. Heparinization should be started and the limb carefully observed. If at the end of six hours muscle paresis has advanced and the ischæmic signs appear more marked, the embolus requires surgery. This is most frequently the case where the embolus has lodged at the common femoral bifurcation. The embolus, it is now known, often lodges at the adductor hiatus level rather than at the popliteal bifurcation, and arteriography before operation may be advisable. Many of the patients are very ill, and local anæsthesia should preferably be employed. The longitudinal arteriotomy incision should be placed directly over the embolus, and vessel handling and dissection should be gentle; suction tubes should not be passed down the vessel lumen. Interrupted mattress sutures are satisfactory for the arterial wound closure. The use of local 1 per cent. papaverine, by polythene tubing is now being tried. Systemic heparinization should continue after clot removal. In the very ill patient, unfit for surgery, massage of the embolus may dislodge it into a more favourable site; this has worked in brachial and common femoral emboli. Occasionally, as Learmonth (1948) pointed out, there may be pseudo-embolism, i.e. arterial arrest, but no clot. These patients are usually very ill and in terminal state.

Spontaneous recovery from aortic embolism is a rare event. The bilateral femoral approach and retrograde freeing of the clot has now been abandoned. For a time, too, the common iliac artery, exposed extraperitoneally, was the route for such embolectomy. Aortic control is, however, easy, and the recently recorded successful cases have been by direct aortic incision via the transperitoneal route. Heparinization is hazardous after such large vessel suture. When limb death is certain, amputation should not be delayed, for toxic symptoms rapidly develop and the mortality is 50 per cent. "Icing" is a very satisfactory painless method of anæsthesia for amputation in the very ill, e.g. when the embolus follows coronary infarction. Such icing is, however, only for the dead limb, and should not be used as a form of therapy.

Pain in the recovering ischæmic limb may be a serious problem, and associated with claudication, and other ischæmic nerve effects, as described on page 340. Intra-arterial injections of papaverine and priscoline had been advocated for such ischæmic states. The physiological studies of Lynn (1950), however, indicate that this route is of no advantage; the limb blood-flow increase does not last any longer than after an intravenous injection.

Functional Conditions
Raynaud's Phenomenon

The term "disease" is no longer used for such cases. Jepson (1951) made a useful contribution by separating them into primary "idiopathic" and secondary types.

In the *idiopathic type,* usually beginning in the late 'teens, sympathectomy—although indicated in a minority of cases—is still the most satisfactory method of treatment. The bad result is now recognized as not related to inadequacy of operation, regeneration or post-ganglionic sensitization. It is due to the "local fault"; i.e. the digital vessel sensitivity to cold is marked and sympathectomy cannot overcome it. The number of attacks are, however, invariably reduced by sympathectomy, and those induced by emotion are abolished. More prolonged or severe cold is now required to initiate such attacks, but they can be induced even after the most adequate operation, if such cold exposure is sufficiently intense.

Sympathectomy gives the best results in the relatively mild case. These are the ones that one hesitates to operate on, and some workers believe that priscoline is as efficient. The particular indications for operation are as follows: increasing attacks with each fresh spell of cold weather; painful finger ulceration; and incapacitating occupational disability due to numbness and finger clumsiness. In quite 50 per cent. of cases the results are first-class, i.e. the patient is satisfied. Relapses occur usually within the first three to six months, at a time when there is no evidence of neurogenic reactivity or "regeneration".

The *secondary* *(acquired) type* of Raynaud's phenomenon is often secondary to occlusive vascular disease, such as thromboangiitis obliterans, and should always be considered in older patients. These cases do well with sympathectomy. Typical Raynaud's attacks have followed also the use of high speed vibrating tools Sympathectomy will not improve them, and an immediate change of employment is the only useful treatment. Raynaud's phenomenon often precedes the onset of scleroderma and sclerodactylia by many years; sympathectomy gives temporary relief. The rheumatoid type of patient with Raynaud's phenomenon should never be operated on whilst the sedimentation rate is raised; as Jepson points out, pericarditis may develop after operation. The last type to be considered is the middle-aged woman, developing her first Raynaud's attacks at the menopause. These cases frequently do well with hormone therapy; a few, however, come to sympathectomy. Patients rarely complain of dry hands after sympathectomy, but this requires consideration in those employed in paper handling or textile (especially nylon) industries.

Acrocyanosis

These cases are often confused with Raynaud's phenomenon. As the name implies, the hands or feet are cold and cyanotic, and associated with marked hyperidrosis. There is increased tone of the arterioles of the skin at ordinary environmental temperature, with stasis in the subpapillary venous plexus and consequent cyanosis. The exact role of the sympathetic system in the ætiology is uncertain. Most cases respond to local iontophoresis measures; severe cases do well with sympathectomy.

Hyperidrosis in itself may be a problem; sympathectomy forthwith cures it, and may be necessary for reasons of occupation, such as clerking, hairdressing, tailoring, etc. Some cases later complain of excessive sweating in other limbs. Quadruple sympathectomies are, however, to be avoided. The sweating mechanism compensates, and these patients then sweat excessively from the trunk; in hot weather their shirts are drenched and they suffer great discomfort.

Erythrocyanosis Frigidorum

This has become a more common problem. The legs are ice cold, with ugly blue-red diffuse patches and often dreadfully painful chilblains. After a time disfiguring fat pads develop around the ankles and lower legs, and the shapeless limbs have been well described as "billiard table" legs. Local fat saponification may lead to ulceration, often mistakenly labelled Bazin's disease (Telford, 1944). Sympathectomy gives a warm limb, cures the chilblains, and halts further fat deposition, but does not influence the fat depots already present. The operation is well worth while, but needs to be undertaken at an early stage.

Poliomyelitis

Sympathectomy gives an excellent result in the cold blue limb with dreadful chilblains, of the paretic case of poliomyelitis. It may be employed to increase the foot blood-supply before foot arthrodesis. Goetz (1950) declares that sympathectomy should not be done for the hopelessly flail limb: vein tone is abolished, and if the muscles are paralysed, blood-pooling in the veins may be followed by œdema. An elastic stocking readily controls this œdema, and relief of the chilblains makes the operation worth while.

Causalgia

This group may be best divided into major and minor causalgias. In the *major type* there is usually associated nerve injury; the pain is burning, comes on in attacks, is diffuse and not localized to any nerve territory. Sympathectomy, preceded by a sympathetic block test, gives an immediate spectacular result. There are no afferent sympathetic fibres, and the dramatic relief of pain cannot be thus explained. Various theories have been put forward, the most attractive being that of Doupe *et al.* (1944). They declare that in such states the insulation of the closely running sensory nerves and sympathetic fibres breaks down (on account of ischæmia) and an "artificial synapse" forms. A constant barrage of sympathetic impulses now streams up along the afferent somatic paths, producing pain. Sympathectomy breaks the vicious circle.

The *minor causalgias*, often called post-traumatic vasomotor dystrophy or Sudeck's atrophy, are a different problem. The limb is found sometimes cold, sometimes hot, and often slightly œdematous; there may be osteoporosis and at times Raynaud's phenomenon. Blood-flow studies show that the circulation is normal or even better-than-normal. The symptoms commonly date to a minor injury, and as the disability appears out of all proportion, the patient is labelled "functional", or a malingerer. Many are certainly maladjusted individuals, but the author's experience, and that shown in the recent literature, indicates that some of these cases are often deprived of such a valuable measure as sympathectomy. The theoretical rationale is interesting. We start with stimulation of a peripheral sensory nerve area; the summation effect of its many neurone connections builds up a barrage within the spinal cord. Circus movements are started in the internuncial pools of Lorente de No, the overflow spills into the spinal sympathetic system, and the vicious circle continues (Livingston, 1943). Preliminary procaine blocks are not conclusive as to the probable value of a sympathectomy. As Shumacker (1947) showed, gratifying results have followed permanent sympathetic interruption, even though the procaine blocks gave unsatisfactory results.

The Collagen Vascular Diseases

There are no frontiers between Surgery and Medicine, and although this group of diseases commonly comes within the province of the physician, the surgeon has a very definite place in their diagnosis and management. The connective tissues of the body, according to the modern concept, can be regarded as an "organ"; alterations in its structure can account for such apparently unrelated diseases as polyarteritis nodosa, scleroderma, and lupus erythematosus, and they are now grouped into one disorder—the collagen diseases. Collagen is an extracellular product of the fibroblast and is present in the collagenous fibres and the homogeneous matrix substance. In polyarteritis nodosa, the collagen fibres in the vessel wall swell, become eosinophilic, later fragment and undergo "fibrinoid necrosis"; associated with this is a fibroblastic proliferation and inflammatory response, i.e. there is both necrosis and repair. This necrotizing arteritis is diffuse, and the term "periarteritis", as commonly used, is therefore incorrect. In scleroderma the proliferative fibroblast reaction is more pronounced, and dense fibrous tissue is laid down, i.e. the fibrosis of repair is paramount. In disseminated lupus erythematosus the proliferative reaction is small and the destruction of collagen fibres great, i.e. destruction and no repair (Mann, 1953).

The clinical features do not require detailed consideration. Polyarteritis nodosa may occur secondary to an allergic reaction and has been reported after serum sickness. This type is less fatal than commonly supposed, and the mortality is said to be only 50 per cent. (Grant, 1940). More commonly the ætiology is obscure, and the disease may present itself as hypertension, as pyrexia of unknown origin, or even as an unexplained peripheral neuritis (mononeuritis multiplex). Small aneurysms may develop, but are rarely found in the limbs; more commonly, they occur on the splenic artery and give rise to intra-abdominal bleeding. In scleroderma, the contracted fingers and rigid facial mask are well known, but widespread visceral manifestations are found in addition. Goetz (1945) has therefore proposed the name "progressive systemic sclerosis". The diagnosis of lupus erythematosus can now be established with certainty by the finding of the characteristic "L.E. cell" in the bone-marrow smear as described by Hargraves (1948). The "L.E. cell" is a polymorphonuclear cell, which shows a peculiar inclusion-body, staining blue with hæmatoxylin.

Cortisone came as a new hope for these cases. A few of the results have been encouraging; healed lesions have been found, and the disastrous effects are now realized as due to obliterative fibrosis healing of affected vessels of the heart and kidneys. Early diagnosis may yet make it possible to abort or ameliorate such fibrous healing.

Sol. M. Cohen

References

ABRAMSON, D. I. (1944) *Vascular Responses in the Extremities of Man in Health and Disease.* Chicago.

ALLEN, A. W. (1953) *Surg. Gynec. Obstet.* **96**, 107.

ANNING, S. T. (1949) *Brit. med. J.* **2**, 458.

ATKINS, H. B. J. (1949) *Lancet* **2**, 1152.

DE BAKEY, M. E., and SEMIONE, F. A. (1946) *Ann. Surg.* **12**, 534.

BARCROFT, H., BOWMAN, W., EDHOLM, O. G., and EFFRON, A. S. (1943) *J. Physiol.* **102**, 21.

BARCROFT, H., and EDHOLM, O. G. (1946) *Lancet* **2**, 513.

BARCROFT, H., and HAMILTON, G. T. C. (1948) *Lancet* **1**, 441.

BARCROFT, H., and DORNHORST, A. C. (1948) *J. Physiol.* **108**, 39.

BARCROFT, H., and WALKER, A. J. (1949) *Lancet* **1**, 1035.

BAUER, G. (1950) *Angiology* **1**, 1.

BAUER, G. (1950) *Brit. med. J.* **2**, 318.

BAZETT, H. C., LOVE, L., NEWTON, M., EISENBERG, L., DAY, R., and FOSTER, R. (1948) *J. Appl. Physiol.* **1**, 1.

BOYD, A. M. (1950) *Brit. med. J.*, **2**, 269.

BOYD, A. M., and ROBERTSON, D. J. (1947) *Brit. med. J.* **2**, 452.

BOYD, A. M., RATCLIFFE, A. H., JEPSON, R. P., and JAMES, G. W. M. (1949) *J. Bone Jt. Surg.* **31**B, 325.

BOYD, A. M., JEPSON, R. P., RATCLIFFE, A. H., and ROSE, S. S. (1952) *Angiology* **3**, 207.

BOYD, J. D., and MONRO, P. A. G. (1949) *Lancet* **2**, 892.

BROCK, R. C. (1953) *Proc. R. Soc. Med.* **46**, 115.

BURTON, A. C. (1939) *Am. J. Physiol.* **127**, 337.

COCKETT, F. B., and JONES, D. E. E. (1953) *Lancet* **1**, 17.

COHEN, S. M. (1944) *Lancet* **1**, 1.

COHEN, S. M., EDHOLM, O. G., HOWARTH, S., McMICHAEL, J., and SHARPEY-SCHAFER, E. P. (1948) *Clin. Sci.* **7**, 35.

*COHEN, S. M. (1952) *Ann. R.C.S.* **11**, 1.

*COHEN, S. M. (1953) *Ibid.*, **12**, 96.

CUMMINE, H., and LYONS, R. N. (1948) *Brit. J. Surg.* **38**, 337.

DORNHORST A. C. and SHARPEY-SCHAFER, E. P. (1951) (*a*) *Clin. Sci.* **10**, 371.

DORNHORST, A. C., and SHARPEY-SCHAFER, E. P. (1951) (*b*) *Lancet* **1**, 81.

DOUPE, J., CULLEN, C. H., and CHANCE, G. Q. (1944) *J. Neurol. Psychiat.* **1**, 33.

DRINKER, C. (quoted by Allen, A. W.) (1953) *Surg. Gynec. Obstet.* **96**, 107.

Editorial (1952) *Brit. med. J.* **1**, 93.

EDWARDS, E. A., and CRANE, C. (1951) *New Engl. J. Med.* **244**, 199.

EJRUP, B. (1948) *Amer. Heart J.* **35**, 41.

ELKIN, D. C. (1946) *Surg. Gynec. Obstet.* **82**, 1.

FORTY, F. (1953) *Proc. R. Soc. Med.* **46**, 125.

FREEMAN, N. E., LEEDS, F. H., and GARDNER, R. E. (1947) *Ann. Surg.* **126**, 873.

* The Author is indebted to the Editor of the *Annals of The Royal College of Surgeons* for permission to use illustrations and material from these articles.

GATCH, W. D. (1950) *Arch. Surg.* **61**, 34.
GOETZ, R. H. (1950) *Circulation* **1**, 56.
GOETZ, R. H., and AMES, F. (1949) *Arch. Int. Med.* **84**, 36.
GROSS, R. E. (1951) *Ann. Surg.* **134**, 753.
GROSS, R. E., BILL, A. H., and PIERCE, E. C. (1949) *Surg. Gynec. Obstet.* **88**, 689.
HAILE, J. (1946) *Lancet* **2**, 85.
HARGRAVES M. M., RICHMOND, H., and MORTON, R. (1948) *Proc. Mayo Clinic*, **23**, 25.
HAXTON, H. A. (1947) *Brit. J. Surg.* **35**, 69.
HAXTON, H. A. (1949) *Brit. med. J.* **1**, 1026.
HOLMAN, E. (1950) *Angiology* **1**, 530.
HUFNAGEL, C. A., and EASTCOTT, H. H. G. (1952) *Lancet* **1**, 541.
INGRAM, P. W. (1936) *Edin. med. J.* **43**, 672.
JEPSON, R. P. (1951) *Ann. R.C.S.* **9**, 35.
JULIAN, O. C., DYE, W. E., OLIVEN, J. H., and JORDAN, P. W. (1952) *Ann. Surg.* **136**, 459.
JULIAN, O. C., DE TAKATS, G., and DEY, W. E. (1953) *Angiology* **4**, 12.
KINMONTH, J. B. (1948) *Lancet* **2**, 717.
KINMONTH, J. B., and HADFIELD, C. B. (1952) *Brit. med. J.* **1**, 1377.
KINMONTH (1952) *Brit. med. J.* **1**, 59.
KIRGIS, H. D., and KUNTZ, A. (1942) *Arch. Surg.* **44**, 95.
KUNKEL, P., and STEAD, E. A. (1938) *J. Clin. Invest.* **17**, 715.
LEARMONTH, J. R. (1948) *Edin. med. J.* **55**, 449.
LEARMONTH, J. R. (1950) *Lancet* **2**, 505.
LEARMONTH, J. R. (1952) Vasc. Congress, Strasbourg.
LERICHE, R., and MOREL, A. (1948) *Ann. Surg.* **127**, 193.
LINTON, R. R. (1952) *Angiology* **3**, 431.
LINTON, R. R., and HARDY, C. B. (1948) *Surgery* **24**, 452.
LIVINGSTON, W. K. (1943) "Pain Mechanisms." Macmillan Co., New York
LOCKHART-MUMMERY, H. E., and SMITHAM, J. H. (1951) *Brit. J. Surg.*, **38**, 284.
LOEWE, L., BERGER, L., and LASSER, R. P. (1951) *Angiology* **2**, 26.
LYNN, R. B. (1950) *Lancet* **2**, 676.
LYNN, R. B., and DARCROFT, H. (1950) *Lancet* **1**, 1109.
MACKENZIE, I., and HAMILTON, H. A. R. (1953) *Brit. J. Surg.* **40**, 442.
MANN, W. N. (1953) *Guy's Hosp. Gaz.* **67**, 175.
MAYBURY, B. C. (1944) *Brit. med. Bull.* **2**, 142.
MURLEY, R. S. (1950) *Ann. R.C.S.*, **6**, 283.
MURLEY, R. S. (1951) *Lancet* **2**, 176.
MUSTARD, W. J. (1946) *Ann. Surg.* **124**, 46.
NORTHFIELD, D. W. C., and MONRO, P. A. G. (1953) *Brit. med J.* **1**, 727.
OCHSNER, A. (1949) *Lancet* **2**, 963.
OUDOT, J. (1953) *Arch. Surg.* **66**, 365.
PARKES, A. R. (1945) *Brit. J. Surg.* **32**, 403.
PICKERING, G. W. (1951) *Lancet* **2**, 845.
PIERCE, E. C. (1952) *Ann. Surg.* **136**, 228.
RAPAPORT, S. I., FRANK, H. A., and MASSEL, T. B. (1950) *Circulation* **2**, 1506.
RAY, B. S., HENSEY, J. C., and GEOHEGAN, W. A. (1943) *Ann. Surg.* **118**, 647.
REBOUL, H., and LAUBURY, P. (1950) *Proc. R. Soc. Med.* **43**, 547.
ROB, C. G. (1953) *Proc. R. Soc. Med.* **46**, 115.
ROSE, S. S. (1953) *Brit. med. J.* **1**, 247.
DOS SANTOS, J. C. (1949) *Presse Med.* **57**, 544.
SEMPLE, R., and WHITESIDE, C. Q. (1951) *Arch. Middlesex Hosp.* **1**, 9.
SHUMACKER, H. B. (1942) *Bull. Johns Hopk. Hosp.* **71**, 1.
SHUMACKER, H. B., and CARTER, K. L. (1946) *Surgery* **20**, 9.
SHUMACKER (1947) *Surg. Gynec. Obstet.* **84**, 739.

SKOOG, T. (1947) *Lancet* **2**, 457.
SILBERT, S. (1945) *J.A.M.A.* **102**, 11.
SZILAGYI, D. E., JAY, G. D., and MUNNEL, E. D. (1951) *Arch. Surg.* **61**, 732.
DE TAKATS, G. (1944) *Surg. Gynec. Obstet.* **79**, 359.
TELFORD, E. D. (1944) *Proc. R. Soc. Med.* **37**, 621.
TOOHEY, M. (1953) *Brit. med. J.*, **1**, 650.
WALKER, A. J. (1950) *Brit. med. J.* **2**, 1307.
WALKER, A. J., and LONGLAND, C. J. (1950) *Clin. Sci.* **9**, 101.
WILKINS, R. W., HALPERIN, M. H., and LITTER, J. (1950) *Circulation* **2**, 373.
WRIGHT, H. P. (1947) *Proc. R. Soc. Med.* **40**, 197.
WRIGHT, H. P., and KUBIK, M. D. (1953) *Brit. med. J.* **1**, 1021.

CHAPTER XXVIII

THE INFECTED HAND

THE loss of his right thumb may be more grievous to a patient than the loss of his right leg. Yet in spite of the pioneer work of Kanavel and Iselin the infected hand has traditionally been the province of the recently qualified houseman, who made a hurried incision under gas anæsthesia in the Casualty Department. Since the second World War, however, the unsatisfactory treatment of the infected hand, with its attendant suffering and economic waste, has been realized, and efforts made to remedy it. The advent of the antibiotics was a spur to this trend, but the greatest advances have been in a reconsideration of the pathology and the principles of treatment and the setting up of special clinics for the treatment of the septic hand.

The commonest infecting organism is the staphylococcus aureus, but various staphylococci, the bacillus coli, and the bacillus proteus are occasionally found. A recent cut, prick, burn or abrasion is often the obvious portal of infection, but more commonly the source of infection cannot be determined. Phage typing has shown that the infecting organisms are often identical with those normally inhabiting the patient's naso-pharynx, but whether they reach the subcutaneous tissues of the hand by the blood stream or through microscopical injuries in the skin is unknown.

Classification

The lesions of the infected hand may be conveniently classified as follows:

1. Paronychia.
2. Apical abscess.
3. Pulp abscess or subcutaneous abscess of the finger.
4. Web space infection.
5. Palmar abscess.
6. Tendon sheath infection.
7. Osteitis and acute arthritis.
8. Carbuncle.
9. Erysipeloid.

Paronychia

Acute paronychia is by far the commonest of the septic lesions of the hand, amounting to about a third of all such lesions. The infection starts under the proximal end of the lateral nail fold, and at first is nearly always subcuticular, being contained by the adherence of the eponychium to the base of the nail; occasionally it burrows more deeply into the subcutaneous tissue of the nail fold. If untreated at this stage the abscess spreads like a collar under the proximal nail fold superficial to the base of the nail, but even more often it extends under the base of the nail. The affected part of the nail is lifted from its bed, and being separated from its growing end, becomes a devitalized foreign body.

Chronic paronychia is an indolent form of paronychia which is common, incapacitating, and resistant to treatment. Its onset is insidious, seldom being associated with an attack of acute paronychia, and the condition may already have been present for months before the patient seeks treatment. By this time the nail fold is fissured and œdematous, and the nail irregular and eroded. In some cases there is an intermittent discharge of thin sero-pus, and in others a mass of granulations between nail and nail fold; frequently the whole attached margin of the nail fold is affected. Many attempts have been made to incriminate a fungus as the cause, but these have not often been successful. The lesion not infrequently is quite dry, and in these circumstances no organisms at all can be recovered.

Apical Abscess

Often misdiagnosed and unsuccessfully incised as a pulp infection, the apical abscess is an exquisitely painful lesion which forms between the distal part of the nail and the dorsum of the terminal phalanx, and points at the tip of the finger immediately under the end of the nail.

Abscess.

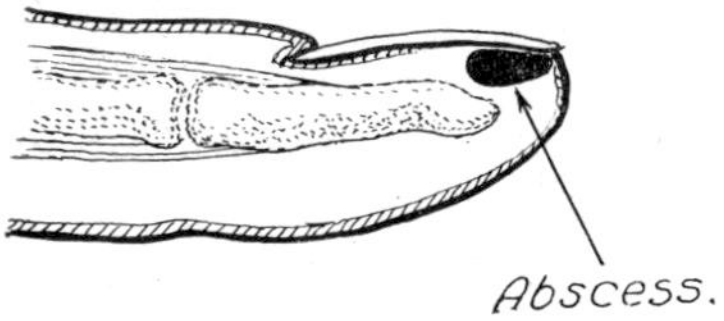

Fig. 28.1. Sagittal section of terminal phalanx to show site of apical abcess.

In the early stages, the terminal segment of the digit is tense, shiny, throbbing, red and very painful, but only a little swollen. Tenderness is greatest just under the end of the nail, where later a patch of discoloration appears; at the same time discoloration is often discernible through the nail itself. The abscess is often very small, out of all proportion to the pain it causes, but frequently it extends proximally some distance under the nail to the dorsum of the distal phalanx.

Pulp Abscess

Pulp infection of the terminal segment is second only to acute paronychia in frequency of occurrence, and together these two lesions account for approximately half of all septic conditions of the hand.

The middle and proximal pulp spaces are less frequently affected. The infection starts in the pulp or subcutaneous tissue on the volar aspect of the finger, and an abscess quickly forms between the skin superfically and the flexor tendon sheath deeply. The fibrous septa traversing the pulp tend to limit the spread of the infection, especially at the interphalangeal creases (Wilkinson, 1950), though it may spread from one phalanx to another. Confined by these septa, tension rises in the abscess and causes the characteristic throbbing pain. In severe cases, the tension may lead to interference with the blood supply and consequent necrosis, resulting in the formation of a slough as well as pus. It is this interference with the blood supply which may also be responsible for the spread of the infection to the underlying tendon sheath and bone. Slough formation may not necessarily be due to interference with the blood supply, however; it may occur in quite small and superficial lesions, and is due to the local virulence of the organism. Disability and loss of function may be severe, and in such cases lymphangitis, spreading up the arm, tender enlargement of the epitrochlear and axillary lymph nodes, and constitutional upset with fever and malaise, are not infrequent. If untreated, a pulp abscess tends to point through a patch of devitalized skin on the volar surface of the finger near the midline, and not laterally; this fact is of considerable importance when planning surgical treatment.

Simple subcuticular abscesses—septic blisters—do occur as a clinical entity, and need no more treatment than removal of the elevated cuticle. More often, however, a subcuticular collection of pus is the result of a pulp abscess which has burst through the true skin to form a collar stud abscess. Such subcuticular abscesses are therefore deceptive, and must be carefully examined for a deep pulp extension.

Web Space Infection

The web space infection is an abscess in the web of the finger between the bases of the proximal phalanges; sometimes it is due to the spread along the lumbrical canal of a pulp abscess of the proximal phalanx. The symptoms are often severe, with separation of the fingers, swelling of the back of the hand, immobility of the hand as a whole, and constitutional disturbance (Fig. 2). Tenderness is maximal either on the dorsum of the web just proximal to its distal edge, or anteriorly opposite the base of the proximal phalanx where blisters commonly occur. It would appear that such a blister becoming infected is often the starting point of a web space abscess. As the lesion progresses, pus reaches the surface at these two sites, or tracks distally along the site of the proximal phalanx.

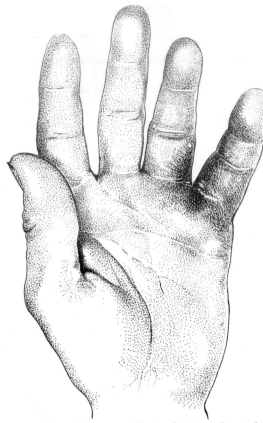

FIG. **28**.2. Web space infection between ring and little fingers.

Anatomically there is direct continuity between the web and the deep palmar spaces, and theoretically infection of the former might easily lead to infection of the latter. In practice, however, this complication seldom occurs.

Palmar Abscess

An abscess may occur anywhere in the subcutaneous tissues of the palm, and even if it originates deep to the palmar aponeurosis it does not necessarily follow that the thenar or mid-palmar spaces are affected. Many palmar abscesses are found in the superficial palmar space between the aponeurosis superficially and the flexor tendons deeply (Birks, 1945). Spontaneous infection of the deep palmar spaces is probably rare; the importance of these spaces lies in the fact that they are liable to infection from penetrating wounds of the hand, and from direct extension along anatomical pathways from tendon sheath and web space infections.

The skin and palmar fascia are firmly adherent, and infection under them is characterized by a dusky painful induration of the affected area, severe œdematous swelling of the dorsum of the hand, immobility of the hand and fingers, and constitutional disturbance.

Tendon Sheath Infection

Acute tenosynovitis appears to be less common than formerly, and it is possible that its previous frequency was the result of unskilful incision of pulp abscesses under gas. In two recent series at a septic hand clinic the incidence was 3 per 1,000 of all cases. Trauma is an important factor in the ætiology, the infection being introduced by a splinter or puncture wound which has pierced the theca.

The clinical picture is well defined. There is usually either a clear history of trauma or there are obvious signs of a severe pulp infection, extension of which has involved the tendon sheath. The whole finger is swollen, red and painful, and presents a fusiform or spindle-shaped appearance. Movements are very painful and it is held immobile. Two physical signs are of great diagnostic importance; excruciating pain on full extension of the terminal phalanx, and tenderness in the palm over the proximal end of the tendon sheath; in the thumb and little finger, tenderness may extend the length of the radial and ulnar bursæ.

Osteitis and Acute Arthritis

Infection of bone is rare except in the terminal phalanx; pyogenic arthritis is rarer still, and probably occurs most frequently in the distal interphalangeal joint as the result of direct spread from osteitis of the terminal phalanx or a penetrating injury. Osteitis is usually considered to be a complication of a neglected pulp abscess, but it is possible that it can arise as a primary blood-borne osteo-myelitis of the phalanx.

Clinically infection of bone is suggested by club-shaped swelling of the terminal phalanx, accompanied by moderate local symptoms. The periosteum and the volar surface of the bone become eroded, and these changes show on an X-ray plate. Sequestrum formation may take place, and finally the terminal phalanx becomes converted into a bag of pus with complete destruction of the pulp and much of the bone. It is not unusual for the skin in such instances to yield, and the patient presents with a discharging sinus at the tip of a club-shaped angry looking phalanx which is, however, comparatively painless owing to the spontaneous relief of tension.

Carbuncle

With the exception of paronychia, nearly all infective lesions on the dorsum of the hand and fingers are carbuncles. They occur on the hair-bearing part of the hand, and most frequently on the dorsum of the proximal phalanx. They differ in pathology and treatment from the other lesions described, and it is therefore important that their true nature is recognized. A carbuncle begins as a localized red patch of painful induration, usually on the back of the proximal phalanx. As the infection spreads the cuticle tends to be lifted off the true skin by thin sero-pus, and if the cuticle at this stage is removed the discharge will be seen issuing from a number of small sinuses deep to which lies a yellow necrotic slough. This slough is at first solid and adherent, and pus discharge is minimal. Later the sinuses tend to coalesce owing to destruction of the overlying skin, and the slough separates and is discharged.

Erysipeloid

Like carbuncle, recognition of erysipeloid is important because its pathology and treatment are different from other infections of the hand; unlike carbuncle, however, its recognition is not always easy. It is due to infection through a skin abrasion by the erysipelothrix rhusiopathiæ of Rosenbach.

It is almost an occupational disease of fishmongers, poultry dealers, cooks and, to a lesser extent, butchers, though it is not exclusively limited to these occupations. The lesion is usually confined to the fingers, though it may spread on to the hand. The affected finger is a little swollen, and dusky red in colour. The swelling, characteristically, has a well defined proximal margin, and this margin advances with the infection. Symptoms are not severe; itching, stiffness and discomfort are more complained of than pain. Tenderness is present, but it also is not severe, and is felt all over the affected part of the finger. It is the contrast between the mildness of the symptoms and the angry appearance of the finger which often first suggests the diagnosis. The healed scar of a recent abrasion can nearly always be found, though the hands of typical sufferers often present with multiple abrasions resulting from handling poultry, fish and game.

Erysipeloid is a low grade infection of the skin and subcutaneous tissue. Pus is never found. It is a self limiting disease, lasting from a few days to three or four weeks, but relapse is common.

Treatment

An infected finger carries with it the menace of prolonged disability, deformity, stiffness or loss of the finger, crippling of the hand, and in extreme cases loss of the arm and even general septicæmia and death. The danger of fatal septicæmia has been greatly reduced since the advent of antibiotics, but it is clear that treatment must be prompt, efficient, and skilful. It must be remembered that a permanent stiff finger is not only useless; it is also a hindrance to the movements of the hand as a whole, and for this reason usually requires amputation.

General principles of treatment

The majority of infected lesions of the hand require surgical intervention for the evacuation of pus, and the general principles of treatment will be discussed (Pilcher *et al.*, 1948; Bailey, 1952; Robins, 1952).

Bloodless Field

Surgical exploration must be carried out at leisure in a bloodless field. Only under these conditions can the lesion be thoroughly explored and dealt with, and damage to other structures, especially tendon sheaths, digital nerves, and arteries, be avoided. To obtain a bloodless field in the fingers and thumb, all that is necessary is a length of thin rubber tubing drawn tightly round the base of the digit and held in position on the dorsum by a pair of Spencer Wells' forceps. For the hand, a sphygmomanometer is applied to the arm above the elbow and, after the whole limb has been elevated for a few moments, inflated to a pressure of 200 mm. of mercury.

Anæsthesia

Proper anæsthesia is essential. It is sometimes tempting to incise an apparently superficial subcuticular abscess without an anæsthetic, only to be confronted with a collar stud abscess extending from the pulp. There is no place for a quick stab under ethyl chloride spray, a method in which the surgery and the anæsthesia are alike deficient. The anæsthetic may be either general or local. For lesions of the hand, web space, and proximal phalanx, it is usually best to employ general anæsthesia, though local anæsthesia can be obtained by injecting round the median, ulnar and radial nerves at the wrist. For the terminal and middle phalanges, however—and it is the terminal phalanx which is affected in over 50 per cent. of all cases—local anæsthesia is ideal. It permits the patient to be treated immediately by the surgeon, and the whole procedure is carried out with both patient and surgeon comfortably sitting down and without hurry. The patient is able to co-operate by moving the finger as required, and the services of an anæsthetist are dispensed with. The procedure is without danger, more than 2,000 local injections of anæsthetic having been given in the writer's clinic over the last four years without ill effect.

The technique is as follows: a thin rubber tourniquet is first applied tightly round the base of the finger and held in place by a pair of Spencer Wells' forceps on the dorsum. The skin at the site of injection is cleaned with cetavlon or surgical spirit. Procaine hydrochloride 2 per cent. without adrenalin is used, and 2 ml. is all that is required. A No. 17 Record needle $\frac{9}{10}$ in. is satisfactory; it is introduced into the lateral side of the proximal phalanx a little anteriorly, and directed towards the digital nerve; $\frac{3}{4}$ to 1 ml. of procaine is injected and then, with the finger held a little flexed, the point of the needle is advanced anterior to the tendon sheath to the opposite side of the finger, and another $\frac{3}{4}$ to 1 ml. injected around the other digital nerve. Anæsthesia is complete in 7 to 10 minutes, and lasts for about half an hour. Except occasionally in the thumb, where each side may require separate injection, it will be noted that only one prick is necessary (Fig. 3).

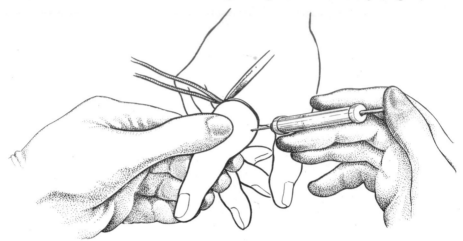

Fig. 28.3.   Technique of anæsthetizing a finger.

Instruments

Fine instruments are essential. The average "casualty" set is too big and cumbersome for hand work. A narrow pointed Bard Parker No. 11 blade is ideal, the only other necessities being fine $4\frac{1}{2}$ in. forceps, toothed and untoothed, a pair of $4\frac{3}{4}$ in. sharp pointed scissors, and a fine blunt probe (Fig. 4).

Incision

The timing, site, and extent of the incision are matters of great importance. If pus is obviously present, it should be evacuated as soon as possible. It is not always easy to be certain, however, whether the infection is still in the early stage of cellulitis or has advanced to pus formation. If in doubt, it is best to make a small exploratory incision, for under such circumstances pus is more often found than not. If pus is not found, the small exploratory incision does no harm; on the other hand, if pus is present but not drained, the patient is condemned to another day's pain, another sleepless night, and longer disability.

Usually the best site for incision is the place where pus is obviously pointing through the skin; if pus is not pointing, incision should be made at the most tender area of the lesion. In the first instance the skin is already partly devitalized by the infection; in the second the pus is nearest the surface at the most tender point. The long classical

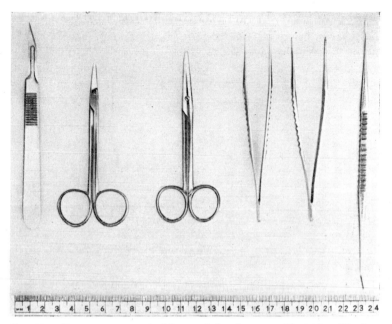

Fig. 28.4. Instruments required for septic hand surgery: No. 11 Bard Parker scalpel, $4\frac{3}{4}$ in. pointed scissors, curved scissors, $4\frac{1}{2}$ in. toothed and plain forceps, and fine Watson Cheyne probe.

lateral incisions are not only unnecessary; many of them are fundamentally unsound because they transgress the natural barriers of the infection, do not drain well, and often leave an unsightly and tender linear scar. The least damage to normal tissues, and the best drainage, is provided by a circular hole in the skin over the centre of the abscess. Unlike a straight incision, the edges do not tend to fall together and prevent drainage, and when the infection has subsided such a wound heals rapidly from the perimeter and leaves a minute scar. Such holes are best made, after determining the extent of the abscess, by removing from its roof a disc of skin, which is often already partly devitalized, with a small pointed scalpel held at right angles to the skin. Alternatively an exploratory incision can be extended to provide adequate drainage by paring its edges to make the wound roughly diamond shaped. All pus and sloughs are carefully and completely removed from the abscess cavity, and when this procedure is adopted there is but little subsequent discharge from the wound.

In some centres formal excision of the whole abscess cavity is practised, followed by suture of the skin incision. The results are claimed to be excellent (Louden *et al.*, 1948; Scott, 1952).

Drainage

There is no room in the fingers, and little in the palm, for the insertion of drains of any kind. They tend to obstruct rather than promote free drainage, and by their very presence they prolong suppuration. They are also painful. If adequate drainage has been provided as described above they are unnecessary, and for these reasons drains should never be used.

Dressings

There is no place for fomentations or frequent wet dressings, for they make the skin soggy and unhealthy, do not absorb discharges, and provide an excellent nidus for the growth of bacteria. Similarly, once the abscess has been evacuated, the local application of antiseptics is unnecessary; even powdered penicillin in lactose tends to clog the wound and obstruct drainage. Vaseline gauze makes the skin of the hand particularly soggy, but it is the kindest dressing to apply initially after removal of a nail and in children. In wounds from which further discharge is anticipated, gauze soaked in hygroscopic glycerine and magnesium sulphate solution is probably the best dressing for a day or two. Otherwise, sterile dry gauze is the best dressing; it is simple, comfortable, absorbs any discharge, and can be removed without pain. Dressings should be infrequent in an ordinary case, on the day after incision and thereafter every two or three days. If the abscess has been properly evacuated initially subsequent discharge is absent or slight, and frequent change of dressing is unnecessary; on the other hand, frequent dressings delay healing and increase the risk of secondary infection. For dressings, as for incisions, the surgeon should always wear a mask.

Movements

Absolute immobilization of the part is practised by some surgeons (Gordon, 1950), a plaster of paris cast being the most efficient means of achieving this. For serious infections of the palm immobilization should be adopted, but for lesions of the fingers the practice is open to criticism. An immobilized finger, especially in older people, very rapidly becomes stiff, and it may be months before full movement is regained; it is remarkable indeed how quickly a finger in which only the terminal phalanx is inflamed will become stiff, and for this reason it is considered that early active movement should be encouraged in uncomplicated lesions of the fingers. The lesion may take a day or two longer to heal, but this is more than offset by the early return of full movement. Sufficient support for the majority of cases is provided by the dressings and a sling.

Antibiotics

It has been customary since its advent to treat all infected lesions of the hand with intramuscular penicillin, which is the antibiotic of choice for staphylococcal and streptococcal infections. Considerable evidence (Harrison *et al.*, 1949; Grossmark *et al.*, 1945) has been produced to show that it modifies the severity of the lesion, reduces complications, and accelerates healing. Penicillin will not, however, cause pus to disappear once it has formed, though it may sterilize a small collection, and in the majority of cases pus is already present when the patient is first seen. Furthermore, penicillin resistant strains of staphylococci and streptococci, which together cause some 95 per cent. of all infections of the hand, are increasing in frequency. In a recent survey (1952) of 271 unselected infective lesions of the hand and fingers, in no less than 77, or 32 per cent., was the infecting organism insensitive to penicillin. Finally, in well localized minor lesions which have been adequately drained, healing in any event is rapid, and the administration of parenteral penicillin is unnecessary, wasteful, and perhaps even dangerous because it might render the patient's habitual staphylococci resistant to the drug.

It is considered, therefore, that systemic penicillin should be reserved for the more severe lesions, such as carbuncles and web space, palmar and tendon sheath infections, and for those cases in which spread of the infection beyond the initial lesion is indicated by lymphangitis, axillary adenitis, and constitutional disturbance. In every case the sensitivities of the infecting organism should be determined as soon as possible. If the organism is resistant to penicillin it may yet be sensitive to other antibiotics, particularly streptomycin, aureomycin and chloramphenicol, and these should then be administered as indicated by the sensitivity tests.

The Treatment of Individual Lesions

Acute Paronychia

The eponychium, or fold of cuticle adhering to the base of the nail, is gently pushed back with a blunt probe towards the base and affected side of the nail. This manœuvre usually liberates the pus. Loose cuticle is excised, all pus mopped away, and the cavity examined. If the abscess is small and well localized, this is often all that is necessary. Frequently, however, the abscess will be found to have extended

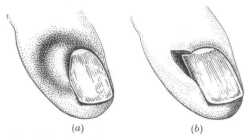

(a)   (b)

FIG. 28.5. Acute localized paronychia (a) and its
treatment by excision of a wedge of nail fold (b).

subcutaneously under the nail fold or under the base of the nail, or both. In the first instance, to prevent pocketing of pus and to provide adequate drainage, a small wedge of the nail fold overlying the abscess must be excised (Fig. 5).

All too often the base of the nail will be found on exploration to be undermined by the infection. This part of the nail is devitalized, and as long as it remains *in situ* the infection will persist, frequently with the formation of a granuloma. Even if only part of the base of the nail is undermined, at least the whole width of the proximal end of the nail must be removed; if only a corner is removed, an irregular, fissured nail results. There is much to be said for total removal of the nail if any part of its root is undermined. Partial removal is less radical and less painful immediately afterwards, but as the new nail grows it grows under and loosens the inert distal end of the old nail, often leading to considerable inconvenience some weeks later.

There is never any need, however severe the paronychia, to make lateral incisions and raise a flap of the skin on the dorsum of the finger.

Chronic Paronychia

The treatment of chronic paronychia is difficult and unrewarding. Occasionally a granuloma or loose nail will need removal, but as a rule there is no indication for surgical interference. Treatment by penicillin, even if a penicillin sensitive staphylococcus has been recovered, is disappointing. The most satisfactory results are obtained by the local application of antiseptics, by irradiation, or by a combination of both these methods. Cetavlon 2 per cent. in 10 per cent. spirit is a suitable antiseptic, and twice a day it should be worked under the nail fold. An orange stick is pared almost to a point, and with it the sulcus between nail fold and nail is opened up as much as possible. Irradiation is given in doses of 100 r. once a week for three or four weeks. This dosage may be repeated after an interval of a month.

Apical Abscess

The only difficulty in treating this painful condition is determining the site of incision, for the collection of pus is characteristically small. Early, however, a patch of devitalized skin appears immediately under the nail, and it is only necessary to remove this and a wedge of the adjoining tip of the nail, the resulting wound being diamond shaped. Occasionally the track of the abscess passes to the dorsum of the bony phalanx, but the bone does not become infected. Healing occurs in two or three days (Fig. 6).

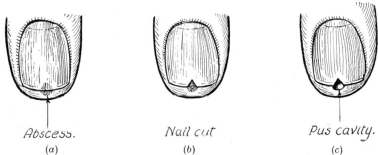

Abscess.	Nail cut	Pus cavity.
(a)	(b)	(c)

FIG. 28.6. Apical abscess (a) and its treatment by excision of the overlying nail (b) and skin (c).

Pulp Abscess

A pulp abscess is incised, as already described, where the skin is already becoming devitalized or where tenderness is greatest. The pus is first located through a small stab wound in the line of the skin creases, and then drainage and complete exploration achieved by removing a small disc of skin over the roof of the abscess. It is important that the full thickness of skin is removed, and the skin edges not merely bevelled. It can be appreciated from the diagram that drainage provided by this simple method is much more efficient and less traumatic to normal tissues than the classical lateral "hockey stick" or "alligator mouth" incision (Fig. 7).

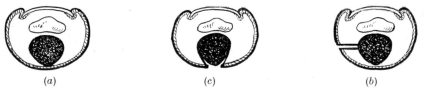

(a)	(c)	(b)

FIG. 28.7. Diagrams to show how a pulp abscess (a) drains better through a hole made directly over it (b) than through a lateral incision (c).

Web Space Infection

Drainage of this abscess depends on where the pus is pointing. If anteriorly, the devitalized skin in the region of the blister over the base of the proximal phalanx is removed. If posteriorly, or if the abscess is not yet pointing, the web is incised in the sagittal plane; this incision, being linear, tends to close spontaneously, so it is necessary to pare away the edges of the wound to a small extent to ensure that it remains open.

Palmar Abscess

Wherever it may lie in the palm, this abscess should be approached by the most direct route. This will be indicated by pus already pointing through the skin, or by the most tender spot. A bloodless field is absolutely essential, as without it not only may the exact situation of the abscess not be determined, but also important structures may be damaged. Initially a small transverse incision in the line of the skin creases is made. This will usually reveal subcutaneous pus which may, however, be found to be coming through a small hole in the palmar aponeurosis from one of the deep spaces. In this instance sufficient of the aponeurosis over the abscess is excised to permit thorough exploration and drainage, and the edges of the skin wound trimmed to a circular or diamond shape to prevent premature healing. If subcutaneous pus is not found, the aponeurosis is carefully incised in the line of the main structures and the same procedure followed.

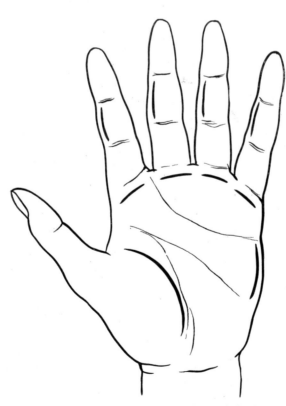

Tendon Sheath Infection

The treatment of acute tenosynovitis is difficult. At best, full function of the finger may result; at worst, the flexor tendons may slough away. Midway between these two extremes, and probably most frequently, the tendons are saved but adhesions form between them and the sheath and movement of the finger is consequently impaired to a greater or a lesser extent.

Any lengthy incision in the sheath will inevitably result in adhesions

FIG. 28.8. Incisions for tendon sheath infections.

and limitation of movement. The aim of surgery is therefore to drain the sheath through as small an incision in it as possible. In the middle three digits, the proximal end of the sheath should first be exposed through a transverse skin incision in the palm over the base of the proximal phalanx, and the sheath opened. Pus is evacuated, aided by "milking" the whole extent of the sheath, and the sheath is then thoroughly irrigated with penicillin solution. This can conveniently be achieved with the use of part of a ureteric catheter. In early cases, especially in those in which the sheath is only mildly distended with clear or semi-purulent fluid, this may be all that is necessary. In severe cases, where there is an obvious wound or a pre-existing pulp infection of the finger, the wound or the pulp abscess should be explored, the sheath exposed, and the same procedure adopted, the sheath being irrigated through from end to end.

The radial bursa is approached through a curved incision over the ball of the thumb, and the ulnar bursa through a lateral incision on the ulnar border of the palm (Fig. 8).

Osteitis

When the terminal phalanx is infected there is usually a sinus already present on the end of the finger; the opening of this should be enlarged and exploration carried out through it. The pulp is characteristically replaced by pus and slough, which must be gently removed. The bone itself should be treated conservatively, for its powers of recovery and regeneration are considerable. Completely detached pieces of bone should be removed, but gentle scraping of the infected portion of the phalanx itself is all that is necessary. Radical removal of all infected bone is likely to result in a formless terminal phalanx.

Carbuncles

Incision has no place in the treatment of carbuncles on the back of the hand and fingers, similar as they are to carbuncles elsewhere. The cuticle early becomes devitalized, and should be removed. Several days later the several sinuses coalesce to form one or two large ones through which the subcutaneous slough may be seen. When it is separated, it can be gently lifted out of its bed; often it comes away with the dressing. Wet hygroscopic dressings, such as compresses of glycerine and magnesium sulphate solution, should be applied daily until the slough separates. Thereafter a dry dressing is all that is necessary until healing has occurred.

Erysipeloid

The most important part of the treatment of this condition is its recognition, and consequently the avoiding of incision. No treatment is necessary, though there is some evidence that systemic penicillin may shorten the course of the disease and prevent relapse (MacDougall, 1951).

HUGH ANDERSON

References:

BAILEY, DAVID (1952) *Lancet* **i,** 167.
BIRKS, P. M. (1945) *Lancet* **ii,** 669.
BOLTON, H., CATCHPOLE, B. N., and JEPSON, R. P. (1947) *Lancet* **ii,** 608.
GORDON, IAN (1950) *Brit. J. Surg.* **38,** 331.
GROSSMARK, G. J., POEWES, L. W. (1945) *Brit. med. J.* **i,** 906.
HARRISON, STEWARD H., TOPLEY, ELIZABETH, and LENNARD-JONES, J. (1949) *Lancet* **i, 425.**
JAMIESON, J. GARDNER (1950) *Brit. J. Surg.* **38,** 193.
LOUDON, J. B., MINIERO, J. D., SCOTT, J. C. (1948) *J. Bone Jt. Surg,* **30B,** 409.
MACDOUGALL, J. A. (1951) *Lancet* **i,** 1345.
PILCHER, R. S., DAWSON, R. L. G., MILSTEIN, B. B., and RIDDELL, A. G. (1948) *Lancet* **i,** 777.
ROBINS, ROBERT H. C. (1952) *J. Bone Jt. Surg.* **34B,** 567.
SCOTT, J. C., and JONES, B. V. (1952) *J. Bone Jt. Surg.* **34B,** 581.
WILKINSON, J. L. (1950-51) *Brit. J. Surg.* **38,** 454.

Books

BUNNELL, S. (1948) "Surgery of the Hand," 2nd ed. Philadelphia, J. B. Lippincott Co.
HANDFIELD-JONES, R. M. (1946) "Surgery of the Hand," 2nd ed. Edinburgh, E. & S. Livingstone, Ltd.
ISELIN, MARC (1940) "Surgery of the Hand," translated by D'Offay, T. M. J., and MOUAT, Thomas B. London, J. & A. Churchill, Ltd.
KANAVEL, ALLEN B. (1939) "Infections of the Hand," 7th ed. Philadelphia, Lea and Febiger.

CHAPTER XXIX

THE INJURED HAND

General Principles

THE general principles governing the treatment of hand injuries differ little from those applicable to general traumatic surgery. Basically, the essentials are:

(1) Efficient surgical cleansing.
(2) Immediate and complete skin cover.
(3) The avoidance of infection by the above means, together with the use of chemotherapy.
(4) Early rehabilitation.

More so than in any other branch of traumatic surgery an immediate assessment of the expected end-result is desirable, for on the primary treatment depends the success of the final result. The hand is a most intricate structure, comprising multiple joints, tendons with their gliding surfaces, small muscles closely co-ordinated for group function, and nerves and skin of a peculiar sensitivity. In a major injury all function cannot be preserved, and it is better to have certain basic functions working well than to try to preserve too much, and so lose mobility by infection or splinting; in the decision as to how much to sacrifice lies the greatest difficulty.

A clear conception of the use to which any hand is to be put is essential. A labourer needs strength of grip, an artisan the ability to grip between index and thumb, and in a musician length and mobility of fingers are essential. Age is an important factor, for in those over 40 procedures involving fixation, such as thenar flaps, lead to joint stiffness; willingness to co-operate is vital where any complicated procedure such as tendon grafting is to be considered, and the mental capacity of the patient, and his economic situation must be borne in mind.

Broadly speaking, the hand has two main functions, the holding of objects between the thumb and fingers—which may be termed the pincers—and the gripping of objects between the fingers and palm—the vice. The pincer action requires an opposable thumb and a digit against which it can move, preferably mobile and preferably on the radial side of the hand, and, it being a fine movement in which tactile discrimination is important, the bearing surfaces should be covered by sensitive hand skin. The vice action is the stronger of the two, and depends for its strength largely on the breadth of the palm. To grip,

379

there must be active flexion and extension of the metacarpo-phalangeal joints of the fingers; the fingers should, if possible, be mobile, but, if this is not possible, they should be flexed at the proximal and distal inter-phalangeal joints; the thumb should, if possible, retain its movement, but, if fixed, should be in the position of function, and out of the way of the flexing fingers.

With these two functional elements in mind, it is possible to lay down certain rules for guidance:

(1) To preserve all possible length of the thumb, and to provide for a free range of active movement at the carpo-metacarpal joint. If the thumb must be fixed, its position must be carefully controlled.

(2) To preserve length of the fingers. The more fingers are involved and the higher the level of amputation, the more important every centimetre of length becomes. Mobility of the fingers is more important on the radial side of the hand, and length on the ulnar.

(3) To preserve breadth of the palm. The fifth finger is the prime mover in clenching and gripping, and even a stump of this finger, unsightly as it may be, adds greatly to the strength of the hand.

(4) Where hand destruction is such that all normal form has been lost, reconstruction is still possible, so long as a mobile thumb stump can be saved. A fixed digit can be built up from the carpus, to provide the second arm of a pincers which is far more useful than any prosthesis.

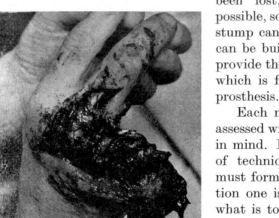

Fig. 29.1. Case 1. Traumatic amputation of the 4th and 5th fingers through the m.p. joints. The wound was grossly contaminated with coal dust. After excision of the wound the 4th and 5th metacarpal shafts were removed to make immediate skin cover possible.

Each major hand injury is first assessed with these broad principles in mind. Before any of the details of technique are considered, one must form a clear idea of the function one is aiming at, and decide what is to be preserved and what may be sacrificed to provide clean healing and early mobility—one must, in fact, make the best of what the press or the rollers have left.

The primary repair of a wound of the hand is essentially no different from that of any other wound—save perhaps that the price paid for inefficient treatment is greater. Functional recovery is dependant upon the avoidance of infection and fibrosis, and this in turn is dependant upon cleansing of the wound and the provision of immediate and complete skin cover (Figs. 1-3). Wound cleansing means a thorough

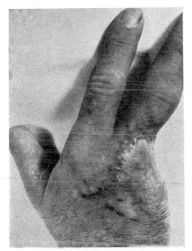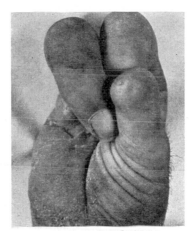

Fig. 29.2-3. Eight weeks later the wounds were soundly healed and the function was excellent, though the narrowing of the palm had resulted in some loss of power.

sterilization of the wound and surrounding skin, and a complete excision of dead and devitalized tissues. In this connection it should be emphasized that it is far better to sacrifice structures which are likely to endanger the rapid healing or hold up the rehabilitation of the rest of the hand, unless their preservation is absolutely essential to the development of the basic hand functions.

Skin Cover

This is undoubtedly the most important single factor in the primary repair. By one means or another complete skin cover *must* be provided at the outset, or infection with its attendant misfortunes is inevitable. The means at our disposal are many. Broadly speaking, the thickest cover consistent with safety should be employed, and where possible, and particularly over the bearing surfaces, full-thickness hand skin cover is most desirable. Nevertheless, it is better to play safe, and, where the blood supply of the base is in any doubt and especially in major crush injuries where œdema and thrombosis of deeper structures may extend far beyond the confines of the primary wound, thin split-skin grafts should be employed, with a view to early full-thickness replacement where necessary later. There will, however, be many cases in which immediate full-thickness repair is safe, or in which split-skin repair is rendered impossible by the presence of structures upon which such grafts will not take; occasionally this last difficulty can be overcome, as when one sacrifices a damaged extensor tendon to make a bed suitable for a thin graft, but there will be many cases in which full-thickness grafting is the method of choice.

Methods of Full-thickness Repair

In general, the wound should be closed wherever possible by rearranging local hand skin, and here some ingenuity may be needed. Where rearrangement is impracticable, skin may be obtained:

(1) by sacrificing damaged phalanges or metacarpals, in order to fillet a finger or narrow a palm;

(2) by rotation or transposition flaps;

(3) by thenar or palmar flaps, where the wound is confined to the terminal phalanges of thumb or fingers, and where not more than two digits are involved.

Sometimes, however, hand skin repair is impossible, and in such cases a direct flap must be obtained from elsewhere. In using direct flaps as a primary procedure the greatest care should be taken to ensure the safety of the flap. There should be no hesitation in sacrificing normal skin to obtain a safe length-breadth ratio, the bed from which the flap was raised and the bare area between bed and insert (the "return-flap") must be completely covered by split-skin graft, and, in the dressing, the flap must be protected from all pressure. The acromio-thoracic flap is by far the best for texture, but it is not suitable in a woman and is not always practicable from a technical point of view. Cross-arm flaps are a good substitute, though they have the disadvantage of growing hair. Abdominal flaps are not successful except in patients with thin abdominal walls, and in children. Neither Wolfe nor dermatome grafts find a place in primary repair, though both may be of value in secondary replacement.

The Treatment of the Underlying Wound

In the treatment of the deeper structures of the hand there are three essentials which must be remembered, and to which all procedures must be contributory:

(1) Complete skin cover. This is so vital a factor that nothing must be done which may prejudice it, and it is frequently

necessary to sacrifice structures in order to make skin cover possible.

(2) Reduction of the risk of infection to a minimum. The débridement must be most careful, and it is better to remove unessential tissue of doubtful viability than hold up the rehabilitation of the hand by slow healing.

(3) Resumption of mobility at the earliest possible moment. This principle, which is of the greatest importance, demands in effect that the primary operation should be as simple as possible, and should consist of excision of tissue, stabilization of bone where necessary, and the provision of skin cover. Tendon repair, though tempting, is more often than not undesirable owing to the increased risk of infection and the need for prolonged post-operative splinting. Where tendon lesions are the major consideration, as in clean wounds of the palm, these principles do not apply, and the methods of repair described by Sterling Bunnell are used.

Nerve repair is well worth while. The amount of buried suture material is negligible, and, unless there is loss of nerve tissue, splinting is unnecessary, so that this repair will not interfere with post-operative movement.

Bone-grafting can be very useful to stabilize a fractured finger or metacarpal, and so permit early active or passive movement; an intra-medullary bone peg made from a discarded phalanx or cut from the ulna takes little time to insert, and is often very useful.

Minor Injuries

Many of these are trivial in character, and require merely adequate cleansing, or excision and suture. Where there is loss of fibro-fatty pulp tissue, partial amputation, or exposure of joint or tendon, other methods must be considered. In many cases, where length of finger or cosmetic reasons are not important, the quickest and most satisfactory treatment will be formal amputation, but as little should be removed in the primary operation as possible—amputation at a higher level can always be done later if desired. In some cases, however, preservation of length is desirable, either for functional or

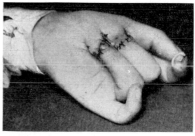

Fig. 29.4. Thenar flaps—skin taken as a direct flap from the thenar eminence to cover defects of the 3rd and 4th fingers. The flap to the 4th finger has been sutured direct to the nail.

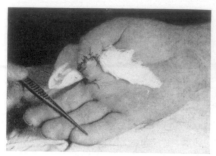

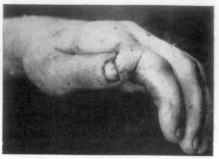

FIG. 29.5. Palmar flap-skin taken from   FIG. 29.6. As an alternative method of
the palm opposite the 2nd m.p. joint to   covering a thumb defect skin may be
cover a defect of the tip of the thumb.   taken from the radial side of the index or
                                           middle finger.

cosmetic reasons, and the use of local skin flaps may be undertaken.
These are:

(1) Thenar flaps (Fig. 4)—skin taken as a direct flap from the
thenar eminence to cover a finger stump. The finger must be
long enough to reach the site of grafting, and the operation
should not be considered in the elderly or arthritic; manual
labourers, in whom the hand skin is thick and horny, are
also unsuitable. Two fingers of the same hand may be treated
by this method.

(2) Palmar flaps (Fig. 5)—skin from the palm over the front of
the second metacarpo-phalangeal joint to cover a thumb
defect; alternately, a defect of the tip of the thumb can be
covered by a skin-flap raised on the radial side of the index
or middle finger (Fig. 6).

(3) Cross-finger flaps—skin from the dorsum of one finger to
cover a defect on the palmar surface of an adjacent finger.
This method has little application, because of the risk of
stiffness in the donor finger.

Free skin-grafts, split-skin or Wolfe, have a smaller field of application.
These grafts are not satisfactory for replacement of the specialized skin
of the pulp surfaces or over exposed joints or tendons, but may be used
for replacement of skin loss on the dorsum or palm of the hand.

Tendon Injuries

In general, the principles of Bunnell are followed, and the exact
method to be recommended will vary according to the tendon involved
and the level of injury.

Flexor Tendons

Fingers. (1) Severed flexor profundus between the distal phalanx and the insertion of flexor sublimis—primary or delayed primary suture by removable stainless steel wire.

(2) Severed flexor profundus between the insertion of flexor sublimis and the distal palmar crease—here the intact sublimis will ensure useful function, and in most cases the condition should be left alone. Occasionally, as in the left index finger of a violinist, it might be worth replacing the profundus tendon by a thin free graft (toe extensor), but the risk would be considerable.

(3) Severed flexor profundus and sublimis tendons between these levels—primary repair is not satisfactory, except under ideal conditions. The primary wound should usually be closed, and secondary free grafting undertaken about five weeks later, when the wound is soundly healed. The sublimis and profundus tendons are excised as far back as the palm, and the excised sublimis portion used as a free graft from the stump of the profundus tendon to the distal phalanx; alternatively, palmaris longus or a toe extensor may be used for the graft material, and these tendons have the advantage of being surrounded by paratenon.

(4) Severed flexor tendons in the palm, proximal to the distal palmar crease—primary or delayed primary suture by a stainless steel basket stitch in each severed tendon is satisfactory.

Thumb. Severed flexor pollicis longus—under ideal conditions primary suture may be undertaken. Alternatively, the proximal stump may be lengthened by a slide at the musculotendinous junction, or a free graft employed.

Extensor Tendons

Primary repair is satisfactory. Direct suture by wire or thread may be undertaken at any level, except for the insertion. Mallet finger is best treated by splinting; where there is an associated fracture of the base of the terminal phalanx which cannot be reduced, or in young people, open repair by removable stainless steel wire may be undertaken, but the operation is by no means universally successful.

Major Hand Injuries

Any combination of injuries may be encountered, and each case must be treated on its merits. A rough classification may be made, however, as an indication of the type of approach which may be used (Fig. 7).

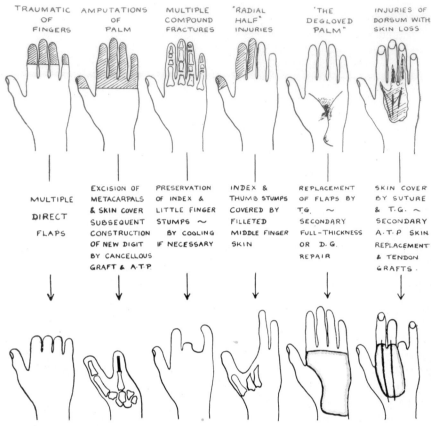

FIG. 29.7. A classification of the commoner types of major hand injury showing some of the methods which may be used in their repair.

Traumatic Amputations

Where several fingers are involved, length should be preserved, and, where local flaps are not available without further bone section, full-thickness cover must be obtained by direct flaps. Where only two fingers are severed distal to the terminal inter-phalangeal joints, hand skin cover is possible by thenar flaps, but in the majority of cases cross-arm or acromio-thoracic flaps will be needed (Figs. 8-14). A hand in which all fingers are amputated at their bases, but in which one or two half-inch stumps can be preserved will still be capable of useful work, provided it is supple and covered with sound pliable skin (Figs. 15-16). The grip between the thumb and a half-inch stump is an efficient pincer, and the broad palm can hold down larger objects for the other hand to work on. Where the amputation is through the palm, the outlook is much worse (Figs. 17-19). The thumb is usually involved in these cases, but, if one can preserve length up to the base of the proximal phalanx and a mobile carpo-metacarpal joint, the hand has possibilities. The essentials are as elsewhere—to get early healing, and, if possible, hand skin cover on the volar aspect. The functional result

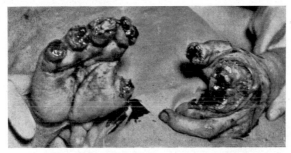

Fig. 29.8. Case 2. Power-press injury.
Right hand—Traumatic amputations of fingers. All fingers and the thumb were amputated through the proximal phalanges.
Left hand—"Radial-half" injury. The thumb was amputated through the i.p. joint and the index through the proximal phalanx, with skin loss over the whole of the dorsum of the 2nd metacarpal. The middle finger was extensively damaged, but had intact skin on its ulnar side, and an intact neuro vascular bundle.

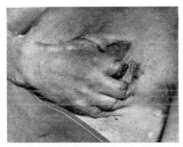

Fig. 29.9. R. hand. Immediate skin cover provided by acromio-thoracic flaps to the thumb, 3rd, 4th, and 5th fingers. The index stump was covered by local flaps.

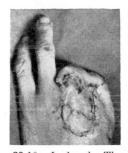

Fig. 29.10. L. hand. The 3rd finger was amputated, and its filleted skin used to cover the stumps of the index finger and thumb. The area of skin loss over the dorsum of the hand was covered by split-skin.

to be expected is a pincer action between the thumb stump and a new fixed digit. To achieve this it is necessary to develop a new web, by removing all finger metacarpals except one, upon which the new digit will eventually be built. This removal of metacarpals is best done as a primary procedure, to increase the amount of hand skin available for

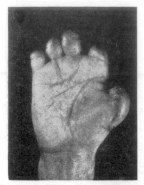

FIG. 11

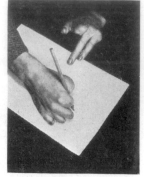

FIG. 12

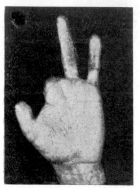

FIG. 13

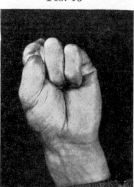

FIG. 14

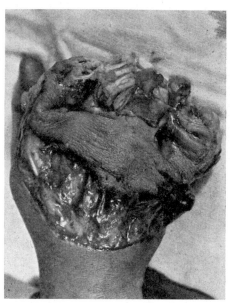

FIGS. 29.11-14. Photographs taken 8 weeks after injury show the degree of function regained. Both hands are supple, and have full ranges of active movement in the joints remaining to them.

FIG. 29.15. Case 3. Power-press injury. Gross destruction of all fingers, amounting to traumatic amputation of index through the proximal phalanx and of the remaining fingers through the m.p. joints. There was an extensive area of skin loss over the dorsum of the hand.

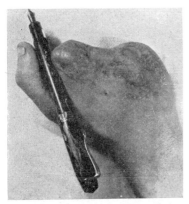

FIG. **29.16.** First intention healing was obtained by split-skin grafting, and hand skin cover was provided over the bearing surface of the index stump (not shown). The index stump provides a useful pincers with the mobile thumb.

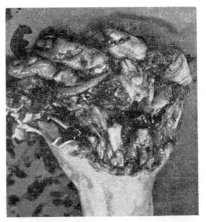

FIG. **29.17.** Case 4. Power-press injury. Traumatic amputation of the palm. The level of amputation was near the bases of the metacarpals, and the thumb was severed through the i.p. joint. The thenar muscles were intact, and there was every prospect of a mobile thumb stump. Skin cover was obtained by excising the 2nd, 4th and 5th metacarpals, and bringing hand skin into the web between the thumb and 3rd metacarpal. Later, a new fixed digit was built up on the stump of the 3rd metacarpal, using a cancellous bone graft covered by acromio-thoracic tube-pedicle skin.

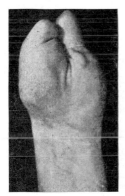

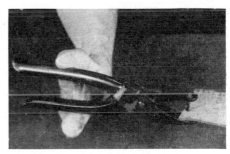

FIG. **29.18-19.** Late photographs show the degree of function obtained. The thumb stump forms an efficient pincers with the fixed digit, and the depth of the new web is adequate.

cover, and the best width for the web is obtained by leaving the 3rd or 4th metacarpal. The new digit is eventually built up by a cancellous graft enclosed in acromio-thoracic skin; it is by no means ideal in that it has a poor circulation and a tendency to break down at the tip, but is to be preferred to a prosthesis.

Multiple Compound Fractures of the Phalanges (Figs. 20-22)

In this type of injury the greatest variation is found between one case and the next. The association of a compound fracture with skin

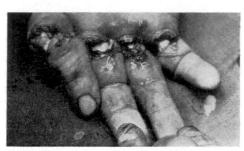

loss, tendon injury, or severance of the neuro-vascular bundles will often decide the issue, but, where all four fingers are involved, something must be saved. In the presence of a mobile thumb, pincer action can be retained by preserving an index or middle finger stump; where these stumps are short, preservation of length is vital, and hand skin cover without further bone loss may be obtained by cross finger or "filleted"

FIG. **29**.20.   Case 5.   Power-press injury. Multiple compound fractures. There was circumferential skin section in all fingers, save for a tenuous bridge on the dorsum of the 4th finger. All fingers had fractures of the proximal phalanges, and all neuro-vascular bundles were severed or badly damaged.

skin flap—for example, the middle finger may be sacrificed to provide cover for the index. On the ulnar side of the hand the fifth finger should be preserved with as much length as possible to give a

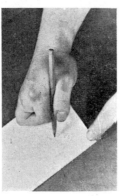
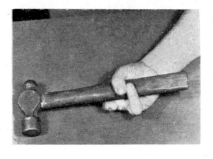

FIG. **29**.21-22. It was decided to rely upon an index stump for the pincers, and to attempt to preserve the 4th finger by cooling in order to give a broad grip to the hand. The final photographs illustrate the pincer and vice elements of hand function.

grip, and, even where its inter-phalangeal movement is likely to be nil, it is well worth preserving with the inter-phalangeal joints fixed in flexion, provided the metacarpal-phalangeal joints can be kept mobile. Even where the neurovascular bundles to all the fingers are severed, an attempt should be made to preserve the fourth or fifth finger for this purpose, if necessary by prolonged cooling. Injuries confined to the radial side of the hand are not uncommon, and here the vital necessity is to provide the thumb with hand skin cover (Figs. 8-14). Where the index is involved, it may well be sacrificed to provide this cover by a direct flap, and occasionally a similar procedure will be indicated with the middle finger—the ring finger can make a useful pincer with a mobile thumb, and the vice action of the hand is preserved.

The "Degloved" Palm (Figs. 23-25)

Degloving injuries of the volar surface of the hand are sometimes encountered. The hand has usually been caught between rollers, and the skin of the palm is severed around the thenar crease and across

the base of the palm, and turned distally in one or more flaps, the line of cleavage being between the subcutaneous tissue and the palmar fascia. These flaps frequently blood when first seen, but in practice they almost always die, the cause of their death being pre-

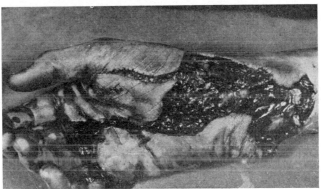

FIG. 29.23. Case 6. The degloved palm. Hand caught by the mudguard of a car. These injuries are important because perfect function can be restored provided it is realized that extensive palmar flaps based distally are seldom viable. They may be retained for a day or two to get a drier bed for grafting, but should be replaced by split skin as soon as possible.

sumably a secondary venous thrombosis. As in degloving injuries elsewhere, the flaps should be stitched back in position, partly because one cannot be certain that they will not survive, and partly because even dead skin is a useful temporary dressing. Against immediate split-skin grafting is the fact that the bed is very vascular, and bleeding difficult to control. Four or five days later it has become clear whether or not the palm is viable, and by this time the bed is more suitable for grafting. The

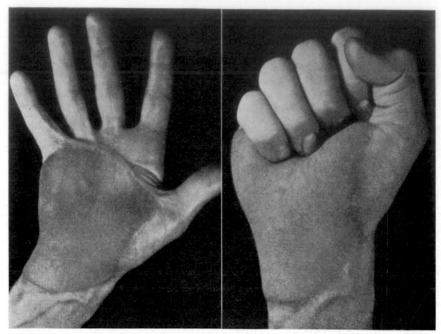

FIG. 29.24-25. The split-skin graft is later replaced by a full-thickness abdominal
flap as in this case, or by a dermatome graft.

split-skin graft in its turn is replaced two or three weeks later by a more
permanent graft. Where the abdominal skin is of a suitable texture, a
direct flap is very satisfactory, though perhaps a dermatome graft will
be the method of choice in many cases.

Injuries of the Dorsum of the Hand with Skin Loss (Figs. 26-27)

Injuries of this type are among the commonest major hand injuries,
and give the least satisfactory results. This is partly due to the
causative agent, which is often a milling or similar machine, and which
causes multiple jagged wounds, often with skin loss and tendon or
joint involvement. The main reason, however, is that, where extensor
tendon and joint capsule are involved, fibrosis and joint stiffness are
likely to occur, particularly when the metacarpo-phalangeal joints are
affected. Immediate skin cover is essential, and one is faced with the
choice between a direct flap and split-skin grafting. Direct flaps have
the advantage that they may be used over damaged tendons and open
joints, but the skin defect is not always in a suitable position, and a
direct flap means a period of immobilization which may cause trouble
later. Furthermore, one can never be certain to what extent œdema

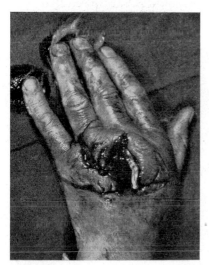

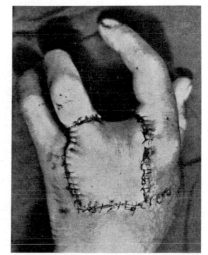

FIG. 29.26. Case 7. Injury of the dorsum of the hand with skin loss. There was, in addition, damage to the 3rd and 4th extensor tendons, together with the fractures of the 2nd, 3rd and 4th metacarpals and of the proximal phalanx of the 3rd finger.

FIG. 29.27. The patient was over 60, and early mobility was essential. Skin cover was provided by sacrificing the fractured 3rd finger and using its filleted skin as a flap, while one of its phalanges provided an intramedullary graft for the 2nd metacarpal. Movements were started at once, and by 5 weeks a full active and passive range was present throughout the whole hand, save for the inability actively to extend the 4th finger.

and thrombosis will devitalize structures outside the immediate wound area, and so endanger the edges or bed of the flap. Split-skin grafting is on the whole more satisfactory; damaged tendons may be excised, and joint capsules repaired to make a suitable bed, and early active and passive movements used to prevent inter-phalangeal and particularly metacarpo-phalangeal joint stiffness. Later, when all wounds are healed and the hand mobile, the split-skin may be replaced by flap or pedicle, under which free tendon grafts will replace the tendons excised at the primary operation. Occasionally full-thickness cover can be obtained by using filleted finger skin; it is in this type of case that intramedullary bone-grafting as a primary procedure can be most valuable. Such a graft will stabilize a phalanx or metacarpal during the early post-operative phase, when active or passive movements are so important, and, by giving rigidity to a hand or finger, may make the application of a flap or split-skin graft easier.

Major Forearm Injuries Affecting the Hand (Figs. 28-30)

Under modern conditions of hazard in industry and on the roads one may be presented with an upper limb injury, which at first sight

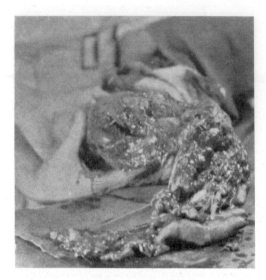

FIG. **29**.28. Case 8. Arm caught in a saw. Multiple compound fractures of the forearm, wrist and carpus, with full-thickness skin loss over the whole of the dorsum of the forearm and hand from the elbow down. All neurovascular bundles were severed, save for those on the radial side of the thumb and the ulnar side of the 5th finger.

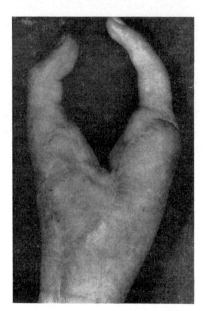

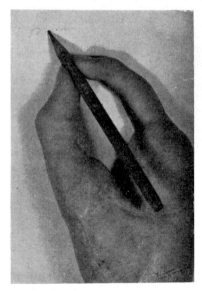

FIG. **29**. 29-30. The hand was converted into a pincer with palm skin in the web and free skin grafts over the dorsum of the hand and forearm. The wounds healed by first intention, and the split skin was later replaced by a full-thickness abdominal flap. The wrist was then arthrodesed, and, finally, extension to the thumb and 5th finger was gained by free tendon grafts. His final photographs show that he has an efficient pincer hand with accurate postural control. He can grip small objects with the tips of the digits, or larger objects by crossing the digits in the manner of scissors.

appears hopeless. On these occasions it is imperative to assess the case on the broadest lines. Skin cover is the first and most vital factor, and can always be achieved—by split-skin grafting, by local rearrangement, by bone shortening, or by direct flaps, coupled perhaps by plate-fixation of the fractures to provide temporary stability. These procedures may not be without risk, and one should always employ the safest method applicable, but with modern therapeutic aids the risks are not great, and the alternative of an upper limb amputation justifies their being taken. Skin cover is not, of course, the only factor. The limb must be viable, and in the presence of a major vascular injury amputation may well be inevitable. Given a viable thumb stump, however, and a digit against which it can later be made to move, it should be possible eventually to reconstruct a pincers of far more value to the patient than a prosthesis. The passive mobility of the remaining joints must be maintained from the start, and this is largely dependant upon immediate and successful skin cover. Later, split-skin may need replacement by full-thickness flap or pedicle; arthrodesis or bone-grafting, tendon transplantation or free tendon grafting, nerve repair may all have to be performed in turn, but, if one can start with sound pliable material upon which to work, the results will fully justify the trouble taken.

Summary

The observance of certain fundamental principles is essential for the successful treatment of hand injuries.

(1) Before any surgery is undertaken, a careful assessment of the injury must be made. From this, and bearing in mind extraneous factors such as the physical and mental capacity of the patient and the type of work for which he can be made fit, a definite plan for treatment is formulated—and only then is the primary operation begun.

(2) The more complete the physical destruction of the hand, the more important is it to reduce hand function to the simplest level in one's consideration of the method of repair to be used. Basically, the hand has two main functions—the pincers and the vice. For the pincers, the minimum requirement is an opposable thumb, with every possible centimetre of length preserved, and a digit against which it can move—preferably mobile, and preferably on the radial side of the hand. The vice depends for its strength upon the breadth of the palm, and, wherever possible, some part of the fourth or fifth fingers should be preserved.

(3) The most important single factor in the surgical repair is the provision of immediate and complete skin cover, and this must take

precedence over all other considerations. The importance of skin cover lies in the fact that infection must be prevented. A wound will inevitably become infected in this field of surgery if left open, and the consequent fibrosis will limit permanently the final function to be expected. The methods of achieving skin cover have been discussed. In general, hand skin cover is the ideal, but, where there is any doubt as to the viability of local flaps, thin split-skin grafts are to be preferred.

(4) Wherever possible, early mobility should be instituted. If active movement of a joint is impossible because of tendon or nerve injury, passive movements should be early and continuous, to preserve a receptive field for the repair. In certain cases it will be desirable to stabilize a phalanx or metacarpal, in order that early movements may be undertaken.

(5) As it is important that the primary repair should be directed towards the provision of a soft and mobile hand for the reparative phase, so also is it essential that reparative surgery should not be undertaken until all the tissues are soundly healed, and the maximum possible joint mobility has been achieved. In this stage also the operative procedures must be planned—first the full-thickness cover where required, secondly operations on bone, and finally tendon repair, and all of them preceded and followed by intensive and continuous rehabilitation.

E. MERVYN EVANS

References

BUNNELL, S. (1944) " Surgery of the Hand." Philadelphia, J. B. Lippincott Co.
EVANS, E. M. (1949) *Brit. J. plast. Surg.* **2,** 150.
HORN, J. S. (1951) *Plast. reconstr. Surg.* **7,** 463.
PULVERTAFT, R. G. (1948) *Ann. R. Coll. Surg. Engl.* **3,** 3.

CHAPTER XXX

AMPUTATIONS

Introduction

FOR some years amputation surgery has become somewhat static and advances have mainly been made in the limb fitting techniques. In the lower limb in particular the surgeon has tended to restrict himself to the two sites of election above and below the knee in accordance with the desires of the limb fitting surgeons.

There are two main reasons why this state of affairs has arisen. The great impetus of two world wars and the ensuing large numbers of limbless young men stimulated limb fitting techniques up to the modern types of mechanical ingeniousness which permit a gait and carriage frequently impossible to differentiate from normal. The limb fitters ask for a certain ideal length of stump above or below the knee for the fitting of these prostheses and operations have been performed primarily with this in view. During these advances in improving the treatment and rehabilitation of the young and relatively young limbless people, the problem of the older patient has been lost sight of and has been absorbed in the whole instead of being regarded as a separate problem. In spite of the large numbers of amputations being performed in wartime, the commonest cause of amputation being necessary is arteriosclerotic disease. It is right that the problem of the young amputee should first be solved but it does not follow that what is a desirable amputation for them is necessarily the best for the older individuals. The second reason is the mistaken belief that the only safe site for amputation in arteriosclerotic gangrene is above the knee at the mid-thigh level. That this is fallacious may easily be shown by reference to older text books of surgery where the supracondylar or Gritti-Stokes amputation was the operation of choice and that below knee amputations were occasionally employed (Burghard, 1909; Thomson and Miles, 1915). Furthermore, little attempt has been made in the past to rehabilitate the elderly amputee and he has frequently been discharged from hospital to his home or to a chronic sick bed as a hopeless cripple to spend the last remaining days in a state of immobility, the expectation of life being thereby greatly shortened.

Within recent years a change has become noticeable in these beliefs. Much interest has been aroused in the surgery of peripheral vascular disease and with this an increased knowledge of the pathology and treatment of the disease processes has become established.

Amputation Surgery in Peripheral Vascular Disease

1. **General.** There are two main reasons for amputation in peripheral vascular disease. Gangrene necessitates the removal of dead tissue sooner or later, and ischæmic pain may be so severe that recourse to amputation is necessary when other methods of treatment have failed. Gangrene is rarely a cause for immediate amputation and it is always advisable to investigate the case thoroughly, meanwhile controlling the infection and attempting to improve the circulation to the limb prior to amputation itself. Although time spent in this fashion is always profitable, too long a time may be harmful. Amputation for vascular disease is uncommon in the upper limb and almost all cases involve removal of a part of the lower limb. The aim must be rapid rehabilitation and early ambulation if the greatest success is to be achieved. It is therefore wrong to keep a patient in bed for prolonged periods with a dry gangrene in the hope and expectation that natural separation will occur.

During the period of investigation, attention should be paid to the following details:

Control of Infection. Infection is always present in cases of gangrene but makes an early appearance in the "wet" types. It is imperative to control this at an early stage in order to improve the patient's general condition, for chronic infection in an elderly patient may have serious consequences. Treatment consists of local drainage of pus whenever present and the intelligent use of antibiotics.

Control of Hæmoglobin Concentration. A degree of anæmia is common and may be severe. It may be secondary to infection, nutritional deficiency or other causes. It is important to correct this and to maintain a high level of hæmoglobin concentration. Transfusions of whole blood may occasionally be necessary.

Local Treatment. The affected limb should be kept as cool as possible in order to reduce the local metabolism and demand for oxygen to a minimum. It is wise to keep the part exposed and if dressings are necessary they should be as light as possible. Local application of surgical spirit assists in cooling and drying the part.

Physiotherapy. It is advisable to give regular physiotherapy to these patients. Stiff joints readily make an appearance unless active and passive exercises are employed. It is of little value to obtain a successful healed amputation stump only to find that the hip joint is stiff and limited in its range of movements. Muscle wasting also may rapidly follow inactivity in bed. The hazards of chest complications and venous thrombosis are now well known and it is important to stress the fact that rehabilitation should start as soon as the patient enters the hospital.

2. **Pathology.** The commonest forms of vascular disease necessitating amputation are:

    (*a*) Arteriosclerosis.
    (*b*) Thrombo-angiitis obliterans.
    (*c*) Embolism.
    (*d*) Chronic ulceration as a result of venous disease.

3. **Investigation.** A full knowledge of the type of disease, the site of arterial obstruction, and the extent of the collateral circulation is important before a decision as to the site of amputation is made. The following methods are of value in making this evaluation:

Oscillometry. This will give information concerning the site of obstruction but little concerning the collateral circulation beyond the block.

Reactive Hyperæmia. This simple test gives valuable information concerning the peripheral circulation.

Skin Temperature Tests.

Arteriography. This is of value in showing the exact site of obstruction, the state of the major vessels and collaterals, and the extent of the circulation to the distal part of the limb. It is of great assistance in deciding the level of amputation.

Plethysmography. Although of great value in giving information about the peripheral circulation it is an expensive and cumbersome method and is of practical importance only in large centres.

Fluorescent Test. Several reports have been made on the use of fluorescein in scratch fluorescence of the skin in order to judge the viability of skin flaps. It may occasionally be of value (Lange, 1942; Neller and Schmidt, 1943; Neller, 1945).

4. **The Use of Sympathectomy.** The aim of amputation surgery should be to amputate as low as possible and there is no doubt that a sympathectomy enhances this possibility. Sympathectomy improves the circulation to the skin and subcutaneous tissues, and what is probably more important, it provides a dry, warm skin which is less likely to harbour pathogenic organisms. This improves the chances of primary wound healing (Telford and Simmons, 1946; Evans, 1950; Edwards and Crane, 1951).

It is sometimes stated that age is a bar to sympathectomy and that, in general, it should not be done over the age of sixty. This is incorrect. Old people stand the operation well and the benefits of the procedure should not be withheld on account of age. In a personal consecutive series of over 50 cases of sympathectomy at all ages and with the majority over the age of sixty there has been one death.

5. **The Site of Amputation,** (Bickel, 1943; McKittrick, 1946; Guttman, 1949; Perlow, 1949; Smith, 1950). In deciding the level of amputation it is important to realize that there is a choice of a number of sites rather than the sites of election above or below the knee. Particularly in the older age groups the lower the level of amputation, the greater the prospects of ambulation. The ideal is the local removal of dead tissues but this is seldom attainable. Other varieties of amputation that may be employed according to the circumstances are amputations of a toe or through the foot, a Syme's or Gritti-Stokes operation. Before amputating at a low level, a very careful assessment is necessary and with the knowledge of the extent of the collateral circulation, the level of amputation may be judged with a reasonable degree of accuracy.

A sympathectomy is almost invariably done before amputation becomes necessary in cases of thrombo-angiitis obliterans. Due consideration should be given to local amputation or a Syme's in spite of the fact that the disease tends to progress and a higher amputation may become necessary at a later date.

In cases of embolism, much depends on the patient's general state and the pathology of the embolic process. Successful embolectomy may be performed with or without sympathectomy. If gangrene ensues a low amputation is usually possible, depending upon the state of the circulation.

It is in the large number of arteriosclerotic patients that the decision becomes more difficult. Boyd (1950) has classified the peripheral manifestations of arteriosclerotic disease into four main types:

  (*a*) Diffuse obliterative arteritis.
  (*b*) Secondary popliteal thrombosis.
  (*c*) Secondary femoral thrombosis.
  (*d*) Distal type.

Gangrene may occur in all the various types and it is impossible to assess the level of block or the state of the collaterals by the extent of the gangrene. Each type does have a fairly typical arteriographic picture but the collateral circulation varies in each individual case and depends to a great extent on the duration of the obliterative process and the number of smaller vessels affected. A clinical examination is not sufficiently accurate in deciding the correct level, but coupled with an arteriogram, a proper choice can be made. The distal type of the disease lends itself particularly to local amputations. In general, the diffuse obliterative arteritis and secondary popliteal thrombosis are more suitable for below knee operations than the secondary femoral thrombosis type.

A Gritti-Stokes amputation is successful in all cases of arteriosclerotic gangrene, and a sympathectomy prior to operation is not always essential. It is a useful operation which results in a sound stump with a posterior scar to which a pylon may be fitted early. It is readily fitted with a prosthesis which entails stiff-legged but stable walking. This is little handicap in the older age groups. The artificial limb is articulated for sitting purposes. In a personal series of 30 cases, sound healing has been achieved in all and no further gangrene has occurred at any time.

If breakdown occurs following amputations below the knee it is usually the anterior flap of skin which is the cause. It is advisable to cut a more generous posterior flap and to make the amputation slightly higher than the classical site of election. A generous bevelling of the anterior surface of the tibia is also wise.

6. **Operative Technique.** Certain variations in technique assist in ensuring sound primary wound healing.

Strict attention to asepsis is fundamental. Wound breakdown is certain if a minor degree of infection is introduced at the time of operation. The gangrenous area should be carefully sealed off from the operation site and antibiotics used as a cover for the operation.

A tourniquet should not be used because it may do damage. Deprivation of blood to the limb during the operative period is prejudicial to sound healing and the tourniquet itself may do further damage to an already diseased main artery. If the main artery is patent at the operation site, digital compression of the femoral artery at the groin may be applied by an assistant during the short period required for the securing of the main vessels.

Drainage should not be necessary. Complete hæmostasis must be achieved prior to wound closure and the presence of a drain may interfere with healing of the skin flaps. It may also be a source of infection.

The scalpel should be used boldly and incisions made down to bone. Numerous small cuts with the knife do unnecessary damage to the tissues.

The skin should be approximated loosely with interrupted sutures but correct apposition is important. The stump should be sealed at the end of the operation and should not be disturbed for 14 days, when the sutures are removed. At this time it may be advisable to leave a few sutures in place for a further period.

Refrigeration Anæsthesia

Refrigeration anæsthesia has been recommended by some, particularly in cases of severe infection. It has the advantage of reducing toxic absorption from the gangrenous area but it also has certain drawbacks. With the latest advances in anæsthetics it is doubtful whether this method will become general practice (Kirz, 1944; Lange, and Heinbecker, 1944; Pratt, 1949; Lange, 1950).

Surgery in Diabetic Gangrene

Infection in the diabetic is common and particularly so if the disease is uncontrolled. Severe sloughing and gangrene may result if treatment is delayed.

Primary treatment should be directed towards control of the diabetes by the usual methods and also the localization of the infection. Extensive whitlows are common, and if pus has formed, adequate drainage should be introduced immediately. Antibiotics should also be employed. The mortality in diabetic gangrene is higher than other forms and this is because of the increased severity of the infective process.

The possibilities of low amputations have been extensively explored and surgical opinion is in some agreement about the prospects of success. Grunberg and his co-workers (Grunberg *et al.*, 1951) recently reported a series of 50 successful cases where a toe or part of the foot had been removed. The below knee amputation is employed frequently by other surgeons (Gilbert and Havinovici, 1950).

If the cases are investigated fully, extensive arteriosclerotic changes are usually found and in fact, the disease is really arteriosclerotic gangrene complicated by diabetes. Grunberg suggests that the diabetic case usually prospers with low amputation because the collateral circulation is fully dilated, but the reason for this is obscure. However, it does suggest that low amputation in the arteriosclerotic subject should be attempted more often, particularly in conjunction with a sympathectomy.

When the diabetes is controlled and the circulation investigated, definitive amputation should be employed. Not infrequently the degree of infection is such that immediate amputation is essential to overcome profound toxæmia which otherwise would cause an early death.

Amputation Surgery in the Upper Limb

In the upper limb advances are steadily made in the development of a satisfactory and useful prosthesis. The difficulties are great and several methods have been introduced in an attempt to afford the patient control over his artificial limb.

In the preparation of the stump it is of great importance to preserve the elbow joint at all costs, for a prosthesis can be fitted to a stump only $1\frac{1}{2}$ in. beyond the insertion of the biceps muscle. When the elbow joint is lost, neoarthrosis of the humerus may be attempted as described by Gillis. To ensure non-union of the humerus the ends of the divided bone are burnt with the electro-cautery.

Amputation may be necessary in brachial plexus injuries and the operation of choice is amputation 6 to 7 in. below the acromium combined with an arthrodesis of the shoulder.

Kineplastic surgery (Henry, 1928; Bergmann, 1946; Magee, 1946; Gillis, 1948) has been employed by many in an attempt to utilize the forearm muscles after a distal amputation has been performed. The object is to make a skin tunnel in the muscle belly and to divide the attachment of the muscle distally. The operation was developed by the Germans under the stimulation of Sauebruch but a number have been performed in England and America. According to Gillis, the degree of control of the prosthesis is impressive. The disadvantages are many; the plastic tunnels are difficult to prepare and the prosthesis is not so well developed as that for the more formal amputations. Furthermore, many amputations are performed in septic cases or sepsis has intervened with consequent muscle destruction and fixation.

Krukenberg's operation converts the radius and ulna into two jaws of a "crocodile" forceps. This again was employed extensively by the Germans and the advantages are that tactile sensation is retained and a prosthesis is unnecessary. The main disadvantage is the unsightliness of the stump and patients themselves are unwilling to have the operation.

The modern prostheses now developed are extremely fine and the amputee is able to hold his own with other workers. A mechanical hand has been developed at Roehampton with remarkable control and ease of function.

ROLAND N. JONES

References

BERGMANN, E. (1946) *J. int. Coll. Surg.* **9**, 99.
BICKEL, W. H. (1943) *Surg. clin. N. Amer.* **23**, 982.
BOYD, A. M. (1950) *Angiology* **1**, 5.
BURGHARD, F. F. (1909) "A System of Operative Surgery," Vol. 1. London.
EDWARDS, E. A., and CRANE, C. (1951) *New Engl. J. Med.* **244**, 199.
EVANS, J. A. (1950) *Canad. med. Ass. J.* **63**, 545.
GILBERT, S., and HAVINOVICI, H. (1950) *J. Amer. med. Ass.* **144**, 454.
GILLIS, L. (1948) *Ann. R. Coll. Surg. Engl.* **3**, 227.

GRUNBERG, A., DAVIES, A. L., and BLAIR, J. L. (1951) *Brit. med. J.* **ii,** 1254.
GUTTMAN, A. P. (1949) *Manitoba med. Rev.* **29,** 361.
HENRY, A. K. (1928) *Brit. J. Surg.* **16,** 188.
KIRZ, E. (1944) *Brit. med. J.* **ii,** 662.
LANGE, A. (1950) *Arch. Surg.* **60,** 683.
LANGE, A., and HEINBECKER, P. (1944) *Ann. Surg.* **120,** 727.
LANGE, K. (1942) *Med. Clin. N. Amer.* **26,** 943.
MAGEE, R. K. (1946) *Lancet* **ii,** 904.
McKITTRICK, L. S. (1946) *New Engl. J. Med.* **235,** 924.
NELLER, J. L. (1945) *Ann. Surg.* **122,** 898.
NELLER, J. L., and SCHMIDT, E. R. (1943) *Ann. Surg.* **117,** 427.
PERLOW, S. (1949) *Surgery* **25,** 547.
PRATT, G. M. (1949) *Postgrad. Med.* **6,** 490.
SMITH, H. G. (1950) *J. Bone Jt. Surg.* **32B,** 392.
TELFORD, E. D., and SIMMONS, H. J. (1946) *Brit. med. J.* **i,** 386.
THOMSON, H. A., and MILES, A. (1915) "Manual of Surgery," Vol. 1, 5th Edition.
    London.

INDEX

405